Amsler's Grid

The chart on the opposite page is patterned after the grid devised by Professor Marc Amsler. It can provide for the rapid detection of small irregularities in the central 20° of the field of vision. The chart is composed of a grid of lines containing a central white fixation spot. The squares on the grid are 5 mm in size and subtend a visual angle of 1° at 30 cm viewing distance.

The chart is to be viewed in modest light monocularly at a distance of 28-30 cm utilizing the correct refraction for this distance. Viewing should be accomplished without previous ophthalmoscopy and without instillation of any drugs affecting pupillary size or accommodation.

A series of questions should be asked while the patient is viewing the central white spot.

1) Is the center spot visible? The absence of the spot may indicate the presence of a central scotoma.

2) While viewing the center white spot can you see all four sides? The inability to perceive these areas may indicate the presence of an arcuate scotoma of glaucoma encroaching upon the central area or a centrocecal scotoma.

3) Do you see the entire grid intact? Are there any defects? If an area of the grid is not visible, then a paracentral scotoma is present.

4) Are the horizontal and vertical lines straight and parallel? If not, then metamorphopsia is present. The parallel lines may "bend" inwards giving rise to micropsia or "bend" outwards giving rise to macropsia.

5) Do you see any blur or distortion in the grid? Any movement? A color aberration? These changes may be present prior to the appearance of a definite scotoma.

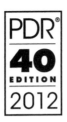

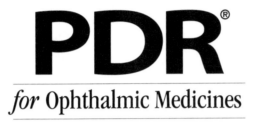

for Ophthalmic Medicines

Editorial Consultants and Contributors

Douglas J. Rhee, MD, Assistant Professor of Ophthalmology, Massachusetts Eye and Ear Infirmary, Harvard Medical School, Boston, MA

Christopher J. Rapuano, MD, Director and Attending Surgeon, Cornea Service, Wills Eye Hospital; Professor of Ophthalmology, Jefferson Medical College of Thomas Jefferson University, Philadelphia, PA

George N. Papaliodis, MD, Instructor, Massachusetts Eye and Ear Infirmary, Harvard Medical School, Boston, MA

F.W. Fraunfelder, MD, Director, Cornea/Refractive Surgery and National Registry of Drug-Induced Ocular Side Effects; and Professor of Ophthalmology, Casey Eye Institute, Oregon Health & Science University, Portland, OR

CEO: Edward Fotsch, MD
President: Richard C. Altus
Chief Medical Officer: Steven Merahn, MD
Chief Technology Officer: David Cheng

Senior Vice President, Publishing & Operations: Valerie E. Berger
Vice President, Emerging Products: Debra Del Guidice
Chief Financial Officer: Dawn Carfora
Senior Vice President, Product Sales, Corporate Development & General Counsel: Andrew Gelman
Senior Vice President, Sales: John Loucks
Vice President, Marketing: Julie Baker
Vice President, Business Development: Tom Dieker

Director of Sales: Eileen Bruno
Senior Business Manager: Karen Fass
Senior Account Executive: Marjorie Jaxel
Account Executives: Nick Clark, Carlos Cornejo, Michael Loechel, Hitesh Mistry, Gary Naccarato
Director, Regulatory Solutions: Chris Thornton

Senior Director, Operations & Client Services: Stephanie Struble
Director, Clinical Services: Sylvia Nashed, PharmD
Director, Marketing: Kim Marich

Client Services Manager: Kathleen O'Brien
Manager, Clinical Services: Nermin Shenouda, PharmD
**Senior Drug Information Specialist,
Database Management:** Christine Sunwoo, PharmD
**Senior Drug Information Specialist,
Product Development:** Anila Patel, PharmD
Drug Information Specialists: Pauline Lee, PharmD; Peter Leighton, PharmD; Kristine Mecca, PharmD
Clinical Editor: Julia Tonelli, MD
Managing Editor: J. Harris Fleming, Jr.
Manager, Art Department: Livio Udina

Senior Director, Content Operations: Jeffrey D. Schaefer
**Associate Director, Manufacturing &
Distribution:** Thomas Westburgh
Senior Production Manager, PDR: Steven Maher
Senior Manager, Content Operations: Noel Deloughery
Senior Index Editor: Allison O'Hare
Index Editor: Julie L. Cross
Senior Production Coordinator: Yasmin Hernández
Production Coordinators: Eric Udina, Christopher Whalen
Project Manager: Gary Lew

ISBN: 978-1-56363-796-4

FOREWORD TO THE 40th EDITION

PDR Network is pleased to provide eyecare professionals with this updated guide to ophthalmic medications. *PDR® for Ophthalmic Medicines* includes FDA-approved guidelines for leading eyecare products, as well as information on newly released medications. In addition, the opening sections feature useful tables summarizing the major pharmaceutical alternatives currently available in ophthalmology, as well as a brief guide to suture materials and information on vision standards and low vision. There are also lens comparison and conversion tables, and a directory of soft-contact lens manufacturers. Four detailed indices help you locate products by manufacturer, product name, product category, and active ingredient; and a full-color product identification section features photos of leading ophthalmic medications.

The special reference sections near the beginning of *PDR for Ophthalmic Medicines* have been prepared with the assistance of Douglas J. Rhee, MD, and George N. Papaliodis, MD, of the Massachusetts Eye and Ear Infirmary, Harvard Medical School in Boston; and Christopher J. Rapuano, MD, of Wills Eye Hospital, Jefferson Medical College of Thomas Jefferson University in Philadelphia. Our thanks also go to F.W. Fraunfelder, MD, of Oregon Health & Science University in Portland, who edited the section on ocular toxicology. The opinions expressed in these sections are those of the authors and are not necessarily endorsed by the publisher.

About This Book

PDR for Ophthalmic Medicines is published by PDR Network, LLC in cooperation with participating manufacturers. *PDR®* contains FDA-approved labeling for drugs as well as prescription information provided by manufacturers for grandfathered drugs and other drugs marketed without FDA approval under current FDA policies. Some dietary supplements and other products are also included. Each full-length entry provides you with an exact formatted copy of the product's FDA-approved or other manufacturer-supplied labeling.

The function of the publisher is the compilation, organization, and distribution of this information. All product information appearing in this title is made possible through the courtesy of the manufacturers whose products appear in it. The information concerning each product has been prepared, edited, and approved by its manufacturer. In organizing and presenting the material in this title, the publisher does not warrant or guarantee any of the products described, or perform any independent analysis in connection with any of the product information contained herein. PDR Network does not assume, and expressly disclaims, any obligation to obtain and include any information other than that provided to it by the manufacturers. It should be understood that by making this material available, the publisher is not advocating the use of any product described herein, nor is the publisher responsible for misuse of a product due to typographical error. Additional information on any product may be obtained from the applicable manufacturer.

Updates to *PDR for Ophthalmic Medicines*

This print/e-book edition of *PDR for Ophthalmic Medicines* contains the latest information available when the printed version of the book went to press. As new drugs are released, and new research data, clinical findings, and safety information emerge throughout the year, it is the responsibility of the manufacturer to provide that information to the medical community and revise that information in the *PDR* database accordingly. These revisions are published six times annually in the *PDR Update Insert Cards*, more regularly on PDR.net and *mobile*PDR, and e-mailed monthly via the eDrug Update. To be certain that you have the most current data, always consult PDR.net, *mobile*PDR, eDrug Update, or the *PDR Update Insert Card* before prescribing or administering any product described in the following pages.

Other products from PDR

PDR for Ophthalmic Medicines enters its 40th year as part of the products and services of **PDR Network, LLC**, the leading distributor of medical product labeling, product safety Alerts, and pharmaceutical Risk Evaluation and Mitigation Strategy (REMS) program communications. PDR Network includes:

- **Physicians' Desk Reference® (PDR®)**, the most trusted and commonly used drug information reference. To ensure that clinicians have the most current available information at their fingertips, PDR also provides:

  - **PDR Update Insert Cards**, a quick reference card designed to make prescribers aware of labeling changes, including newly approved labeling, that have occurred since the publication of *PDR*. Mailed every other month, each card lists changes that have occurred in the past 60 days. These updates and the full product information can be viewed at PDR.net/updates.

  - **PDR eDrug Updates**, a monthly electronic newsletter that provides specialty-specific drug information, including FDA alerts, new drug approvals, and labeling changes that have occurred in the past 30 days. To sign up for this free e-newsletter, send an e-mail to customerservice@pdr.net.

- **PDR.net®**, the online home of *PDR*, with weekly updates to FDA-approved full product labeling, manufacturer-supplied product information, and concise drug information based on FDA-approved labeling. Earn free CME credits for reading product labels and product safety Alerts viewed on PDR.net.

- **PDR Drug Alerts,** delivered via the Health Care Notification Network (HCNN), a Service of PDR Network, and free to all licensed U.S. physicians and their staff. This is the only specialty-specific service providing immediate electronic delivery of FDA-approved safety Alerts to physicians and other prescribers. Register at PDR.net to receive these Alerts.

- **mobilePDR®**, which provides the only source for FDA-approved full product labeling and concise point-of-care information from *PDR* directly on your mobile device. Information on over 2,400 drugs, full-color images and weekly updates provide the most up-to-date drug information available. *mobilePDR* is FREE to US-based MDs, DOs, NPs, and PAs in full-time patient practice and can be downloaded at PDR.net.

- A wide range of prescribing references and clinical decision publications, including the *2011 PDR® for Nonprescription Drugs, Dietary Supplements, and Herbs* and *2012 PDR® Nurse's Drug Handbook*. For more information, a complete list of titles, or to order, visit **PDRBooks.com**.

- For more information on these or any other members of the growing family of *PDR* products, please call, toll-free, 800-232-7379; fax 201-722-2680; or e-mail customerservice@pdr.net.

For more information about licensing PDR Network content, please contact Andrew Gelman at 201-358-7540 or andrew.gelman@pdr.net.

CONTENTS

SECTION 1

INDICES

This section offers four ways to locate the product information you need:

1. Manufacturers' Index: Gives the location of each participating manufacturer's product information. If two page numbers appear, the first refers to photographs in the Product Identification Guide, the second to product information. Also listed are the addresses and telephone numbers of the company's headquarters and regional offices.

2. Product Name Index: Lists page numbers of product information alphabetically by brand name. A diamond symbol to the left of a name indicates that a photograph of the item appears in the Product Identification Guide. For these products, the first page number refers to the photograph, the second to an entry in one of the Product Information Sections. All pharmaceuticals, equipment, and intraocular products are included.

3. Product Category Index: Lists products alphabetically by type or category, such as "Anti-Infectives" or "Hypertonic Agents." All pharmaceuticals, equipment, and intraocular products are included.

4. Active Ingredients Index: Groups products alphabetically by generic name or material, such as "Atropine Sulfate" or "Dexamethasone." Equipment is not included.

PART I/MANUFACTURERS' INDEX

ALCON LABORATORIES, INC.   201
and its Affiliates
Corporate Headquarters
6201 South Freeway
Fort Worth, TX 76134

Address Inquiries to:
(800) 757-9195
Outside the US call (817) 568-6725
medinfo@alconlabs.com

ALLERGAN, INC.   103, 214
2525 Dupont Drive
P.O. Box 19534
Irvine, CA 92623-9534

For Medical Information, Contact:
Outside CA: (800) 433-8871
CA: (714) 246-4500
Sales and Ordering:
Outside CA: (800) 377-7790
CA: (714) 246-4500

BAUSCH & LOMB INCORPORATED   103, 224
One Bausch & Lomb Place
Rochester, NY 14604

7 Giralda Farms
Madison, NJ 07940

Direct Inquiries to:
(800) 323-0000
Consumer Affairs
1-800-553-5340

FOCUS LABORATORIES, INC.   104, 240
7645 Counts Massie Rd.
North Little Rock, AR 72113

Direct Inquiries to:
(501) 753-6006
Fax: (501) 753-6021
www.focuslaboratories.com

MERCK   104, 241
One Merck Drive
P.O. Box 100
Whitehouse Station, NJ 08889

For Medical Information Contact:
Generally:
Product and service information:
Call the Merck National Service Center,
8:00 AM to 7:00 PM (ET), Monday
through Friday:
(800) NSC-MERCK (800) 672-6372
FAX: (800) MERCK-68
FAX: (800) 637-2568

Adverse Drug Experiences:
Call the Merck National Service Center,
8:00 AM to 7:00 PM (ET), Monday
through Friday:
(800) NSC-MERCK (800) 672-6372
Pregnancy Registries
(800) 986-8999

In Emergencies:
24-hour emergency information for
healthcare professionals:
(800) NSC-MERCK (800) 672-6372

Sales and Ordering:
For product orders and direct account
inquiries only, call the Order Management
Center, 8:00 AM to 6:00 PM (ET),
Monday through Friday:
(800) MERCK RX (800) 637-2579

PART II/PRODUCT NAME INDEX

PART III/PRODUCT CATEGORY INDEX

PART IV/ACTIVE INGREDIENTS INDEX

Italic Page Number **Indicates Brief Listing**

SECTION 2

PHARMACEUTICALS IN OPHTHALMOLOGY

Douglas J. Rhee, MD,[1] Christopher J. Rapuano, MD,[2] and George N. Papaliodis, MD,[1] with a section on ocular toxicology by F.W. Fraunfelder, MD[3]

We are pleased to present this updated overview of pharmaceutical options in ophthalmology. In all, this section offers 30 reference tables presenting therapeutic alternatives in all major categories of ophthalmic treatment, as well as a survey of recently identified adverse drug reactions encountered in ophthalmology. The material is divided into 14 parts as follows:

1. Mydriatics and Cycloplegics
2. Antimicrobial Therapy
3. Ocular Anti-inflammatory Agents
4. Anesthetic Agents
5. Agents for Treatment of Glaucoma
6. Medications for Dry Eye
7. Ocular Decongestants
8. Ophthalmic Irrigating Solutions
9. Hyperosmolar Agents
10. Diagnostic Agents
11. Viscoelastic Materials Used in Ophthalmology
12. Anti-Angiogenesis Treatments
13. Off-Label Drug Applications in Ophthalmology
14. Ocular Toxicology

There are a number of excellent references related to pharmacology and treatment regimens in ophthalmology. Listed below are some of the ones we regard as particularly useful.

GENERAL REFERENCES

American Medical Association. *Drug Evaluations Annual.* Milwaukee, WI: AMA Department of Drugs, Division of Toxicology.

Ehlers JP, Shah CP, Fenton GL, Hosking EN, Shelsta HN. *The Wills Eye Manual, Fifth Edition, for PDA* (Palm OS, Windows CE, and Pocket PC). Philadelphia, PA: Wolters Kluwer, Lippincott Williams & Wilkins; 2008.

Fraunfelder FT, Fraunfelder FW. *Drug-Induced Ocular Side Effects,* ed 5. Woburn, MA: Butterworth-Heinemann; 2001.

Fraunfelder FT, Roy FH. *Current Ocular Therapy,* ed 5. Philadelphia, PA: WB Saunders; 1999.

Rhee DJ, Colby KA, Rapuano CJ, Sobrin L. *Ocular Drug Guide,* ed 2. New York, NY: Springer; 2010.

Tasman W, Jaeger EA. *Duane's Clinical Ophthalmology on CD-ROM, 2004 Edition.* Philadelphia, PA: Lippincott Williams & Wilkins; 2004.

Vaughan D, Asbury T, Riordan-Eva P. *General Ophthalmology,* ed 15. Norwalk, CT: Appleton & Lange; 1999.

1. Massachusetts Eye and Ear Infirmary; Boston, MA.

2. Wills Eye Institute; Philadelphia, PA.

3. Casey Eye Institute; Portland, OR.

1. MYDRIATICS AND CYCLOPLEGICS

The autonomic drugs that produce mydriasis (pupillary dilation) and cycloplegia (paralysis of accommodation) are among the most frequently used topical medications in ophthalmic practice. The most commonly used mydriatic is the direct-acting adrenergic agent phenylephrine hydrochloride, usually in a 2.5% concentration. Phenylephrine is used alone or, more commonly, in combination with a cycloplegic agent for refraction or pupillary dilation. The 2.5% concentration is favored for most cases. There is an increased possibility of severe adverse systemic effects from the use of the 10% solution.

Anticholinergic agents have both cycloplegic and mydriatic activity. They are usually used for refraction, pupillary dilation, and relief of photosensitivity during intraocular inflammation (by minimizing movement of the inflamed iris).

It is important to remember that the effect of these medications depends on many factors, including age, race, and eye color. For example, the mydriatics and cycloplegics tend to be less effective in dark-eyed individuals than in those with blue-eyes.

When using mydriatics and cycloplegic drugs, it is important to instruct the patient to wear sunglasses to protect against bright lights, use caution when driving, and avoid operating dangerous machinery.

TABLE 1

MYDRIATICS AND CYCLOPLEGICS

GENERIC NAME	TRADE NAMES	CONCENTRATION	ONSET/DURATION OF ACTION
Atropine sulfate	Atropine-Care Isopto Atropine Available generically	Soln, 1% Soln, 1% Soln, 1% Ointment, 1%	45–120 min/7–14 days
Cyclopentolate HCl	AK-Pentolate Cyclogyl Available generically	Soln, 1%, 2% Soln, 0.5%, 1%, 2% Soln, 1%	30–60 min/6–24 h
Homatropine HBr	Isopto Homatropine Available generically	Soln, 2%, 5% Soln, 2%, 5%	30–60 min/3 days
Hydroxyamphetamine HBr/tropicamide	Paremyd	Soln, 1%/0.25%	15 min/60 min
Phenylephrine HCl	AK-Dilate Mydfrin Neo-Synephrine Available generically	Soln, 2.5%, 10% Soln, 2.5% Soln, 2.5% Soln, 2.5%, 10%	30–60 min/1–3 h
Proparacaine HCl	Alcaine	Soln, 0.5%	Rapid acting: 10-20 min
Scopolamine HBr	Isopto Hyoscine	Soln, 0.25%	30–60 min/4–7 days
Tropicamide	Mydriacyl Tropicacyl Available generically	Soln, 0.5%, 1% Soln, 0.5%, 1% Soln, 0.5%, 1%	15-30 min/3-8 h

2. ANTIMICROBIAL THERAPY

Antibiotics are routinely used in ophthalmology for both treatment and prophylaxis. They are used prophylactically in the management of foreign bodies and corneal abrasions and in preoperative and postoperative care, administered as an ophthalmic solution, ointment, or subconjunctival injection (see **Table 2**).

Many ophthalmic institutions have been using a solution of 5% povidone-iodine (Betadine) preoperatively to "sterilize" the eye, lids, and brow. Another development is the use of collagen shields (usually 12-hour) soaked in antibiotic, with or without steroid, in place of a patch and/or subconjunctival injection after surgery. While more expensive, the shields do have the advantage of being more comfortable for the patient and are less likely to cause tissue degeneration.

Also noted in the literature is another prophylactic measure: the addition of antibiotics to the irrigating solution. This technique is being used in several hospitals and high-volume surgicenters throughout the country. The maximum nontoxic concentrations of antibiotics are listed in **Table 3**. For prophylaxis, however, clinicians advise using half these amounts. Note that concentrations are given in micrograms per milliliter. It is critical that these medications be prepared by well-trained technicians, nurses, or pharmacists. The Centers for Disease Control has issued a statement discouraging the prophylactic use of antibiotics in irrigating solution due to inability to achieve MIC and the potential for selection of drug resistant microorganisms. The results of the European Society of Cataract and Refractive Surgeons' Endophthalmitis Study Group found a significant reduction in the risk of postoperative endophthalmitis following cataract surgery when cefuroxime 1 mg/1 mL was given at the end of surgery. This policy has not been widely adopted in the United States.

Whether treating an external or intraocular infection, slides for gram and Giemsa stain and aerobic and anaerobic cultures should be secured prior to initiating therapy if the severity, history, or site of infection dictates the necessity of culturing. When fungal, acanthamoebal, or atypical mycobacterial involvement is a possibility, additional stains to consider are: methenamine silver, periodic acid-Schiff (PAS), acridine orange, and calcofluor white. You can also consider using Lowenstein-Jensen culture medium. When an active or suspected superficial ocular infection is accompanied by inflammation, a variety of combination agents may be considered (see **Table 4**).

Corneal ulcers and intraocular infections require vigorous management. Most physicians and hospitals have protocols for their treatment. One such protocol for treating endophthalmitis, modified from Mandelbaum and Forster, is given in **Table 5**. Serious ocular infections are usually treated by the topical, subconjunctival, and intravitreal routes of administration (see **Table 6**). Corneal ulcers are usually treated with one or more of the topical solutions listed in **Table 6**, usually given every $\frac{1}{2}$ to 1 hour, in alternating doses if more than one solution is used. In severe cases, such as impending or actual perforation and scleral extension, medication is given by the topical, subconjunctival, oral, and/or intravenous route.

Fungal keratitis (keratomycosis) is relatively uncommon, but should be suspected in patients who have previously received topical steroids and/or antibiotics or have experienced ocular trauma, and in patients whose corneal ulcer does not respond to antibiotics. A recent outbreak of Fusarium keratitis in soft-contact lens wearers highlights the fact that contact lens disinfecting solutions are not 100% effective at preventing infections. Corneal scraping often permits correct clinical diagnosis. Natamycin 5% ophthalmic suspension (Natacyn) is recognized as one of the most potent broad-spectrum antifungal agents available for use in the eye. Amphotericin B 0.15%

ophthalmic solution, which is extemporaneously prepared, is another commonly used antifungal agent. Topical voriconazole 1%, made from the IV solution, is gaining popularity for treating recalcitrant fungal corneal ulcers.

Endogenous fungal endophthalmitis can be seen in intravenous drug users, patients with indwelling catheters, and patients with compromised immune systems. For these infections, amphotericin B has been used subconjunctivally, intravenously, and, where indicated, intravitreally. Prior to intravitreal use, a small portion of the vitreous abscess should be aspirated for microbiologic study. In addition to amphotericin B, flucytosine has also been used to treat fungal endophthalmitis. For more on treatment of fungal infections, see **Table 7**.

There has been an increase, within the last decade, in the incidence of Acanthamoeba keratitis. This has been linked, in many cases, to use of contaminated solutions for soft-contact lenses — especially tap water and homemade saline solutions. Current therapy includes the concurrent use of polyhexamethylene biguanide (PHMB) compounded with Baquacil or chlorhexidine digluconate (CHX) (found in Boston Rewetting Drops) plus propamidine (Brolene).

In bacterial endophthalmitis, the use of intraocular and periocular antimicrobial therapy has significantly improved the final visual outcome. A diagnosis of bacterial endophthalmitis should be strongly suspected in a patient who is postoperative or posttraumatic, or when the intraocular inflammation is out of proportion to the situation. Ocular pain is often present before obvious inflammation. Preoperative and postoperative antibiotics may decrease the incidence of postoperative endophthalmitis.

Once endophthalmitis is suspected, prompt intervention is required. Promptly secure samples of the aqueous and vitreous humors and initiate treatment quickly with antimicrobials appropriate to the suspected organism(s). Fungal or anaerobic organisms should be considered in cases where inflammation occurs several weeks or more after surgery or in cases of trauma or immunosuppression.

Once the aqueous and vitreous humors have been cultured, directly inject antimicrobial agents into the vitreous. To prevent retinal toxicity, medications injected slowly into the anterior vitreous cavity, with particular caution after vitrectomy. Vitrectomy and intravitreal antibiotics should always be considered when treating endophthalmitis.

In a study by Pavan and Brinser, the use of intravenous antibiotics was found to make no difference in final visual acuity or media clarity. The authors concluded that "omission of systemic antibiotic treatment can reduce toxic effects, costs, and length of hospital stay." Despite advances in antimicrobial therapy, this premise is still supported by current publications documenting the efficacy of intravitreal antibiotics without the need for intravenous antibiotics, assuming the infection is limited to the eye.

REFERENCES

Anonymous. Results of endophthalmitis vitrectomy study. *Arch Ophthalmol.* 1995;113:1479.

Axelrod AJ, Peyman GA. Intravitreal amphotericin B treatment of experimental fungal endophthalmitis. *Am J Ophthalmol.* 1973;76:584.

Barza M. Antibacterial agents in the treatment of ocular infections. *Infect Dis Clin North Am.* 1989;3:533.

Baum JL. Antibiotic use in ophthalmology. In: Tasman W, Jaeger EA, eds. *Duane's Clinical Ophthalmology.* Vol. 4. Philadelphia, PA: JB Lippincott; 1989:chap 26.

Ellis P. *Ocular Therapeutics and Pharmacology.* 7th ed. St. Louis, Mo: CV Mosby; 1985.

Endophthalmitis Study Group. Prophylaxis of postoperative endophthalmitis following cataract surgery: results of the ESCRS multicenter study and identification of risk factors. *J Cataract Refract Surg.* 2007;33:978.

Forster RK. Endophthalmitis. In: Tasman W, Jaeger EA, eds. *Duane's Clinical Ophthalmology.* Vol. 4. Philadelphia, PA. JB Lippincott; 1989:chap 24.

Gardner S. Treatment of bacterial endophthalmitis. *Ocular Therapeutics and Management.* 1991;2(1):3.

Lamberts DW, Potter DE, eds. *Clinical Ocular Pharmacology.* Boston, MA: Little, Brown; 1987.

Lemp MA, Blackman HJ, Koffler BH. Therapy for bacterial and fungal infections. *Int Ophthalmol Clin.* 1980;20(3):135.

Pavan PR, Brinser JH. Exogenous bacterial endophthalmitis treated without systemic antibiotics. *Am J Ophthalmol.* 1987;104:121.

Peyman GA. Antibiotic administration in the treatment of bacterial endophthalmitis. II. Intravitreal injections. *Surv Ophthalmol.* 1977;21:332,339.

Tabbara KF, Hyndiuk RA, eds. *Infections of the Eye.* Boston, MA: Little, Brown; 1986.

TABLE 2

COMMERCIALLY AVAILABLE OPHTHALMIC ANTIBACTERIAL AGENTS

GENERIC NAME	TRADE NAME	CONCENTRATION	
		OPHTHALMIC SOLUTION	OPHTHALMIC OINTMENT
INDIVIDUAL AGENTS			
Azithromycin	AzaSite	1%	Not available
Bacitracin	Available generically	Not available	500 units/g
Besifloxacin	Besivance	0.6%	Not available
Ciprofloxacin HCl	Ciloxan	0.3%	0.3%
	Available genericallly	0.3%	Not available
Erythromycin	Available generically	Not available	0.5%
Gatifloxacin	Zymaxid	0.5%	Not available
	Zymar	0.3%	Not available
Gentamicin sulfate	Genoptic	0.3%	Not available
	Genoptic S.O.P.	Not available	0.3%
	Gentak	0.3%	0.3%
	Available generically	0.3%	0.3%
Levofloxacin	Iquix	1.5%	Not available
	Quixin	0.5%	Not available
Moxifloxacin	Moxeza, Vigamox	0.5%	Not available
Ofloxacin	Ocuflox	0.3%	Not available
	Available generically	0.3%	Not available
Sulfacetamide sodium	Bleph-10	10%	Not available
	Sulf-10 (15-mL bottle or preservative-free dropperettes)	10%	10%
	Available generically	10%	10%
Tobramycin sulfate	AK-Tob	0.3%	Not available
	Tobrex	0.3%	0.3%
	Tobrasol	0.3%	Not available
	Available generically	0.3%	Not available
MIXTURES			
*Bacitracin/Hydrocortisone/ Neomycin/Polymyxin	Available generically	Not available	400 units-1%
Polymyxin B/Bacitracin Zinc	AK-Poly-Bac Available generically	Not available	10,000 units - 500 units/g

(*continued on the following page*)

TABLE 2

COMMERCIALLY AVAILABLE OPHTHALMIC ANTIBACTERIAL AGENTS (continued)

GENERIC NAME	TRADE NAME	CONCENTRATION	
		OPHTHALMIC SOLUTION	OPHTHALMIC OINTMENT
MIXTURES (continued from the previous page)			
Polymyxin B/Neomycin/Bacitracin	Neosporin Available generically	10,000 units - 1.75 mg - 0.025 mg/mL	10,000 units - 3.5 mg - 400 units/g
Polymyxin B/Neomycin/Gramicidin	Neosporin Available generically	10,000 units - 1.75 mg - 0.025 mg/mL	Not available
Polymyxin B/Trimethoprim	Polytrim Available generically	10,000 units - 1 mg/mL	Not available

*Suspension available; same concentration as ointment.

TABLE 3

ANTIBIOTICS IN INFUSION FLUID

AGENT	MAXIMUM NONTOXIC DOSE (mcg/mL)	AGENT	MAXIMUM NONTOXIC DOSE (mcg/mL)
Amikacin	10	Oxacillin	10
Ceftazidime	40	Tobramycin	10
Clindamycin	9	Vancomycin*	30
Gentamicin	8		

*Routine usage for prophylaxis is discouraged by CDC because of increased resistant organisms.
Adapted from Peyman GA, Daun M. Prophylaxis of endophthalmitis. *Ophthalmic Surg.* 1994;25:673.

TABLE 4

COMBINATION OCULAR ANTI-INFLAMMATORY AND ANTIBIOTIC AGENTS

GENERIC NAME	TRADE NAME	PREPARATION & CONCENTRATION
Dexamethasone - Neomycin - Polymyxin B	Dexasporin Maxitrol Poly-Dex Available generically AK-Trol Maxitrol Poly-Dex Available generically	Suspension, 0.1% - 3.5 mg/mL - 10,000 units/mL Ointment, 0.1% - 3.5 mg/g - 10,000 units/mL Ointment, 0.1% - 3.5 mg/g - 10,000 units/g
Dexamethasone - Tobramycin	Tobradex Tobradex Available generically	Suspension, 0.1% - 0.3% Ointment, 0.1% - 0.3%
Fluorometholone - Sulfacetamide	FML-S	Suspension, 0.1% - 10%
Gentamicin - Prednisolone acetate	Pred-G Pred-G S.O.P.	Suspension, 0.3% - 1.0% Ointment, 0.3% - 0.6%
Loteprednol etabonate - Tobramycin	Zylet	Suspension, 0.5% - 0.3%
Prednisolone acetate - Neomycin - Polymyxin B	Poly-Pred Available generically	Suspension, 0.5% - 0.35% - 10,000 units/mL
Prednisolone acetate - Sulfacetamide	Blephamide Blephamide S.O.P.	Suspension, 0.2% - 10% Ointment, 0.2% - 10%
Prednisolone sodium phosphate - Sulfacetamide	Vasocidin Available generically	Solution, 0.23% - 10% Solution, 0.23% - 10%

TABLE 5

REGIMEN FOR ENDOPHTHALMITIS

1. Diagnostic anterior chamber and vitreous aspiration; diagnostic vitrectomy when liquid vitreous fails to aspirate or in cases of suspected fungal endophthalmitis.

2. Initial therapy (in operating room after diagnostic technique).
A. Intraocular: gentamicin 100 mcg or amikacin 400 mcg and vancomycin 1000 mcg or ceftazidime 2000 mcg; the injection of intraocular triamcinolone or decadron remains controversial.
B. Subconjunctival: gentamicin 40 mg and triamcinolone acetonide [Trivaris (Allergan)] 40 mg.*
C. Topical: gentamicin 9.1 or 13.4 mg/mL and cefazolin 50 mg/mL and prednisolone acetate 1%; alternatively; a 3rd or 4th generation fluoroquinolone (along with prednisolone acetate 1%).
D. Systemic: cefazolin (Ancef or Kefzol) 1000 mg every 6 to 8 hours or Imipenem/Cilastatin 500 mg IV q 6 hours. (Ceftriaxone has good penetration of the blood-ocular barrier and may be used as an alternative.) The use of systemic antibiotics is controversial; many practitioners do not employ them.

3. If cultures are positive for virulent bacteria, consider repeating the above intraocular injections at the bedside on the second and fourth postoperative days. Continue topical treatment every half hour, subconjunctival treatment daily, and systemic therapy. Consider therapeutic vitrectomy with repeat intraocular antibiotics.

4. If cultures are negative after 48 hours, do not repeat intraocular antibiotics. Consider tapering topical, subconjunctival, and systemic antibiotic therapy while continuing topical and subconjunctival corticosteroids.

5. If endophthalmitis presents as a delayed inflammation in which a fungal etiology is considered, the vitreous sample should be obtained by a vitreous instrument using membrane filters; intraocular amphotericin B (Fungizone) at a dosage of 5 mcg should be considered.

6. If endophthalmitis presents as a delayed inflammation or chronic indolent infection, a *Propionibacterium acnes* infection should be considered.

Source: Mandelbaum S, Forster RK.
Anonymous. Results of endophthalmitis vitrectomy study. *Arch Ophthalmol.* 1995;113:1479.

*Subconjunctival corticosteroids should be deferred 48 to 72 hours to await culture growth and confirmation if a fungal etiology is suspected or the inflammation is delayed.

TABLE 6

CONCENTRATIONS AND DOSAGE OF PRINCIPAL ANTIBIOTIC AGENTS

DRUG NAME*	TOPICAL	SUBCONJUNCTIVAL	INTRAVITREAL	INTRAVENOUS†
Amikacin sulfate	10 mg/mL	25 mg	400 mcg	15 mg/kg daily in 2–3 doses
Ampicillin sodium	50 mg/mL	50–150 mg	5 mg	4–12 g daily in 4 doses
Azithromycin	1%	. . .	. . .	500 mg IV
Bacitracin zinc	10,000 units/mL	5000 units	. . .	. . .
Besifloxacin	0.6%	. . .	. . .	. . .
Cefazolin sodium	50 mg/mL	100 mg	2250 mcg	2–4 g daily in 3–4 doses
Ceftazidime	50 mg/mL	100 mg	2000 mcg	1 g daily in 2–3 doses
Ceftriaxone	50 mg/mL	. . .	. . .	1–4 g daily in 1–2 doses
Ciprofloxacin	0.3%	. . .	. . .	400 mg IV q 8 hours
Clarithromycin	10 mg/mL	. . .	. . .	. . .
Clindamycin	50 mg/mL	15–50 mg	1000 mcg	900–1800 mg daily in 2–3 doses
Colistimethate sodium	10 mg/mL	15–25 mg	100 mcg	2.5–5 mg/kg daily in 2–4 doses
Erythromycin	50 mg/mL	100 mg	500 mcg	. . .
Gatifloxacin	0.3%–0.5%	. . .	. . .	. . .
Gentamicin sulfate	8–15 mg/mL	10–20 mg	100–200 mcg	3–5 mg/kg daily in 2–3 doses
Imipenem/Cilastatin sodium	5 mg/mL	. . .	. . .	2 g daily in 3–4 doses
Kanamycin sulfate	30–50 mg/mL	30 mg	500 mcg	. . .
Levofloxacin	0.5–1.5%	0.5%	. . .	500 mg IV q 24 hours
Moxifloxacin	0.50%	. . .	. . .	400 mg IV q 24 hours
Neomycin sulfate	5–8 mg/mL	125–250 mg	. . .	. . .
Ofloxacin	0.3%	. . .	. . .	. . .
Penicillin G	100,000 units/mL	0.5–1.0 million units	300 units	12–24 million units daily in 4–6 doses
Piperacillin	12.5 mg/mL	100 mg	. . .	. . .
Polymyxin B sulfate	10,000 units/mL	100,000 units	. . .	. . .
Ticarcillin disodium	6 mg/mL	100 mg	. . .	200–300 mg/kg daily 3 x in 4–6 doses
Tobramycin sulfate	8–15 mg/mL	10–20 mg	100–200 mcg	3–5 mg/kg daily in 2–3 doses
Vancomycin HCl‡	12.5–25 mg/mL	25 mg	1000 mcg	15–30 mg/kg daily in 1–2 doses

*Most penicillins and cephalosporins are physically incompatible when combined in the same bottle with aminoglycosides such as amikacin, gentamicin, or tobramycin. †Adult doses. ‡Usage discouraged by CDC because of increased resistant organisms.

TABLE 7

ANTIFUNGAL AGENTS

GENERIC (TRADE) NAME	ROUTE	DOSAGE	SPECTRUM
Amphotericin B (AmBisome)	Intravenous	3-5 mg/kg/day IV	Candida, Aspergillus, Cryptococcus
Amphotericin B	Topical	0.1–0.5% solution (most commonly 0.15%); dilute with water for injection or dextrose 5% in water	Blastomyces (Fungizone), Candida, Coccidioides, Histoplasma
	Subconjunctival	0.8–1.0 mg	
	Intravitreal	5 mcg	
	Intravenous	*	
Anidulafungin (Eraxis)	Intravenous	100 mg daily	Candida
Caspofungin (Cancidas)	Intravenous	50 mg daily	Candida, Aspergillus
Clotrimazole	Oral	One troche 5 times a day	Candida
Fluconazole (Diflucan)	Oral	150 mg single dose 200 mg on day 1, then 100 mg once daily 400 mg on day 1, then 200 mg once daily	Candida, Cryptococcus
	Intravenous	100-400 mg IV daily*	
Flucytosine (Ancobon)	Oral	50–150 mg/kg daily in 4 divided doses*	Candida, Cryptococcus
Griseofulvin	Oral	500 mg daily	Trichophyton, Microsporum, Epidermophyton
Gris-PEG (Griseofulvin ultramicrosize)	Oral	375 mg daily 750 mg daily (divided doses)	Trichophyton, Microsporum, Epidermophyton
Itraconazole (Sporanox)	Oral	200–400 mg daily*	Blastomyces, Histoplasma, Aspergillus, Onychomyces
	Intravenous	200 mg IV twice a day for 4 doses, then 200 mg IV daily for 14 days*	
Ketoconazole (Nizoral)	Oral	200–400 mg daily*	Candida, Cryptococcus, Histoplasma
Mycafungin (Mycamine)	Intravenous	100 mg IV daily (usual range: 10-47 days)	Candida
Natamycin (Natacyn)	Topical	5% suspension dosing ranges from hourly to two-hourly as determined by the clinician.	Candida, Aspergillus, Cephalosporium, Fusarium, Penicillium
Posaconazole (Noxafil)	Oral	200 mg three times a day 100 mg (2.5mL) twice a day on day 1, then 100 mg daily for 13 days. Also 400 mg twice a day	Candida, Aspergillus
Terbinafine (Lamisil)	Oral	250 mg daily	Tinea
Voriconazole (Vfend)	Topical	1% (made from IV solution); dosing ranges from hourly to bid as determined by the clinician.	Aspergillus, Blastomyces, Candida, Cryptococcus, Fusarium, Histoplasma, Penicillium, Scedosporium
	Oral	200 mg twice a day	
	Intravenous	3-6 mg/kg every 12 hours*	

TABLE 8

ANTIVIRAL AGENTS

GENERIC (TRADE) NAME	TOPICAL CONC.	INTRAVIT. DOSE	SYSTEMIC DOSAGE*
Trifluridine (Viroptic) Available generically	1.0% (oph. solution)	. . .	. . .
Acyclovir sodium (Zovirax) Available generically	. . .	. . .	Oral–Herpes simplex keratitis, acute infection: 400 mg 5 times daily for 7–14 days; prophylactic dose: 400 mg 2 times daily. Oral–Herpes zoster ophthalmicus: 800 mg 5 times daily for 7-10 days; IV therapy†
Cidofovir (Vistide)	. . .	. . .	IV–Induction: 5 mg/kg constant infusion over 1 hour administered once weekly for 2 consecutive weeks. Maintenance: 5mg/kg constant infusion over 1 hour administered once every 2 weeks
Famciclovir (Famvir)	. . .	. . .	Oral–Herpes zoster ophthalmicus: 500 mg 3 times daily for 7 days
Foscarnet sodium (Foscavir)	. . .	. . .	IV–by controlled infusion only, either by central vein or by peripheral vein. Induction: 60 mg/kg (adjusted for renal function) given over 1 h every 8 h for 14–21 days. Maintenance: 90–120 mg/kg given over 2 hours once daily
Ganciclovir sodium (Cytovene)	. . .	200 mcg	IV–Induction: 5 mg/kg every 12 h for 14–21 days over 1 h. Maintenance: 5 mg/kg daily for 7 days/week or 6 mg/kg once daily for 5 days/week.
Ganciclovir sodium (Zirgan)		0.15% topical ophthalmic gel	Treatment of herpes dendritic keratitis: 5 x day until the ulcer heals then 3 x day for 7 days
Ganciclovir sodium (Vitrasert)	. . .	4.5 mg	Sterile intravitreal insert designed to release the drug over a 5- to 8-month period
Valacyclovir (Valtrex)	. . .	. . .	Oral–Herpes zoster ophthalmicus: 1 gram 3 times daily for 7 days
Valganciclovir (Valcyte)	. . .	. . .	Oral–CMV retinitis: Induction: 900 mg every 12 hours for 21 days. Maintenance: 900 mg once a day

*Because of potential side effects and toxicity, the practitioner should consult the main edition of PDR for possible dosage adjustments and warnings.
†IV therapy should be considered if the patient is immunocompromised.

3. OCULAR ANTI-INFLAMMATORY AGENTS

A wide variety of medications is available for the treatment of ocular inflammatory disorders, and the list expands annually. At one time, it was felt that corticosteroids were contraindicated in infectious disease states. However, it is now appreciated that, when used synchronously with antibiotics and/or with other appropriate antimicrobial, antifungal, or antiviral medications, these agents may help prevent more serious ocular damage. They are listed in **Table 9**.

TABLE 9

TOPICAL ANTI-INFLAMMATORY AGENTS

NAME AND DOSAGE FORM	TRADE NAME	CONCENTRATION
Cyclosporine Ophthalmic Emulsion	Restasis	0.05%
Dexamethasone Sodium Phosphate Ophthalmic Solution or Ointment	Ocu-Dex, Maxidex Ointment	0.1%, 0.5%
Dexamethasone Sodium Phosphate Ophthalmic Suspension	Maxidex	0.1%
Difluprednate Ophthalmic Emulsion	Durezol	0.05%
Fluorometholone Ophthalmic Ointment	FML S.O.P.	0.1%
Fluorometholone Ophthalmic Suspension	Fluor-Op FML FML Forte Available generically	0.1% 0.1% 0.25% 0.1%
Fluorometholone Acetate Ophthalmic Suspension	Flarex	0.1%
Loteprednol Etabonate Ophthalmic Ointment	Lotemax	0.5%
Loteprednol Etabonate Ophthalmic Suspension	Alrex Lotemax	0.2% 0.5%
Medrysone Ophthalmic Suspension	HMS	1%
Prednisolone Acetate Ophthalmic Suspension	Econopred Plus Omnipred Pred Forte Pred Mild Available generically	1% 1% 0.12% 1%
Prednisolone Sodium Phosphate Ophthalmic Solution	AK-Pred Available generically	1% 0.125%, 1%
Rimexolone Ophthalmic Suspension	Vexol	1%
NONSTEROIDAL ANTI-INFLAMMATORY DRUGS		
Bromfenac Ophthalmic Solution	Bromday	0.09%
Diclofenac Sodium Ophthalmic Solution	Voltaren Available generically	0.1% 0.1%
Flurbiprofen Sodium Ophthalmic Solution	Ocufen Available generically	0.03% 0.03%
Ketorolac Tromethamine Ophthalmic Solution	Acular LS Acular Acular PF Acuvail Available generically	0.4% 0.5% 0.5% 0.45% 0.5%
Nepafenac Ophthalmic	Nevanac	0.1%
INTRAOCULAR STEROIDS		
Fluocinolone acetonide	Retisert	0.59 mg
Ozurdex	Dexamethasone	0.7 mg
Triamcinolone	Triesence Trivaris	40 mg/mL 80 mg/mL

Steroids may be administered by four different routes in the treatment of ocular inflammation. **Table 10** lists the preferred route in various conditions.

Topical corticosteroids can elevate intraocular pressure and, in susceptible individuals, can induce glaucoma. Some corticosteroids, such as fluorometholone acetate, medrysone, and loteprednol cause less elevation of intraocular pressure than others but are lower potency. Corticosteroids, particularly intravitreal and topically administered forms, may also cause cataract formation. However, long-term systemic use can also accelerate cataract formation.

In addition to topical, subtenons, and singular intravitreal dosing of triamcinolone acetonide 4 mg per 0.05 mL (Trivaris; Allergan) or 40 mg/mL (Triesence; Alcon), sustained-release dosing of fluocinolone acetonide 0.59 mg (Retisert) is also available. Additionally, a sustained-release intravitreal implant, dexamethasone 0.7 mg (Ozurdex; Allergan), was approved by the FDA. Ozurdex is approved for the treatment of macular edema following branch retinal vein occlusion or central retinal vein occlusion, and also for the treatment of posterior, non-infectious uveitis.

There are also five nonsteroidal anti-inflammatory drugs (NSAIDs) available. They are: bromfenac (Bromday), diclofenac (Voltaren); flurbiprofen (Ocufen); ketorolac (Acular, and Acuvail) and nepafenac (Nevanac). Flurbiprofen is indicated solely for inhibition of intraoperative miosis. Diclofenac has an official indication for the postoperative prophylaxis and treatment of ocular inflammation. Ketorolac is indicated for the treatment of postoperative inflammation and for relief of ocular itching due to seasonal allergic conjunctivitis. It has also shown some success in alleviating the pain associated with keratotomy, although unapproved for this use. Both diclofenac and ketorolac have also been used successfully to prevent and treat cystoid macular

TABLE 10

USUAL ROUTE OF STEROID ADMINISTRATION IN OCULAR INFLAMMATION

CONDITION	ROUTE
Anterior uveitis	Topical and/or peribulbar
Blepharitis	Topical
Conjunctivitis	Topical
Cranial arteritis	Systemic
Endophthalmitis	Systemic-periocular, and/or intravitreal
Episcleritis	Topical
Keratitis	Topical
Optic neuritis	Systemic or periocular
Posterior uveitis	Systemic and/or periocular, and/or intravitreal
Scleritis	Topical, regional, and/or systemic
Sympathetic ophthalmia	Systemic and periocular, and intravitreal

edema. Bromfenac and nepafenac are both indicated for the treatment of postoperative inflammation and reduction of ocular pain in patients who have undergone cataract extraction. NSAIDs cause little, if any, rise in intraocular pressure. However, in rare instances, topical NSAIDs have been associated with corneal melts and perforations, especially in older patients with ocular surface disease such as dry eyes.

Other useful agents include mast-cell inhibitors, antihistamines, low-concentration steroids, and decongestants to treat vernal conjunctivitis or allergic keratoconjunctivitis. Tetracycline, taken orally, in doses of 250 mg 4 times daily for 4 weeks, then 250 mg once daily, is useful in treating ocular rosacea. Alternatively, doxycycline or minocycline, taken orally, in doses of 100 mg twice daily for 1 to 2 weeks, then 40-100 mg once daily or in divided doses may be used.

Agents useful in treatment of seasonal allergic conjunctivitis are listed in **Table 11**.

TABLE 11

AGENTS FOR RELIEF OF SEASONAL ALLERGIC CONJUNCTIVITIS

GENERIC NAME	TRADE NAME	CLASS	TYPICAL DAILY DOSE
Alcaftadine	Lastacaft	H$_1$-Antagonist/Mast-cell inhibitor	1
Azelastine HCl	Optivar Available generically	H$_1$-Antagonist/Mast-cell inhibitor	2
Bepotastine besilate	Bepreve	H$_1$-Antagonist/Mast-cell inhibitor	2
Cromolyn sodium	Crolom Available generically	Mast-cell inhibitor	4-12
Emedastine difumarate	Emadine	H$_1$-Antagonist	4
Epinastine HCl	Elestat Available generically	H$_1$- and H$_2$-Antagonist/Mast-cell inhibitor	2
Ketorolac tromethamine	Acular, Acular LS, Acular PF	NSAID	4
Ketotifen fumarate	Alaway (OTC), Zaditor (OTC) Available generically	H$_1$-Antagonist/Mast-cell inhibitor	2
Lodoxamide tromethamine	Alomide	Mast-cell inhibitor	4
Loteprednol etabonate	Alrex	Corticosteroid	4
Naphazoline/antazoline	Vasocon-A (OTC)	Antihistamine/decongestant	4
Naphazoline/pheniramine	Naphcon-A (OTC) Opcon-A (OTC) Visine-A (OTC)	Antihistamine/decongestant	4-8
Nedocromil sodium	Alocril	Mast-cell inhibitor	2-4
Olopatadine HCl 0.1%	Patanol	H$_1$-Antagonist/Mast-cell inhibitor	2
Olopatadine HCl 0.2%	Pataday	H$_1$-Antagonist/Mast-cell inhibitor	1
Pemirolast potassium	Alamast	Mast-cell inhibitor	4-8

4. ANESTHETIC AGENTS

A. Topical anesthetics

The agents listed in **Table 12** permit the clinician to perform ocular procedures such as tonometry, removal of foreign bodies from the surface of the eye, and lacrimal canalicular manipulation and irrigation. Cocaine, the prototype topical anesthetic, is a natural compound; the others are synthetic.

Cocaine is rarely used as an anesthetic agent because it causes damage to the corneal epithelium, produces pupillary dilation, and may affect intraocular pressure. However, it is considered useful when removal of the corneal epithelium is desired, as in epithelial debridement for dendritic keratitis.

The table lists available agents and concentrations. Most begin working within a minute and continue acting for 10 to 20 minutes. A transient, superficial punctate keratitis may develop rapidly after instillation of the agent.

B. Regional anesthetics

The actions, benefits, and drawbacks of the most common regional anesthetic agents used in ophthalmic surgery are summarized in **Table 13**.

TABLE 12

TOPICAL ANESTHETIC AGENTS

USP OR NF NAME	TRADE NAME	CONCENTRATION
Cocaine HCl*	. . .	1%–4%
Lidocaine HCl	Akten	3.5%
Proparacaine HCl	Alcaine	0.5%
	Ocu-Caine	0.5%
	Ophthetic	0.5%
	Paracaine	0.5%
	Available generically	0.5%
Tetracaine HCl	Available generically	0.5%

*Extemporaneous formulation.

TABLE 13

REGIONAL ANESTHETICS*

USP OR NF NAME	CONCENTRATION/ MAXIMUM DOSE	ONSET OF ACTION	DURATION OF ACTION	MAJOR ADVANTAGES/ DISADVANTAGES
Bupivacaine[†,‡]	0.25%–0.75%	5–11 min	480–720 min (with epinephrine)	
Etidocaine[†]	1%	3 min	300-600 min	
Lidocaine[†]	1%–2%/500 mg	4–6 min	40–60 min 120 min (with epinephrine)	Spreads readily without hyaluronidase
Mepivacaine[†]	1%–2%/500 mg	3–5 min	120 min	Duration of action greater without epinephrine[2]
Prilocaine	1%-2%/600 mg	3-4 min	90-120 min	Duration of action greater without epinephrine[2]
Procaine[§]	1%–2%/500 mg	7–8 min	30–45 min 60 min (with epinephrine)	Short duration. Poor absorption from mucous membranes
Tetracaine[§]	0.25%	5–9 min	120–140 min (with epinephrine)	

*Retrobulbar injection has been reported to cause apnea.
[†]Amide type compound.
[‡]A mixture of bupivacaine, lidocaine, and epinephrine has been shown to be effective in retinal detachment surgery under local anesthesia.[1]
[§]Ester type compound.

REFERENCES
1. Holekamp TLR, Arribas NP, Boniuk I. Bupivacaine anesthesia in retinal detachment surgery. *Arch Ophthalmol.* 1979;97:109.
2. Everett WG, Vey EK, Finlay JW. Duration of oculomotor akinesia of injectable anesthetics. *Trans Am Acad Ophthalmol.* 1961;65:308.

5. AGENTS FOR TREATMENT OF GLAUCOMA

A. α₂ Selective agonists — see **Table 14**
There are two medications in this class: apraclonidine and brimonidine. Apraclonidine is available as a single-dose applicator of a 1% solution for suppression of the acute intraocular pressure spikes that occur after laser treatments. A 0.5% concentration is also available, supplied in a multiple-dose bottle for use with other glaucoma medications to control pressure in patients who are not responding adequately to maximally tolerated glaucoma therapy. The medication is generally useful only for short-term therapy, since it has been associated with tachyphylaxis within 3 months in up to 48% of patients. Brimonidine, the second agent in this class, is 23 to 32 times more selective for alpha₂ versus alpha₁ adrenoreceptors than is apraclonidine. This allows the medication to be used on a chronic basis with reduced risk of tachyphylaxis. Brimonidine ophthalmic solution is available in concentrations of 0.2% (generic), 0.15% (Alphagan-P and generic), and 0.1% (Alphagan-P).

B. β-Adrenergic blocking agents — see **Table 15**
These medications work by blocking β-adrenergic receptor sites and decreasing aqueous production, thereby reducing intraocular pressure. Because β-adrenergic receptors occur in a number of organ systems, systemic side effects of these drugs may include slowed heart rate, decreased blood pressure, and exacerbation of intrinsic bronchial asthma and emphysema. These agents can also enhance the effects of a number of systemic medications including β-blockers, digitalis alkaloids, and reserpine. Since betaxolol is a cardioselective β-blocker, it has significantly less effect on the respiratory system and can be used in some patients with respiratory illnesses.

C. Carbonic anhydrase inhibitors — see **Table 16**
Used both topically and systemically, these drugs decrease the formation and secretion of aqueous humor. The systemic forms are usually used to supplement various topical agents (but not topical (CAIs). Use of the systemic agents is limited by their side effects, which include paresthesias, anorexia, gastrointestinal disturbances, headaches, altered taste and smell, sodium and potassium depletion, ureteral colic, a predisposition to form renal calculi, and, rarely, bone marrow suppression. The most commonly reported adverse effects of the topical solution are superficial punctate keratitis and ocular allergic reactions. Less frequently reported are blurred vision, tearing, ocular dryness, and photophobia. Infrequent are headache, nausea, asthenia, and fatigue. Rarely, skin rashes, urolithiasis, and iridocyclitis may occur.

CAIs have a sulfonamide moiety and should be avoided in patients with known drug allergies to sulfonamides. In addition to hypersensitivity mediated allergic reactions, systemic CAIs have been associated with bilateral acute angle-closure glaucoma and acute myopia.

D. Hyperosmotic agents — see **Table 17**
These medications decrease intraocular pressure by creating an osmotic gradient between the blood and intraocular fluid, causing fluid to move out of the aqueous and vitreous humors into the bloodstream. They are used for acute situations and are not to be used chronically. These agents are employed to decrease pressure in an attack of acute-closure glaucoma, and to give a "soft" eye during surgery. Increased intravas-cular osmolarity increases the intravascular fluid volume and has the potential to increase cardiovascular stress. Therefore, these agents should be used with caution in patients with a history of cardiac disease.

E. Miotics — see **Table 18**
Parasympathomimetic agents (miotics) are used primarily as topical therapy for glaucoma. A secondary use is the control of accommodative esotropia. This class of agents mimics the effect of acetylcholine on parasympathomimetic postganglionic nerve endings within the eye. The class is subdivided into direct-acting (cholinergic) agents and indirect-acting (anticholin-esterase) agents, based on their respective abilities to bind acetylcholine receptors and inhibit the enzymatic hydrolysis of acetylcholine. **Table 18** lists the parasympathomimetics approved for topical use in the United States. In addition, two agents are available for intraocular use: Miochol-E, a 1% solution of acetylcholine, and Miostat or Carbastat, a 0.01% solution of carbachol.

F. Prostaglandins — see **Table 19**
A single evening dose of latanoprost, travoprost, or bimatoprost has each been shown to be more effective in reducing intraocular pressure than timolol 0.5% administered twice daily. Ocular side effects—hyperemia, itching, foreign-body sensation, and stinging—appear to be minimal, and systemic side effects have not been observed. An increase in pigmentation in the iris occurs in approximately 10% of patients; the rate is higher in eyes with mixed-color irises and lower in blue or brown irises. Changes in periocular skin pigmentation have also been noted.

G. Sympathomimetics — see **Table 20**
These medications work by improving aqueous outflow and, to a lesser extent, improving uveoscleral output. The prodrug dipivefrin causes fewer systemic side effects than epinephrine and can sometimes be used in patients who have developed a sensitivity to epinephrine.

H. Combination agents — see **Table 21**
Other options for the treatment of glaucoma are the brand Cosopt (Merck), which is a combination of the β-adrenergic blocker timolol with the carbonic anhydrase inhibitor dorzolamide (available as a generic) and Combigan (Allergan), which is a combination of timolol and the selective β-adrenergic medication brimonidine. Cosopt and Combigan are the only combination agents available in the United States.

Other combination agents may be available in some countries. These include: Duotrav by Alcon (timolol 0.5% with travoprost 0.004%), Gantfort by Allergan (timolol 0.5% with bimatoprost 0.03%), and Xalacom by Pfizer (timolol 0.5% and latanoprost 0.005%).

I. Preservatives
Which allow for multidose bottles, can have a deleterious effect on the ocular surface. Timolol maleate is available in preservative-free single-dose vials. The typical preservative used in topical glaucoma medications is benzalkonium chloride. Other preservatives, such as purite (Alphagan-P) and sofzia (Travatan-Z), are also used.

REFERENCES
Fiscella RG, Winarko T. Glaucoma new therapeutic options. *U.S. Pharmacist*, December 1996.
Rhee DJ, Colby KA, Rapuano CJ, Sorbin L. *Ophthalmic Drug Guide*, New York, NY: Springer. 2007.

TABLE 14

α₂ SELECTIVE AGONISTS

GENERIC NAME	TRADE NAME	CONCENTRATION	SIZES (mL)
Apraclonidine HCl	Iopidine	0.5%, 1.0%	5, 10, 0.1 mL single-use container
		Available generically 0.5%	5, 10
Brimonidine tartrate	Alphagan P	0.1%, 0.15%	5, 10, 15
	Available generically	0.15%, 0.2%	5, 10, 15

TABLE 15

β-ADRENERGIC BLOCKING AGENTS

GENERIC NAME	TRADE NAME	CONCENTRATION	SIZES (mL)
Betaxolol HCl	Betoptic-S	0.25%	2.5, 5, 10, 15
	Available generically	0.5%	5, 10, 15
Carteolol HCl	Available generically	1%	5, 10, 15
Levobunolol HCl	Betagan	0.25%, 0.5%	5, 10, 15
	Available generically	0.25%, 0.5%	5, 10, 15
Metipranolol	OptiPranolol	0.3%	5, 10
	Available generically	0.3%	5, 10
Timolol hemihydrate	Betimol	0.25%, 0.5%	5, 10, 15
Timolol maleate	Timoptic	0.25%, 0.5%	5, 10
	Available generically	0.25%, 0.5%	5, 10, 15
	Available as preservative-free		
Timolol maleate (gel)	Timoptic - XE	0.25%, 0.5%	5
	Available generically	0.25%, 0.5%	5

TABLE 16

CARBONIC ANHYDRASE INHIBITORS

USP OR NF NAME	TRADE NAME	PREPARATION	ONSET/DURATION OF ACTION
Acetazolamide	Diamox	500 mg (extended-release) capsules	. . ./18-24 h
	Available generically	125, 250 mg tablets	2 h/8-12 h
Brinzolamide	Azopt	1% ophthalmic suspension	. . .
Dorzolamide HCl	Trusopt	2% ophthalmic solution	. . .
	Available generically		
Methazolamide	Available generically	25, 50 mg tablets	2-4 h/10-18 h

TABLE 17

HYPEROSMOTIC AGENTS

USP OR NF NAME	TRADE NAME	PREPARATION	DOSE	ROUTE	ONSET/DURATION OF ACTION
Glycerin	Osmoglyn	50%	1–1.5 g/kg	Oral	60-90 min
Mannitol*	Osmitrol	5%–20%	0.5–2 g/kg	IV	30-60 min/4-6 h
Urea	Ureaphil	Powder (4 g) for reconstitution to 30% solution	0.5-2 g/kg	IV	30-45 min/5-6 h

*Do not confuse with mannitol hexanitrate, an antianginal agent.

TABLE 18

MIOTICS

GENERIC NAME	TRADE NAME	STRENGTHS	SIZES
CHOLINERGIC AGENTS			
Carbachol	Isopto Carbachol	1.5%, 3%	15, 30 mL
	Miostat	0.01%	1.5 mL x 12
Pilocarpine HCl	Isopto Carpine	1%, 2%, 4%	15, 30 mL
	Pilopine-HS gel	4%	3.5 g
	Available generically	0.5%, 1%, 2%, 3%, 4%, 6%	15 mL

TABLE 19

PROSTAGLANDINS

GENERIC NAME	TRADE NAME	CONCENTRATION	SIZES (mL)
Bimatoprost	Lumigan	0.01%, 0.03%	2.5, 5, 7.5
Latanoprost	Xalatan	0.005%	2.5
	Available generically		2.5, 3.0
Travoprost	Travatan, Travatan-Z	0.004%	2.5, 5

TABLE 20

SYMPATHOMIMETICS

GENERIC NAME	TRADE NAME	CONCENTRATION	SIZES (mL)
Dipivefrin HCl	Propine	0.1%	5, 10, 15
	Available generically	0.1%	5, 10, 15
Epinephrine hydrochloride	Available generically	0.5%, 1%, 2%	5, 10, 15

TABLE 21

COMBINATION AGENTS (AVAILABLE IN THE U.S.)

GENERIC NAME	TRADE NAME	CONCENTRATION	SIZES (mL)
Brimonidine tartrate and timolol maleate	Combigan	0.2% brimonidine/0.5% timolol	5, 10
Dorzolamide HCl and timolol maleate	Cosopt	2% dorzolamide/0.5% timolol	5, 10
	Available generically	2% dorzolamide/0.5% timolol	5, 10

6. MEDICATIONS FOR DRY EYE

Dry eye refers to a deficiency in either the lipid, aqueous, or mucin components of the precorneal tear film. The most commonly encountered aqueous-deficient dry eye in the United States is keratoconjunctivitis sicca, while mucin-deficient dry eyes may be seen in cases of hypovitaminosis A, Stevens-Johnson syndrome, ocular pemphigoid, extensive trachoma, and chemical burns. Posterior blepharitis (meibomitis) accounts for the vast majority of lipid-deficient dry eye symptoms. Dry eye is treated with artificial tear preparations (see **Table 22**), prescription medications (see **Table 23**) and ophthalmic lubricants (see **Table 24**). The lubricants form an occlusive film over the ocular surface and protect the eye from drying. Administered as a nighttime medication, they are useful both for dry eye and in cases of recurrent corneal erosion. Topical cyclosporin A 0.05% is very helpful in many patients with mild-to-severe dry eyes. Punctal occlusion with plugs or cautery can also be helpful in some patients with dry eyes.

TABLE 22

ARTIFICIAL TEAR PREPARATIONS

MAJOR COMPONENT(S)	CONCENTRATION	TRADE NAME	PRESERVATIVE/EDTA*
Carboxymethylcellulose	0.25% 0.5% 0.5% 1% 0.25%	GenTeal Gel Drops Refresh Plus Refresh Tears Refresh Liquigel TheraTears	Sodium perborate None Purite Purite Sodium perborate
Carboxymethylcellulose, Glycerin	0.5%, 0.9%	Optive/Optive Sensitive	Purite/None
Glycerin	1.0%	Computer Eye Drops	Benzalkonium chloride, None
Glycerin, Propylene glycol	0.3%, 1.0% 0.6%, 0.6% 0.55%, 0.55%	Moisture Eyes Soothe Soothe Xtra Hydration	Benzalkonium chloride None Butylated hydroxyanisole
Hydroxypropyl cellulose	5 mg/insert	Lacrisert (biodegradable insert)	None
Hydroxypropyl methylcellulose (Hypromellose)	0.2% 0.3% 0.5%	GenTeal Mild GenTeal Moderate GenTeal Gel GenTeal PF Tearisol	Sodium perborate Sodium perborate Sodium perborate None Benzalkonium chloride, EDTA
Hydroxypropyl methylcellulose, dextran 70	0.3%, 0.1%	Tears Renewed Tears Naturale Free	Benzalkonium chloride, EDTA None
Hydroxypropyl methylcellulose, glycerin, dextran 70	0.3%, 0.2%, 0.1%	Tears Naturale Forte	Polyquaternium-1
Hydroxypropyl methylcellulose, glycerin, PEG-400	0.2%, 0.2%, 1%	Visine Tears Visine Pure Tears	Benzalkonium chloride
Hypromellose, dextran 70	0.8%, 0.1%	Moisture Eyes	None
Hypromellose, glycerin		Clear Eyes CLR Visine for Contacts	Sorbic acid, EDTA Potassium sorbate, EDTA
Hypromellose/Glycerin Polyethylene glycol 400	0.2%, 0.36%, 1%	Visine Tears	Benzalkonium chloride
Methylcellulose	1%	Murocel	Methylparabens, propylparabens
Mineral oil, light mineral oil	4.5%, 1.0%	Soothe XP	Polyhexamethylene biguanide
Mineral oil, white petrolatum	15%, 85% 3%, 94%	GenTeal PM Tears Naturale P.M.	None None
PEG-400, sodium hyaluronate	0.25%	Blink Tears, Blink Gel Tears	Sodium chlorite
Polysorbate 80	1%	VIVA Lubricating	None
Polysorbate 80, hypromellose, glycerin, zinc sulfate	1%, 0.3%, 0.125%, 0.25%	VIVA Ultra Tears Lubricating + MR	None
Polyvinyl alcohol	1.4%	AKWA Tears	Benzalkonium chloride, EDTA
Polyvinyl alcohol, PEG-400	1%, 1%	HypoTears	Benzalkonium chloride
Polyvinyl alcohol, povidone	0.5%, 0.6%	Murine Tears	Benzalkonium chloride
Polyvinyl alcohol, povidone, Tetrahydrozoline HCl	0.5%, 0.6%, 0.05%	Murine Tears Plus	Benzalkonium chloride
Propylene glycol	0.6%	Systane Balance	Polyquaternium-1
Propylene glycol	0.95%	Moisture Eyes Preservative Free	None
Propylene glycol, PEG-400	0.3%, 0.4%	Systane, Systane Ultra, Systane Gel Drops, Systane Preservative Free	Polyquaternium-1, also available as preservative free

EDTA = ethylenediaminetetraacetic acid.

TABLE 23

PRESCRIPTION MEDICATIONS FOR DRY EYE SYNDROME

MAJOR COMPONENT	CONCENTRATION	DOSE	TRADE NAME	PRESERVATIVE
Cyclosporine	0.05%	q 12h	Restasis	None
Polyvinyl pyrrolidone, polyvinyl alcohol (87%/99% hydrolyzed)	2%, 0.9%/1.8%	3-4 x day	FreshKote	Disodium edetate dihydrate, polixetonium

TABLE 24

OPHTHALMIC LUBRICANTS

TRADE NAME	COMPOSITION OF STERILE OINTMENT
AKWA Tears Ointment	White petrolatum, liquid lanolin, and mineral oil
Genteal PM Ointment	85% white petrolatum, 15% mineral oil
HypoTears Ointment Tears Renewed	White petrolatum and light mineral oil
Lacri-Lube S.O.P.	56.8% white petrolatum and mineral oil
Puralube Ophthalmic Ointment	85% white petrolatum, 15% mineral oil, preservative-free
Refresh P.M.	57.3% white petrolatum, 42.5% mineral oil, and lanolin alcohols
Soothe Night Time Lubricant Eye Ointment	80% white petrolatum, 20% mineral oil
Systane Nighttime Lubricant Eye Ointment	94% white petrolatum, 3% mineral oil, preservative-free

7. OCULAR DECONGESTANTS

These topically applied adrenergic medications are commonly used to whiten the eye. Those containing naphazoline and tetrahydrozoline are more stable than those with phenylephrine. Usual dosage is 1 or 2 drops no more than 4 times a day (see **Table 25**).

TABLE 25

OCULAR DECONGESTANTS

DRUG	TRADE NAME	ADDITIONAL COMPONENTS
Naphazoline HCl	AK-Con (0.1%)	Benzalkonium chloride, edetate disodium
	Albalon (0.1%)	Benzalkonium chloride, edetate disodium
	All Clear (0.012%)	Benzalkonium chloride, edetate disodium, PEG-300, polyethylene glycol
	All Clear AR (0.03%)	Benzalkonium chloride, edetate disodium, hydroxypropyl methylcellulose 0.5%
	Clear Eyes (0.012%)	Benzalkonium chloride, edetate disodium
	Available generically	Benzalkonium chloride, EDTA[†]
Oxymetazoline HCl	Visine L.R. (0.025%)	Benzalkonium chloride, edetate disodium
Phenylephrine HCl	AK-Nefrin (0.12%) Available generically	Benzalkonium chloride, edetate disodium
Tetrahydrozoline HCl	Murine Tears Plus (0.05%)	Benzalkonium chloride, edetate disodium, polyvinyl alcohol, povidone
	Visine (0.05%)	Benzalkonium chloride, edetate disodium
	Visine Advanced Relief (0.05%)	Benzalkonium chloride, edetate disodium, PEG-400, povidone, dextran 70
	Available generically	Benzalkonium chloride, edetate disodium, PEG-400, povidone, dextran 70
DECONGESTANT/ASTRINGENT COMBINATIONS		
Naphazoline HCl plus antazoline phosphate	Vasocon-A	Benzalkonium chloride, edetate disodium
Naphazoline HCl plus pheniramine maleate	Visine-A Naphcon-A	Benzalkonium chloride, edetate disodium Benzalkonium chloride, edetate disodium
Naphazoline HCl plus zinc sulfate	Clear Eyes ACR (0.0125%) (allergy/cold relief)	Benzalkonium chloride, edetate disodium, glycerin
Tetrahydrozoline plus zinc sulfate	Visine A.C.	Benzalkonium chloride, edetate disodium
Naphazoline hydrochloride, Polysorbate 80	VIVA Lubricating Redness Relief	Citric acid, edetate disodium, sodium chloride

†EDTA = ethylenediaminetetraacetic acid.

8. OPHTHALMIC IRRIGATING SOLUTIONS

Listed in **Table 26** are sterile isotonic solutions for general ophthalmic use. They are all over-the-counter products. There are also intraocular irrigating solutions available for use during surgical procedures.

They include prescription medications such as Bausch & Lomb's Balanced Salt Solution, Alcon's BSS and BSS Plus, and Iolab's Iocare Balanced Salt Solution.

TABLE 26

OPHTHALMIC IRRIGATING SOLUTIONS

TRADE NAME	COMPONENTS	ADDITIONAL COMPONENTS
Collyrium Fresh Eyes	Boric acid and sodium borate	Benzalkonium chloride
Dacriose	Sodium and potassium chlorides, and sodium phosphate	Benzalkonium chloride, edetate disodium
Eye Wash Solution	Boric acid, sodium borate, and sodium chloride	EDTA*, sorbic acid

*EDTA = ethylenediaminetetraacetic acid.

9. HYPEROSMOLAR AGENTS

Hyperosmolar (hypertonic) agents are used to reduce corneal edema. They act through osmotic attraction of water through the semipermeable corneal epithelium.

TABLE 27

HYPEROSMOLAR AGENTS

GENERIC NAME	TRADE NAME	CONCENTRATION
Sodium chloride	Muro-128	2% or 5% (solution), 5% (ointment)
	Available generically	5% (solution and ointment)

10. DIAGNOSTIC AGENTS

Some of the more common diagnostic agents and tests used in ophthalmologic practice are listed below.

A. Examination of the Conjunctiva, Cornea, and Lacrimal Apparatus

Fluorescein, applied primarily as a 2% alkaline solution, and with impregnated paper strips, is used to examine the integrity of the conjunctival and corneal epithelia. Defects in the corneal epithelium will appear bright green in ordinary light and bright yellow when a cobalt blue filter is used in the light path. Similar lesions of the conjunctiva appear bright orange-yellow in ordinary illumination.

Fluorescein has also come into wide use in the fitting of rigid contact lenses, though it cannot be used for soft lenses, which absorb the dye. Proper fit is determined by examining the pattern of fluorescein beneath the contact lens.

In addition, fluorescein is used in performing applanation tonometry. Also, one test of lacrimal apparatus patency (Jones test) uses 1 drop of 1% fluorescein instilled into the conjunctival sac. If the dye appears in the nose, drainage is normal.

Rose bengal, available as 1% solution or in impregnated strips, is particularly useful for demonstrating abnormal conjunctival or corneal epithelium. Devitalized cells stain bright red, while normal cells show no change. *Lissamine green*, available as 1% solution or in impregnated strips, also stains abnormal conjunctival and corneal cells. It is less irritating to the eye than rose bengal. The abnormal epithelial cells that present in dry eye disorders are effectively revealed by these stains.

The *Schirmer* test is a valuable method of assessing tear production. It employs prepared strips of filter paper 5 by 30 mm in size. The strips are inserted into the topically anesthetized conjunctival sac at the junction of the middle and outer third of the lower lid, with approximately 25 mm of paper exposed. After 5 minutes, the strip is removed and the amount of moistening measured. The normal range is 10 to 25 mm. If inadequate production of tears is found on the initial test, a Schirmer II test can be performed by repeating the procedure while stimulating the nasal mucosa. A number of variations of the Schirmer test can be found in textbooks and journals.

B. Examination of Acquired Ptosis or Extraocular Muscle Palsy

To confirm myasthenia gravis as the cause of ptosis or muscle palsy, an IV injection of 2 mg of *edrophonium chloride* is administered, followed 45 seconds later by an additional 8 mg if there is no response to the first dose. (In case of a severe reaction to the edrophonium, immediately give atropine sulfate, 0.6 mg IV.) Alternatively, a non-invasive, low-risk test, such as the "ice test" may be used. The ice test has approximately a 0.94 sensitivity for ocular myasthenia and 0.82 sensitivity for generalized disease. The ice test also has a 0.97 specificity for ocular myasthenia and 0.96 specificity for generalized disease.

C. Examination of the Retina and Choroid

Sodium fluorescein solution, in concentrations of 5%, 10%, and 25%, is injected intravenously to study the retinal and choroidal circulation. It has been used primarily in examination of lesions at the posterior pole of the eye, but anterior segment fluorescein angiography (wherein the vessels of the iris, sclera, and conjunctiva are studied) is also a useful clinical tool.

Intravascular fluorescein is normally prevented from entering the retina by the intact retinal vascular endothelium (blood-retinal barrier) and the intact retinal pigment epithelium. Defects in either the retinal vessels or the pigment epithelium will allow leakage of fluorescein, which can then be studied by either direct observation or photography. For good results, appropriate filters are needed to excite the fluorescein and exclude unwanted wavelengths. The peak frequencies for excitation lie between 485 and 500 nm and, for emission, between 520 and 530 nm.

Fluorescein has proved to be a safe diagnostic agent, the most common side effects being nausea and vomiting. However, occasional allergic and vagal reactions do occur, so oxygen and emergency equipment should be readily available when angiography is performed. Patients should also be warned that the dye will temporarily stain their skin and urine; in the average patient this lasts no more than a day.

Indocyanine green (IC-Green) has been used in recent years, either alone or with fluorescein, to obtain better frames of choroid neovascularization.

D. Examination of Abnormal Pupillary Responses

Methacholine, as a 2.5% solution instilled into the conjunctival sac, will cause the tonic pupil (Adie's pupil) to contract, but will leave a normal pupil unchanged. A similar pupillary response is seen following instillation of 2.5% methacholine in patients with familial dysautonomia (Riley-Day syndrome).

Table 28 shows the effects of several drugs on miosis due to interruption of the sympathetic nervous system (Horner's syndrome). The effect depends on the location of the lesion in the sympathetic chain.

TABLE 28

HORNER'S SYNDROME

TOPICAL DROP (CENTRAL)	NEURON III (POST-GANGLIONIC)	NEURON II (PRE-GANGLIONIC)	NEURON I
Cocaine 2%–10%	–	–	+/–
Epinephrine (Adrenalin) 1:1000	+++	+	–
Phenylephrine 1%	+++	+	+/–

Pilocarpine may be used to determine whether a fixed dilated pupil is due to an atropine-like drug or interruption of the pupil's parasympathetic innervation. If an atropine-like drug is involved, the pupil will not react to pilocarpine. If dilation is due to interruption of the parasympathetic innervation (compression by aneurysm, Adie's tonic pupil) instillation of pilocarpine will cause the pupil to constrict.

REFERENCES

Benatar M. A systemic review of diagnostic studies in myasthenia gravis. *Neuromus Dis*. 2000;16:459.

Hecht SD. Evaluation of the lacrimal drainage system. *Ophthalmology*. 1978;85:1250.

Thompson HS, Mensher JH. Adrenergic mydriasis in Horner's syndrome: Hydroxyampheta mine test for diagnosis of post-ganglionic defects. *Am J Ophthalmol*. 1971;72:472.

Thompson HS, Newsome DA, Lowenfeld IE. The fixed dilated pupil. Sudden iridoplegia or mydriatic drops; a simple diagnostic test. *Arch Ophthalmol*. 1971;86:12.

11. VISCOELASTIC MATERIALS USED IN OPHTHALMOLOGY

Viscoelastic substances are used in ophthalmic surgery to maintain the anterior chamber, hydraulically dissect tissues, act as a vitreous substitute/tamponade, and prevent mechanical damage to tissue, especially the corneal endothelium. The individual characteristics of the various viscoelastic materials are the result of the chain length and intra- and interchain molecular interactions of the compounds comprising the viscoelastic substance. All viscoelastic materials have the potential to produce a large postoperative increase in pressure if they are not adequately removed from the anterior chamber following surgery.

AMVISC (Bausch and Lomb) – Composed of sodium hyaluronate 1.2% in physiologic saline. The viscosity is 40,000 cSt (@25°C, 1/sec shear rate), and molecular weight is ≥2,000,000 daltons. Its shelf life is estimated at 2 years.

AMVISC PLUS (Bausch and Lomb) – Composed of sodium hyaluronate 1.6% in physiologic saline. The viscosity is 55,000 cSt (@25°C, 1/sec shear rate), and molecular weight is approximately 1,500,000 daltons. The greater viscosity is obtained by increasing total concentration and using sodium hyaluronate of lower molecular weight. Its shelf life is estimated at 1 year.

BIOLON (Akorn) – Composed of sodium hyaluronate 1%. The viscosity is 215,000 cps, and the molecular weight is approximately 3,000,000 daltons. The product does not require refrigeration and its shelf life is estimated to be approximately 2 years.

DUOVISC (Alcon) – Package contains two separate syringes. One syringe containing Provisc; the other containing Viscoat. Please see individual descriptions below for details of each.

HEALON (Abbott Medical Optics) – Composed of sodium hyaluronate 1% in physiologic saline. The viscosity is 300,000 mPas (@ 0/sec shear rate), and the molecular weight is approximately 4,000,000 daltons.

HEALON GV (Abbott Medical Optics) – Composed of sodium hyaluronate 1.4% in physiologic saline. The viscosity is 3,000,000 mPas (@ 0/sec shear rate), and the molecular weight is approximately 5,000,000 daltons. In the presence of high positive vitreous pressure, Healon GV has 3 times more resistance to pressure than does Healon.

HEALON5 (Abbott Medical Optics) – Composed of sodium hyaluronate 2.3%. The viscosity is 7,000,000 cP (@ 25°C, 1/sec shear rate), and the molecular weight is 4,000,000 daltons.

OCUCOAT (Storz – Bausch and Lomb) – Composed of hydroxypropylmethylcellulose 2% in balanced salt solution (BSS). The viscosity is 4,000 cSt (@ 37°C measured on Cannon-Fenske Viscometer), and the molecular weight is approximately 80,000 daltons. Ocucoat is termed a viscoadherent rather than a viscoelastic because of its coating ability, which is related to its contact angle and low surface tension.

PROVISC (Alcon) – Composed of sodium hyaluronate 1% in physiologic saline. The viscosity is 39,000 cps (@ 25°C, 2/sec shear rate) and the molecular weight is approximately 1,900,000 daltons. Clinical studies demonstrate that ProVisc functions in a similar fashion to Healon.

VISCOAT (Alcon) – Composed of a 1:3 mixture of chondroitin sulfate 4% (CS) and sodium hyaluronate 3% (SH) in physiologic saline. The viscosity is 40,000 cps (@ 25°C, 2/sec shear rate), and the molecular weight is 22,500 daltons for CS and 500,000 daltons for SH.

VITRAX (Allergan) – Composed of sodium hyaluronate 3% in balanced salt solution (BSS). The viscosity is 30,000 cps (@ 2/sec shear rate) and the molecular weight is 500,000 daltons. It is highly concentrated to produce a significantly viscous material. It does not require refrigeration and has a shelf life of 18 months.

12. ANTI-ANGIOGENESIS TREATMENTS

These medications are generally used for the treatment of wet age-related macular degeneration. A significant warning of potential risk for thromboembolic events with their use has been issued.
TABLE 29

ANTI-ANGIOGENESIS TREATMENTS

GENERIC NAME	TRADE NAME	DOSAGE	FDA-APPROVED INDICATION
Verteporfin for injection	Visudyne	6 mg/m^2 intravenously over 10 min at 3 mL/min.*	Treatment of predominantly classic subfoveal CNV due to AMD, pathologic myopia, or presumed ocular histoplasmosis
Pegaptanib sodium	Macugen	0.3 mg intravitreal q 6 weeks	Treatment of wet AMD (all subtypes, including predominantly classic, minimally classic, and occult)
Ranibizumab	Lucentis	0.5 mg intravitreal q month	Treatment of wet AMD (all subtypes, including predominantly classic, minimally classic, and occult)

*Initiate photoactivation with laser light therapy with nonthermal diode laser 15 minutes after starting intravenous infusion. Re-evaluate every 3 months and repeat if CNV leakage is detected on fluorescein angiography.

AMD = age-related macular degeneration; CNV = choroidal neovascularization.

Note: Bevacizumab is often used off label as an anti-VEGF agent. More detail is provided in the off-label drug applications (Section 13) below.

REFERENCE
Gragoudas ES, et al. Pegaptanib for neovascular age-related macular degeneration. *N Engl J Med.* 2004;351:2805.

13. OFF-LABEL DRUG APPLICATIONS IN OPHTHALMOLOGY

A. Acetylcysteine
Used to treat corneal conditions (eg, alkali burns, corneal melts, filamentary keratitis, and keratoconjunctivitis sicca), this agent is thought to improve healing by inhibiting the action of collagenase, which may contribute to delay in healing. Though none of the commercially available solutions is FDA approved for use in ophthalmology, they have been administered as frequently as hourly in acute cases, and up to 4 times a day in maintenance therapy.

B. Alteplase (tissue plasminogen activator)
This thrombolytic agent, available under the trade name Activase, is used to treat fibrin formation in postvitrectomy patients. Initial studies were based on intraocular injections of 25 mcg; more recent work has shown doses as low as 3 to 6 mcg to be effective. Because byproducts of alteplase activity may mediate endothelial cell toxicity, the lower doses are preferred. This agent

has also been used for submacular hemorrhage, but this use is controversial.

Alteplase injections, 6-12 mcg, have been used to remove fibrin membranes that occlude the intraocular portion of tube shunts. However, caution should be used, as this is a potent thrombolytic agent and there is a significant risk of hyphema formation. A careful examination of the anterior chamber should be made preoperatively and the product avoided if there is any evidence of neovascularization.

C. Antimetabolites
5-Fluorouracil (5-FU). This drug inhibits fibroblast proliferation and diminishes scarring after glaucoma filtering surgery. Initial recommendations of the 5-FU study group called for subconjunctival injections of 5 mg twice daily for 7 days postoperatively and once daily for the next 7 days (total 21 injections). Other physicians achieve

success with five injections over 15 days. Many use an intraoperative application of 50 mg/mL solution soaked into a murocell sponge lasting for 3 to 5 minutes, with a body of literature supporting its effectiveness (see references at the end of this section). Complications associated with this drug include conjunctival wound leak, corneal epithelial defects, hypotony associated with permanently reduced vision acuity, serious corneal infections in eyes with preexistent corneal epithelial edema, and increased susceptibility to late-onset bleb infections. The drug should be considered only when there is a high risk of surgical failure.

Mitomycin C. This potent chemotherapeutic agent is being used in glaucoma filtering surgery for the same purpose and on the same type of patients as 5-FU, with similar reported side effects. It is applied once during surgery on a small piece of Gelfilm or Weck cell sponge in a concentration of 0.2 mg/mL (0.02%) to 0.4 mg/mL (0.04%). With a possibility of delayed reactions 6 to 24 months after surgery, some serious side effects may go unreported. Mitomycin has also been administered in a concentrated solution of 0.2 mg/mL (0.02%) to 0.4 mg/mL (0.04%) 2 to 4 times a day — and more recently as a one-time application in the operating room — to prevent recurrence after pterygium surgery and reduce scarring after corneal surgery, especially excimer laser surgery. Serious side effects associated with this therapy include corneal melts and scleral ulceration and calcification.

The possibility of major side effects exists with all antineoplastic agents. Remember, too, that these agents should always be handled and discarded in accordance with OSHA, AMA, ASHP, and hospital policies.

D. Bevacizumab
This humanized monoclonal antibody inhibits vascular endothelial growth factor-A and is available under the trade name Avastin (Genentech/Roche). Bevacizumab is approved to treat many cancers; however, there is significant use of it off-label to treat age-related macular degeneration, macular edema after retinal vein occlusion, and diabetic retinopathy. When used for AMD, dosing is generally the same as with ranibizumab (Lucentis; Genentech/Roche)—usually 1.25 mg for intravitreal injection. The Comparison of Age-Related Macular Degeneration Treatment Trials (CATT) concluded that "at 1 year, bevacizumab and ranibizumab had equivalent effects on visual acuity when administered according to the same schedule." The CATT study did find that the proportion of patients with serious systemic adverse events was higher with bevacizumab than with ranibizumab.

Bevacizumab has also been used as a surgical adjunct for procedures to treat neovascular glaucoma to decrease subsequent bleeding. It is given either intraoperatively or one week ahead of surgery when possible.

E. Cyclosporine
This potent immunosuppressant has a high degree of selectivity for T lymphocytes. Available under the trade name Sandimmune, it has been used in a 0.5–2% topical solution as prophylaxis against rejection in high-risk, penetrating keratoplasty and for treating severe vernal conjunctivitis resistant to conventional therapy, ligneous conjunctivitis unresponsive to other topical therapy, and noninfectious peripheral ulcerative keratitis associated with systemic autoimmune disorders.

F. Doxycycline and Minocycline
These tetracycline derivatives are used to treat ocular rosacea meibomianitis, and certain conditions involving corneal melting. Usual dose is 100 mg PO 1-2 times per day for 2 to 12 weeks, after which the dose is often reduced. Lower doses (eg, 40-50 mg/day) may provide a similar anti-inflammatory effect, but without the same antibiotic effect. They have the same side effects, contraindications, and interactions as tetracycline, although doxycycline may be taken with food.

G. Edetate disodium
This chelating agent plays a role in treating band keratopathy. After removal of the corneal epithelium, it is used to remove calcium from Bowman's membrane.

REFERENCES
CATT Research Group, Martin DF, Maguire MG, Ying GS, Grunwald JE, Fine SL, Jaffe GJ. Ranibizumab and bevacizumab for neovascular age-related macular degeneration. *N Engl J Med.* 2011;364;1897.

Dietze PJ, Feldman RM, Gross RL. Intraoperative application of 5-fluorouracil during trabeculectomy. *Ophthalmic Surg Lasers.* 1992;23(10):662.

Dunn J, Seamone S, Ostler H. Development of scleral ulceration and calcification after pterygium excision and mitomycin therapy. *Am J Ophthalmol.* 1991;112:343.

Feldman RM, Dietze PJ, Gross RL, et al. Intraoperative 5-fluorouracil administration in trabeculectomy. *J Glaucoma.* 1994;3:302.

Frucht-Perry J, et al. The effect of doxycycline on ocular rosacea. *Am J Ophthalmol.* 1989;170(4):434.

Jaffe G, Abrams G, et al. Tissue plasminogen activator for post vitrectomy fibrin formation. *Ophthalmology.* 1990;97:189.

Goldenfeld M, Krupin T, Ruderman JM, et al. 5-Fluorouracil in initial trabeculectomy. A prospective, randomized, multicenter study. *Ophthalmology.* 1994;101(6):1024.

Lanigan L, Sturmer J, Baez KA, Hitchings RA, Khaw PT. Single intraoperative applications of 5-fluorouracil during filtration surgery: early results. *Br J Ophthalmol.* 1994;78(1):33.

Lish A, Camras C, Podos S. Effect of apraclonidine on intraocular pressure in glaucoma patients receiving maximally tolerated medications. *Glaucoma.* 1992;1:19.

McDermott M, Edelhauser H, et al. Tissue plasminogen activator and corneal endothelium. *Am J Ophthalmol.* 1989;108:91-92.

Mora JS, Nguyen N, Iwach AG, et al. Trabeculectomy with intraoperative sponge 5-fluorouracil. *Ophthalmology.* 1996;103(6):963. Review.

Perry HD, Donnenfeld ED. Medications for dry eye syndrome: a drug-therapy review. *Manag Care.* 2003;12(suppl 12):26.

Pflugfelder SC. Antiinflammatory therapy for dry eye. *Am J Ophthalmol.* 2004;137:337.

Quarterman MJ, et al. Signs, symptoms, and tear studies before and after treatment with doxycycline. *Arch Dermatol.* 1997;133:89.

Rothman RF, Liebmann JM, Ritch R. Low-dose 5-fluorouracil trabeculectomy as initial surgery in uncomplicated glaucoma: long-term followup. *Ophthalmology.* 2000;107(6):1184.

Rubinfeld R, Pfister R, et al. Serious complications of topical mitomycin-C after pterygium surgery. *Ophthalmology.* 1992;99:1647.

Sall K, Stevenson OD, Nundorf TK, Reis BL. Two multicenter, randomized studies of the efficacy and safety of cyclosporine ophthalmic emulsion in moderate to severe dry eye disease. CsA Phase 3 Study Group. *Ophthalmology.* 2000;107:631. Erratum in: *Ophthalmology.* 2000;107:1220.

Smith MF, Sherwood MB, Doyle JW, Khaw PT. Results of intraoperative 5-fluorouracil supplementation on trabeculectomy for open-angle glaucoma. *Am J Ophthalmol.* 1992;114(6):737.

Stevenson D, Tauber J, Reis BL. Efficacy and safety of cyclosporine A ophthalmic emulsion in the treatment of moderate-to-severe dry eye disease: a dose-ranging, randomized trial. The Cyclosporin A Phase 2 Study Group. *Ophthalmology.* 2000;107:967.

Three-year follow-up of the Fluorouracil Filtering Surgery Study. *Am J Ophthalmol.* 1993;115(1):82.

Williams D, Benett S, et al. Low-dose intraocular tissue plasminogen activator for treatment of postvitrectomy firbrin formations. *Am J Opthalmol.* 1990;109:606.

14. OCULAR TOXICOLOGY — F. W. FRAUNFELDER, MD

The table on the following pages lists recently reported ocular side effects of drugs as they relate to the eye. The list is not intended to be comprehensive but should provide clinicians with an overview of some of the more clinically relevant side effects that have been reported. For more extensive information, please consult our book *Clinical Ocular Toxicology* or our website at www.eyedrugregistry.com.

Toxicology data are cataloged by the National Registry of Drug-Induced Ocular Side Effects. To report a suspected adverse drug response, or to obtain references for the information listed in the table, please contact:

F.W. Fraunfelder, MD, Director, Cornea/Refractive Surgery and National Registry of Drug-Induced Ocular Side Effects; and Professor of Ophthalmology
Casey Eye Institute
Oregon Health & Science University
3375 SW Terwilliger Blvd.
Portland, OR 97239-4197
Phone: (503) 494-4318
Fax: (503) 418-2284
E-mail: eyedrug@ohsu.edu
Website: www.eyedrugregistry.com

REFERENCES

Fraunfelder FT, Fraunfelder FW. *Drug-Induced Ocular Side Effects*, ed 5. Woburn, Mass: Butterworth-Heinemann; 2001.

Fraunfelder FT, Fraunfelder FW, Edwards R. Ocular side effects possibly associated with isotretinoin usage. *Am J Ophthalmol.* 2001;132(3):299-305.

Fraunfelder FT, Fraunfelder FW, Chambers WA. *Clinical Ocular Toxicology*. Saunders Elsevier Philadelphia, PA, USA, 2008.

Fraunfelder FT, Fraunfelder FW. Trichomegaly and other external eye side effects associated with epidermal growth factor inhibitors. *Cornea.* (In press.)

Fraunfelder FW. Corneal toxicity from topical ocular and systemic medications. *Cornea.* 2006 Dec;25(10):1133-8.

Fraunfelder FW. Ocular side effects associated with bisphosphonates. *Drugs of Today.* 2003;39(11):829-835.

Fraunfelder FW. Ocular side effects associated with COX-2 inhibitors. *Arch Ophthalmol.* 2006 Feb; 124(2):277-9.

Fraunfelder FW. Twice-yearly exams not necessary for patients taking quetiapine. *Am J Ophthalmol.* 2004;138(5):870-871.

Fraunfelder FW. Visual side effects associated with erectile dysfunction agents. *Am J Ophthalmol.* 2005 Oct; 140(4):723-4.

Fraunfelder FW, Fraunfelder FT. Topiramate associated acute, bilateral, secondary angle-closure glaucoma. *Ophthalmol.* 2004;111(1):109-111.

Fraunfelder FW, Fraunfelder FT. Oculogyric crisis in patients taking cetirizine. *Am J Ophthalmol.* 2004;137(2):355-57.

Fraunfelder FW, Fraunfelder FT. Scleritis associated with pamidronate disodium use. *Am J Ophthalmol.* 2003;135(2):219-222.

Fraunfelder FW, Fraunfelder FT. Interferon Alfa Associated Anterior Ischemic Optic Neuropathy. Accepted by *Ophthalmology.* February 2010.

Fraunfelder FW, Fraunfelder FT, Corbett JJ. Isotretinoin-associated intracranial hypertension. *Ophthalmology.* 2004;111(6):1248-1250.

Fraunfelder FW, Fraunfelder FT. Diplopia associated with fluoroquinolones. *Ophthalmology.* 2009;116(9):1814-1817.

Fraunfelder FW, Fraunfelder FT. Central serous chorioretinopathy associated with sildenafil *Retina.* 2008;28(4):606-609.

Fraunfelder FW, Harrison D. Peripheral ulcerative keratitis-like findings associated with filgrastim. *Cornea.* 2007 Apr;26(3):368-9.

Fraunfelder FW, Pomeranz H, Egan RA. Nonarteritic ischemic optic neuropathy and sildenafil. *Arch Ophthalmol.* 2006 May; 124(5): 733-4.

Fraunfelder FW, Rich LF. Possible adverse effects of drugs used in refractive surgery. *J Cataract Refractive Surg.* 2003;29(1):170-175.

Fraunfelder FW, Richards AB. HMG-CoA reductase inhibitors (statins), and ptosis, ophthalmoplegia, and diplopia. Accepted to *Ophthalmology July 2008.*

Wheeler D, Fraunfelder FW. Ocular motility dysfunction associated with chemotherapeutic agents. *J Am Assoc Pediatr Ophthalmol Strabismus.* 2004;8(1):15-17.

TABLE 30

ADVERSE DRUG EFFECTS

GENERIC NAME	PRINCIPAL GENERAL USE	POSSIBLE ADVERSE EFFECTS
I. MEDICATION BY INJECTION		
Adrenal Corticosteroids		
Depo-steroids	Allergic disorders Anti-inflammatory disorders	If injected into a blood vessel, eg, the tonsillar fossa, may cause unilateral or bilateral retinal arterial occlusions due to emboli of depo-steroid. Permanent bilateral blindness may ensue.
Triamcinolone	Allergic disorders Anti-inflammatory disorders	Fatty atrophy in area of injection, ie, enophthalmus if given retrobulbar or, if given in periocular skin, some deformity can occur in area due to loss of fat. 50% chance of an IOP elevation.
Alpha-blocker		
Tamsulosin	Benign prostatic hyperplasia	Intraoperative floppy iris syndrome
Antifungals		
Amphotericin B	Aspergillosis, blastomycosis, candidiasis, coccidioidomycosis, histoplasmosis	Ischemic necrosis after subconjunctival injection Subconjunctival nodule, yellow discoloration

GENERIC NAME	PRINCIPAL GENERAL USE	POSSIBLE ADVERSE EFFECTS
Antineoplastics		
Carmustine	Brain tumors	Optic neuritis
	Multiple myeloma	Retinal vascular disorders
Cisplatin	Metastatic testicular or ovarian tumors. Advanced bladder carcinoma	Cortical blindness Papilledema, retrobulbar or optic neuritis
Epithelial growth factor receptor (EGFR)	Treats solid tumors	Conjunctivitis, blepharitis, meibomitis, periocular skin rash, periocular erythema and edema, corneal superficial punctate keratitis, corneal erosions, trichiasis, trichomegaly, and dry eye.
Fluorouracil	Carcinoma of the colon, rectum, breast, stomach, and pancreas	Ocular irritation with tearing, conjunctival hyperemia, canalicular fibrosis, ocular motility dysfunction
Ophthalmic Dyes		
Fluorescein	Ocular diagnostic tests	Nausea, vomiting, urticaria, rhinorrhea, dizziness, hypotension, pharyngoedema, anaphylactic reaction
Parasympathomimetics		
Acetylcholine	Produces prompt, short-term miosis	Hypotension and bradycardia with intraocular injection
Vaccinations		
Hepatitis B vaccine	Used to prevent HBV infection	Uveitis
II. ORAL		
Antiarrhythmics		
Amiodarone HCl	Cardiac abnormalities	Keratopathy
	Ventricular arrhythmias	Lens opacities, optic neuropathy, color vision defects Discoloration of conjunctiva and eyelids
Propranolol	Cardiovascular abnormalities	May precipitate latent myotonia
	Certain hypertensive states	May mask hyperthyroidism; when taken off drug, thyroid stare and exophthalmos may occur
Antibiotics and Antituberculars		
Chloramphenicol	Typhoid fever	Aplastic anemia
Ethambutol HCl	Pulmonary tuberculosis	Optic neuropathy
Fluoroquinolones	Used to treat a variety of bacterial infections; inhibits DNA replication and transcription.	Diplopia Uveitis
Rifampin	Asymptomatic carriers of meningococcus	Conjunctival hyperemia
	Many gram-negative and gram-positive cocci, including *Neisseria* and *Haemophilus influenzae*	Exudative conjunctivitis Increased lacrimation
	Pulmonary tuberculosis	
Minocycline	Useful against gram-negative and gram-positive bacteria	Pseudotumor cerebri and papilledema as early as 3 days after onset of medication in infants and in young adults
	Members of lymphogranuloma-psittacosis group *Mycoplasma*	Transient myopia
	Acne rosacea	Permanent pigmentation of sclera
Anticholesterol Agents		
HMG-CoA reductase inhibitors (statins)	Used to treat hyperlipidemia and hypercholesterolemia	Blepharoptosis, diplopia, and ophthalmoplegia
Antihelmintics		
Levamisole HCl	Connective tissue disorders *Ascaris* infestation	Patients with Sjögren's syndrome and possibly keratitis sicca have marked increase in systemic side effects, including pruritus and muscle weakness
Antihistamines		
Cetirizine	Treatment of perennial allergic rhinitis, chronic urticaria, and allergic rhinitis	Oculogyric crisis (primarily in children)
Antihypertensives		
Sodium nitroprusside	Provides controlled hypotension during anesthesia	Contraindicated in Leber's hereditary optic atrophy and tobacco amblyopia
	Management of severe hypertension	
Antileprotics		
Clofazimine	Dermatologic diseases—psoriasis, pyoderma gangrenosum	Conjunctival, corneal, and macular pigmentation
	Leprosy	

GENERIC NAME	PRINCIPAL GENERAL USE	POSSIBLE ADVERSE EFFECTS
Antimalarials and Anti-inflammatories		
Hydroxychloroquine	Malaria Lupus erythematosus Rheumatoid arthritis	Disturbance of accommodation Corneal changes Bull's-eye maculopathy—central, pericentral, or paracentral scotomas
Antineoplastics		
Busulfan	Chronic myelogenous leukemia	Cataracts Decreased lacrimation
Tamoxifen	Metastatic breast carcinoma	Corneal opacities Refractile retinal deposits Posterior subcapsular cataracts Decreased color perception
Bisphosphonates	Osteoporosis Hypercalcemia of malignancy	Scleritis, uveitis, conjunctivitis, episcleritis (reversible)

Imatinib mesylate	Treatment of chronic myelogenous leukemia,
	   gastrointestinal stromal tumors,
	   mastocytosis, and myelodysplastic syndrome
		Periorbital edema,
		epiphora, conjunctivitis

Antipsychotics		
Lithium carbonate	Manic phase of manic/depressive psychosis	Exophthalmos, oculogyric crisis, myoclonus
Quetiapine fumarate	Schizophrenia and Bipolar disorder	Cataracts unlikely
Antiseizure		
Topiramate	Refractory epilepsy	Acute angle-closure glaucoma, myopia, uveal effusion
Antispasmodics		

Baclofen	Muscle spasms in multiple sclerosis and
	   disorders associated with increased
	   muscular tone
		Blurred vision
		Hallucinations

Carbonic Anhydrase Inhibitors		

Acetazolamide
Methazolamide
	Glaucoma	Aggravation of metabolic acidosis, primarily in
		   known CO_2-retaining diseases such as
		   emphysema and bronchiectasis, and in
		   patients with poor vital capacity
		Aplastic anemia, various blood disorders
		Decreased libido
		Impotency

Chelating Agents		

Penicillamine	Cystinuria
	Heavy metal antagonist—iron, lead,
	   copper, mercury poisoning
	Wilson's disease
		Facial or ocular myasthenia, including extraocular
		   muscle paralysis, ptosis, and diplopia
		Ocular pemphigoid
		Optic neuritis and color-vision problems

Erectile Dysfunction Agents		

Sildenafil
Tadalafil
Vardenafil
	Erectile dysfunction	Transitory changes in color perception, blurred
		   vision, changes in light perception,
		   electroretinography (ERG) changes,
		   conjunctival hyperemia, ocular pain,
		   photophobia, subconjunctival hemorrhages,
		   optic neuropathy possible, central serous retinopathy

Hormonal Agents		
Oral contraceptives	Amenorrhea Dysfunctional uterine bleeding Dysmenorrhea Hypogonadism Oral contraception Premenstrual tension	Contraindicated in patients with preexisting retinal vascular diseases Decrease in color vision with chronic use Macular edema
Hydantoins		

Phenytoin	Chronic epilepsy	Optic nerve hypoplasia in infants with epileptic mothers
		   on the drug; ocular teratogenic effects, including
		   strabismus, ptosis, hypertelorism, epicanthus

Interferon Alfa	Used to treat hepatitis B & C Malignant melanoma Renal cell carcinoma and other malignancies	Anterior ischemic optic neuropathy

GENERIC NAME	PRINCIPAL GENERAL USE	POSSIBLE ADVERSE EFFECTS
Nonsteroidal Anti-inflammatory Drugs		
COX-2 inhibitors (celecoxib)	Rheumatoid arthritis Osteoarthritis	Blurred vision Irritative conjunctivitis
Ibuprofen	Rheumatoid arthritis Osteoarthritis	Decreased color vision Optic neuritis, visual field defects
Naproxen	Rheumatoid arthritis Osteoarthritis Ankylosing spondylitis	Corneal opacity Periorbital edema
Sulindac	Rheumatoid arthritis Osteoarthritis Ankylosing spondylitis	Keratitis Stevens-Johnson syndrome
Psychedelics		
Marijuana	Cerebral sedative or narcotic	Conjunctival hyperemia; decreased lacrimation; decreased intraocular pressure; dyschromatopsia with chronic long-term use
Sedatives and Hypnotics		
Ethanol	Antiseptic Used as a beverage	Fetal alcohol syndrome: offspring of alcoholic mothers may have epicanthus, small palpebral fissures, and microphthalmia
Synthetic Retinoids		
Isotretinoin	Severe recalcitrant nodular acne	Permanent night blindness, color vision defects, keratitis sicca. **Note:** All retinoids, in rare instances, can cause intracranial hypertension.
III. TOPICAL		
Anticholinergics		
Cyclopentolate HCl	Used as a cycloplegic and mydriatic	Central nervous system toxicity, including slurred speech, ataxia, hallucinations, hyperactivity, seizures, syncope, and paralytic ileus
Tropicamide	Used as a cycloplegic and mydriatic	Cyanosis, muscle rigidity, nausea, pallor, vomiting, vasomotor collapse
Parasympathomimetics or Anticholinesterases		
Echothiophate iodide Pilocarpine	Glaucoma	Retinal detachments primarily in eyes with peripheral retinal or retinal-vitreal disease. (Patients need to be warned of this possible effect when first placed on this medication.) Miotic upper respiratory infection—rhinorrhea, sensa- tion of chest constriction, cough, conjunctival hyperemia; seen primarily in young children on anticholinesterase agents
Prostaglandins		
Latanoprost	Open-angle glaucoma	Flulike syndrome; increased pigmentation of iris, eyelid skin, eyelid and eyelash; eyelashes—increased number, growth, and curling; iritis
Sulfonamides		
Carbonic anhydrase inhibitors	Open-angle glaucoma and ocular hypertension	Ciliary body and uveal effusion causing acute and myopia and bilateral angle-closure glaucoma
Sympathomimetics		
Dipivefrin	Open-angle glaucoma	Follicular blepharoconjunctivitis, keratitis
Epinephrine	Used as a bronchodilator Open-angle glaucoma Used as a vasoconstrictor to prolong anesthetic action	Cicatricial pemphigoid Stains soft-contact lenses black Hypertension, headache
10% Phenylephrine	Used as a mydriatic and vasoconstrictor	Cardiac arrhythmias and cardiac arrests with pledget form or subconjunctival injection, possible myocardial infarcts, systemic hypertension
Betaxolol Levobunolol HCl Timolol	Open-angle glaucoma	Cardiac syncope, bradycardia, lightheadedness, fatigue, congestive heart failure; in diabetics—hyperglycemia or hypoglycemia; in myasthenia gravis—severe dysarthria

SECTION 3

SUTURE MATERIALS

Although *sutureless* cataract surgery is diminishing the need for certain sutures, there is still no other discipline that requires as many specialized needles and suture materials as ophthalmic surgery. To meet this need, manufacturers offer the ophthalmologist a comprehensive array of precisely manufactured reverse-cutting and spatula needles swaged to suture materials of collagen (plain and chromic), silk (black and white braided), virgin silk (black and white twisted), Nylon, Dacron, and synthetics.

Suture material intended for use in ophthalmic surgery can be either absorbable or nonabsorbable. Following is a list of various suture materials available with a brief description of each.

Absorbable
The absorption of sutures occurs in two distinct phases. After implantation, the suture's tensile strength diminishes during the early postoperative period. When most of the strength is lost, the remaining suture mass

begins to decrease in what may be termed as the second phase of absorption. The mass-loss phase then proceeds until the entire suture has been absorbed.

Plain Catgut—Prepared from the submucosal or mucosal layers of sheep or beef intestine, respectively, this material consists primarily of collagen—a fibrous protein—which is absorbed by the body. The material is chemically purified to minimize tissue reaction. Available in sizes 4–0 through 6–0.

Chromic Catgut—same as plain catgut except that it is treated with chromium salts to delay the absorption time. Available in sizes 4–0 through 7–0.

Plain Collagen—prepared from bovine deep flexor tendon. The tendon is purified and converted to a uniform suspension of collagen fibril. This fibrillar suspension is then extruded into suture strands and chemically treated to accurately control absorption rate. Available in sizes 4–0 through 7–0.

TABLE 1

COMPARISON OF OPHTHALMIC SUTURE MATERIALS

SUTURE MATERIAL	RELATIVE TENSILE STRENGTH*	RELATIVE HOLDING DURATION†	RELATIVE TISSUE REACTION‡	EASE OF HANDLING	SPECIAL KNOT REQUIRED	BEHAVIOR OF EXPOSED ENDS	AVAILABLE SIZES§
ABSORBABLE							
Surgical gut or collagen							
Plain	6	1 week	4+	Fair	No	Stiff	4–0 to 7–0
Chromic	6	<2 weeks	3+	Fair	No	Stiff	4–0 to 8–0
SYNTHETIC ABSORBABLE							
Polyglactin 910							
Braided	9	2 weeks	2+	Good	Yes	Stiff	4–0 to 9–0
Monofilament	9	2 weeks	2+	Good	Yes	Stiff	9–0 to 10–0
Polyglycolic acid	9	2 weeks	2+	Good	Yes	Stiff	4–0 to 10–0
NONABSORBABLE							
Silk							
Virgin	7	2 months	3+	Excellent	No	Softest	8–0 to 9–0
Braided	8	2 months	3+	Good	No	Soft	4–0 to 9–0
Polyamide (Nylon)	9	6 months	1+	Fair	Yes	Stiff, sharp	8–0 to 11–0
Polypropylene	10	>12 months	1+	Fair	Yes	Stiff, sharp	4–0 to 6–0
							9–0 to 10–0

* The higher the number, the greater the relative tensile strength. Strength varies with size of material; estimates apply mainly to size 8–0 sutures.

† Holding duration will vary with location and size of suture, health of patient, medications employed, etc. The time given in this table is an average of the time at which about 30% of tensile strength is lost.

‡ 1+ indicates least inflammatory response, 4+ greatest.

§ With needles appropriate for ophthalmic use. Sizes available will vary from time to time.

Adapted from Spaeth GL. *Ophthalmic Surgery, Principles and Practice.* Philadelphia, Pa: WB Saunders; 1982:64.

Chromic Collagen—prepared in the same way as plain collagen except that chromium salts are added during the chemical treatment to further delay absorption. Available in sizes 4–0 through 8–0.

Synthetic Absorbable Sutures—Products include Vicryl (Polyglactin 910, a copolymer of lactide and glycolide) and Dexon (polyglycolic acid). These materials offer high tensile strength and minimal tissue reaction during the critical postoperative healing period, followed by predictable absorption. Coated Vicryl sutures are also available. Manufactured in size 4–0 through 10–0 (coated 4–0 through 8–0).

Nonabsorbable
Virgin Silk—twisted with the individual silk filaments still embedded in their natural sericin coating, providing a smooth, uniform suture in very fine sizes. The suture is offered in black or white, permitting optimum contrast with tissues. Available in sizes 8–0 and 9–0.

Black Braided Silk Suture—braided under controlled conditions to maximize strength and ensure resistance to breaking while knots are tied. Gums and other impurities are removed, resulting in a suture that remains tightly braided, with virtually no loose filaments and minimal tendency to broom. Available in sizes 4–0 through 9–0.

Monofilament Nylon Sutures (Ethilon, Dermalon, and Supramid)—These sutures offer high tensile strength and minimal tissue reaction. Nylon has been reported to lose tensile strength postoperatively at a rate of approximately 15% per year. Available in sizes 8–0 through 11–0.

Polypropylene Suture (Prolene)—a monofilament suture with high tensile strength and minimal tissue reaction. The material is not degraded or weakened by tissue enzymes. Available in sizes 4-0 to 6-0 and 9-0 to 10-0.

Polyester Fiber Sutures—Products include Mersilene and Ti Cron. They exhibit minimal tissue reaction and are braided by a special method for tightness, uniformity, and a smooth surface that minimizes trauma. Available in sizes 4–0 through 6–0.

A variety of physical characteristics of different sutures have been published. In addition, the United States Pharmacopeia has established specifications for various suture materials. Some of the useful parameters measured have been: (1) tensile strength, (2) elasticity, (3) suture diameters, and (4) weight per unit length. Data are summarized in **Tables 1** through **3**.

TABLE 2

ELASTICITY OF SELECTED SUTURES

SUTURE MATERIAL	ELONGATION OF STANDARD 30.5-cm SEGMENT	INCREASE IN LENGTH	WEIGHT AT BREAKING POINT
6–0 plain gut	4.7 cm	15.4%	264 g
6–0 chromic gut	4.3 cm	14.1%	257 g
6–0 Mersilene	1.9 cm	6.3%	254 g
6–0 braided silk	1.2 cm	3.9%	237 g
7–0 chromic gut	3.6 cm	1.8%	118 g
7–0 braided silk	0.9 cm	3.0%	126 g
8–0 virgin silk	0.8 cm	2.6%	53 g
10–0 Nylon	8.7 cm	28.5%	23 g

From Middleton DG, McCulloch C. *Adv Ophthalmol.* 1970;22:35.

TABLE 3

WEIGHT OF SELECTED SUTURE MATERIAL

SUTURE MATERIAL	WEIGHT/LENGTH (MG/CM)
6–0 plain gut (wet)	0.170
6–0 chromic gut (wet)	0.176
6–0 Mersilene	0.116
6–0 braided silk	0.165
7–0 chromic gut (wet)	0.062
7–0 braided silk	0.065
8–0 virgin silk	0.025
10–0 Nylon	0.007

SECTION 4

OPHTHALMIC LENSES

1. COMPARISON AND CONVERSION TABLES

TABLE 1

RELATIVE MAGNIFICATION PRODUCED BY CONTACT AND SPECTACLE LENSES

The percentage increase (or decrease) in the size of the retinal image afforded by contact lenses in comparison with orthodox spectacles fitted at 12 mm from the cornea.

SPECTACLE REFRACTION	EQUIVALENT POWER OF CONTACT LENS SYSTEM	PERCENTAGE INCREASE AFFORDED BY CONTACT LENS	SPECTACLE REFRACTION	EQUIVALENT POWER OF CONTACT LENS SYSTEM	PERCENTAGE INCREASE AFFORDED BY CONTACT LENS	SPECTACLE REFRACTION	EQUIVALENT POWER OF CONTACT LENS SYSTEM	PERCENTAGE INCREASE AFFORDED BY CONTACT LENS
−20	−15.73	27.2	−8	−7.07	12.9	+6	+6.10	−4.7
−18	−14.41	24.8	−6	−5.42	10.5	+8	+8.29	−7.4
−16	−13.06	22.5	−4	−3.69	7.8	+10	+10.62	−10.3
−14	−11.65	20.1	−2	−1.88	5.4	+12	+13.07	−13.8
−12	−10.19	17.8	+2	+1.96	1.2	+14	+15.64	−17.3
−10	−8.66	15.3	+4	+3.99	−1.7			

Bennet AG. *Optics of Contact Lenses*, ed 4. London: Hatton Press; 1966.

TABLE 2

INDEX OF REFRACTION OF LENS MATERIAL

	CROWN GLASS	1.6-INDEX CROWNLITE GLASS	HILITE GLASS	8-INDEX GLASS	CR–39 PLASTIC	HIRI PLASTIC	1.6-INDEX PLASTIC	POLY–CARBONATE THIN–LITE PLASTIC
INDEX OF REFRACTION The higher the number, the thinner the material	1.523	1.601	1.701	1.805	1.498	1.56	1.6	1.586
SPECIFIC GRAVITY The higher the number, the heavier the material	2.5	2.67	2.99	3.37	1.32	1.216	1.34	1.20
DISPERSION The higher the number, the less chromatic aberration (Abbe value)	59	42.24	31	25	58	38	37	31
PERSONALITY	Temperable, coatable, ease in handling, vast availability	Chemically temperable, ease in handling, limited availability	Chemically temperable, fairly easy to handle, SV and multifocals; vacuum coatings cause lens to become highly sensitive to scratching	SV, difficult to temper, highly reflective so A/R coatings recommended, but have same problems as hilite; mfrs suggest having patient sign liability waiver when ground thin. Multifocal available in laminate.	Strong, tintable, coatable, ease in handling, vast availability	SV and bifocal, tints well before SRC, edges well, must be SRC, extremely brittle	SV only, tints well before SRC, edges well, must be SRC	SV and multifocal, strongest lens material available, limited tintability, must be SPC, no fast fabrication, special edging equipment needed, a must for children and athletes

SV = single-vision lenses. A/R = antireflective. SRC = scratch-resistant coating. SPC = scratch-proof coating.

TABLE 3

CORNEAL RADIUS EQUIVALENCE DIOPTERS/MILLIMETERS

DIOPTERS	mm	DIOPTERS	mm	DIOPTERS	mm	DIOPTERS	mm	DIOPTERS	mm	DIOPTERS	mm	DIOPTERS	mm	DIOPTERS	mm
20.00	16.875	36.00	9.375	39.00	8.653	42.00	8.035	45.00	7.500	48.00	7.031	51.00	6.617	54.00	6.250
22.00	15.340	36.12	9.343	39.12	8.627	42.12	8.012	45.12	7.480	48.12	7.013	51.12	6.602	54.12	6.236
24.00	14.062	36.25	9.310	39.25	8.598	42.25	7.988	45.25	7.458	48.25	6.994	51.25	6.585	54.25	6.221
26.00	12.980	36.37	9.279	39.37	8.572	42.37	7.965	45.37	7.438	48.37	6.977	51.37	6.569	54.37	6.207
27.00	12.500	36.50	9.246	39.50	8.544	42.50	7.941	45.50	7.417	48.50	6.958	51.50	6.553	54.50	6.192
28.00	12.053	36.62	9.216	39.62	8.518	42.62	7.918	45.62	7.398	48.62	6.941	51.62	6.538	54.62	6.179
29.00	11.638	36.75	9.183	39.75	8.490	42.75	7.894	45.75	7.377	48.75	6.923	51.75	6.521	54.75	6.164
29.50	11.441	36.87	9.153	39.87	8.465	42.87	7.872	45.87	7.357	48.87	6.906	51.87	6.506	54.87	6.150
30.00	11.250	37.00	9.121	40.00	8.437	43.00	7.848	46.00	7.336	49.00	6.887	52.00	6.490	55.00	6.136
30.50	11.065	37.12	9.092	40.12	8.412	43.12	7.826	46.12	7.317	49.12	6.870	52.12	6.475	55.12	6.123
31.00	10.887	37.25	9.060	40.25	8.385	43.25	7.803	46.25	7.297	49.25	6.852	52.25	6.459	55.25	6.108
31.50	10.714	37.37	9.031	40.37	8.360	43.37	7.781	46.37	7.278	49.37	6.836	52.37	6.444	55.37	6.095
32.00	10.547	37.50	9.000	40.50	8.333	43.50	7.758	46.50	7.258	49.50	6.818	52.50	6.428	55.50	6.081
32.50	10.385	37.62	8.971	40.62	8.308	43.62	7.737	46.62	7.239	49.62	6.801	52.62	6.413	55.62	6.068
33.00	10.227	37.75	8.940	40.75	8.282	43.75	7.714	46.75	7.219	49.75	6.783	52.75	6.398	55.75	6.054
33.50	10.075	37.87	8.912	40.87	8.257	43.87	7.693	46.87	7.200	49.87	6.767	52.87	6.383	55.87	6.041
34.00	9.926	38.00	8.881	41.00	8.231	44.00	7.670	47.00	7.180	50.00	6.750	53.00	6.367	56.00	6.027
34.25	9.854	38.12	8.853	41.12	8.207	44.12	7.649	47.12	7.162	50.12	6.733	53.12	6.353	56.50	5.973
34.50	9.783	38.25	8.823	41.25	8.181	44.25	7.627	47.25	7.142	50.25	6.716	53.25	6.338	57.00	5.921
34.75	9.712	38.37	8.795	41.37	8.158	44.37	7.606	47.37	7.124	50.37	6.700	53.37	6.323	57.50	5.869
35.00	9.643	38.50	8.766	41.50	8.132	44.50	7.584	47.50	7.105	50.50	6.683	53.50	6.308	58.00	5.819
35.25	9.574	38.62	8.738	41.62	8.109	44.62	7.563	47.62	7.087	50.62	6.667	53.62	6.294	58.50	5.769
35.50	9.507	38.75	8.708	41.75	8.083	44.75	7.541	47.75	7.068	50.75	6.650	53.75	6.279	59.00	5.720
35.75	9.440	38.87	8.682	41.87	8.060	44.87	7.521	47.87	7.050	50.87	6.634	53.87	6.265	60.00	5.625

TABLE 4

VERTEX DISTANCE CONVERSION SCALE (mm)

SPECTACLE LENS POWER	PLUS LENSES								MINUS LENSES							
	8	9	10	11	12	13	14	15	8	9	10	11	12	13	14	15
4.00	4.12	4.12	4.12	4.12	4.25	4.25	4.25	4.25	3.87	3.87	3.87	3.87	3.87	3.75	3.75	3.75
4.50	4.62	4.75	4.75	4.75	4.75	4.75	4.75	4.87	4.37	4.37	4.25	4.25	4.25	4.25	4.25	4.25
5.00	5.25	5.25	5.25	5.25	5.25	5.37	5.37	5.37	4.75	4.75	4.75	4.75	4.75	4.75	4.62	4.62
5.50	5.75	5.75	5.75	5.87	5.87	5.87	6.00	6.00	5.25	5.25	5.25	5.12	5.12	5.12	5.12	5.12
6.00	6.25	6.37	6.37	6.37	6.50	6.50	6.50	6.62	5.75	5.62	5.62	5.62	5.62	5.50	5.50	5.50
6.50	6.87	6.87	7.00	7.00	7.00	7.12	7.12	7.25	6.12	6.12	6.12	6.00	6.00	6.00	6.00	5.87
7.00	7.37	7.50	7.50	7.62	7.62	7.75	7.75	7.75	6.62	6.62	6.50	6.50	6.50	6.37	6.37	6.37
7.50	8.00	8.00	8.12	8.12	8.25	8.25	8.37	8.50	7.12	7.00	7.00	6.87	6.87	6.87	6.75	6.75
8.00	8.50	8.62	8.75	8.75	8.87	8.87	9.00	9.12	7.50	7.50	7.37	7.37	7.25	7.25	7.25	7.25
8.50	9.12	9.25	9.25	9.37	9.50	9.50	9.62	9.75	8.00	7.87	7.87	7.75	7.75	7.62	7.62	7.50
9.00	9.75	9.75	9.87	10.00	10.12	10.25	10.37	10.37	8.37	8.37	8.25	8.25	8.12	8.00	8.00	8.00
9.50	10.25	10.37	10.50	10.62	10.75	10.87	11.00	11.12	8.87	8.75	8.62	8.62	8.50	8.50	8.37	8.37
10.00	10.87	11.00	11.12	11.25	11.37	11.50	11.62	11.75	9.25	9.12	9.12	9.00	8.87	8.87	8.75	8.75
10.50	11.50	11.62	11.75	11.87	12.00	12.12	12.25	12.50	9.62	9.62	9.50	9.37	9.37	9.25	9.12	9.12
11.00	12.00	12.25	12.37	12.50	12.75	12.87	13.00	13.12	10.12	10.00	9.87	9.75	9.75	9.62	9.50	9.50
11.50	12.62	12.87	13.00	13.12	13.37	13.50	13.75	13.87	10.50	10.37	10.37	10.25	10.12	10.00	9.87	9.87
12.00	13.25	13.50	13.62	13.87	14.00	14.25	14.50	14.62	11.00	10.87	10.75	10.62	10.50	10.37	10.25	10.12
12.50	13.87	14.12	14.25	14.50	14.75	15.00	15.25	15.37	11.37	11.25	11.12	11.00	11.00	10.75	10.62	10.50
13.00	14.50	14.75	15.00	15.25	15.50	15.62	16.00	16.12	11.75	11.62	11.50	11.37	11.25	11.12	11.00	10.87
13.50	15.12	15.37	15.62	15.87	16.12	16.37	16.62	16.87	12.25	12.00	11.87	11.75	11.62	11.50	11.37	11.25
14.00	15.75	16.00	16.25	16.50	16.75	17.12	17.50	17.75	12.62	12.50	12.25	12.12	12.00	11.87	11.75	11.50
14.50	16.50	16.75	17.00	17.25	17.50	17.87	18.25	18.50	13.00	12.75	12.62	12.50	12.37	12.25	12.00	11.87
15.00	17.00	17.37	17.75	18.00	18.25	18.62	19.00	19.37	13.37	13.25	13.00	12.87	12.75	12.50	12.37	12.25
15.50	17.75	18.00	18.25	18.75	19.00	19.37	19.75	20.25	13.75	13.62	13.50	13.25	13.00	12.87	12.75	12.62
16.00	18.25	18.75	19.00	19.37	19.75	20.25	20.50	21.00	14.25	14.00	13.75	13.62	13.25	13.25	13.00	12.87
16.50	19.00	19.37	19.75	20.25	20.50	21.00	21.50	21.87	14.50	14.37	14.12	14.00	13.75	13.62	13.50	13.25
17.00	19.75	20.25	20.50	21.00	21.50	22.00	22.25	22.87	15.00	14.75	14.50	14.25	14.12	14.00	13.75	13.50
17.50	20.50	20.75	21.25	21.75	22.25	22.75	23.25	23.75	15.37	15.12	14.87	14.75	14.50	14.25	14.00	13.87
18.00	21.00	21.50	22.00	22.50	23.00	23.50	24.00	24.62	15.75	15.50	15.25	15.00	14.75	14.62	14.37	14.12
18.50	21.75	22.25	22.75	23.25	23.75	24.50	25.00	25.62	16.12	15.87	15.62	15.37	15.12	14.87	14.75	14.50
19.00	22.50	23.00	23.50	24.00	24.75	25.25	26.00	26.50	16.50	16.25	16.00	15.75	15.50	15.25	15.00	14.75

TABLE 5

MJK SPHEROCYLINDRICAL VERTEX CHART

VERTEX DISTANCE = 13.00 mm					SPHERE INCREMENT = 0.125 DIOPTER						CYLINDER INCREMENT = 0.25 DIOPTER		
SR	SRV	−0.25	−0.50	−0.75	−1.00	−1.25	−1.50	−1.75	−2.00	−2.25	−2.50	−2.75	−3.00
−3.00	−2.87	−0.25	−0.50	−0.75	−1.00	−1.25	−1.25	−1.50	−1.75	−2.00	−2.25	−2.50	−2.75
−3.25	−3.12	−0.25	−0.50	−0.75	−1.00	−1.25	−1.25	−1.50	−1.75	−2.00	−2.25	−2.50	−2.75
−3.50	−3.37	−0.25	−0.50	−0.75	−1.00	−1.25	−1.25	−1.50	−1.75	−2.00	−2.25	−2.50	−2.75
−3.75	−3.62	−0.25	−0.50	−0.75	−1.00	−1.00	−1.25	−1.50	−1.75	−2.00	−2.25	−2.50	−2.75
−4.00	−3.75	−0.25	−0.50	−0.75	−1.00	−1.00	−1.25	−1.50	−1.75	−2.00	−2.25	−2.50	−2.50
−4.25	−4.00	−0.25	−0.50	−0.75	−1.00	−1.00	−1.25	−1.50	−1.75	−2.00	−2.25	−2.50	−2.50
−4.50	−4.25	−0.25	−0.50	−0.75	−1.00	−1.00	−1.25	−1.50	−1.75	−2.00	−2.25	−2.25	−2.50
−4.75	−4.50	−0.25	−0.50	−0.75	−1.00	−1.00	−1.25	−1.50	−1.75	−2.00	−2.25	−2.25	−2.50
−5.00	−4.75	−0.25	−0.50	−0.75	−0.75	−1.00	−1.25	−1.50	−1.75	−2.00	−2.25	−2.25	−2.50
−5.25	−4.87	−0.25	−0.50	−0.75	−0.75	−1.00	−1.25	−1.50	−1.75	−2.00	−2.25	−2.25	−2.25
−5.50	−5.12	−0.25	−0.50	−0.75	−0.75	−1.00	−1.25	−1.50	−1.75	−2.00	−2.00	−2.25	−2.50
−5.75	−5.37	−0.25	−0.50	−0.75	−0.75	−1.00	−1.25	−1.50	−1.75	−2.00	−2.00	−2.25	−2.50
−6.00	−5.62	−0.25	−0.50	−0.75	−0.75	−1.00	−1.25	−1.50	−1.75	−2.00	−2.00	−2.25	−2.50
−6.25	−5.75	−0.25	−0.50	−0.75	−0.75	−1.00	−1.25	−1.50	−1.75	−1.75	−2.00	−2.25	−2.50
−6.50	−6.00	−0.25	−0.50	−0.75	−0.75	−1.00	−1.25	−1.50	−1.75	−1.75	−2.00	−2.25	−2.50
−6.75	−6.25	−0.25	−0.50	−0.75	−0.75	−1.00	−1.25	−1.50	−1.75	−1.75	−2.00	−2.25	−2.50
−7.00	−6.37	−0.25	−0.50	−0.50	−0.75	−1.00	−1.25	−1.50	−1.75	−1.75	−2.00	−2.25	−2.50
−7.25	−6.62	−0.25	−0.50	−0.50	−0.75	−1.00	−1.25	−1.50	−1.75	−1.75	−2.00	−2.25	−2.50
−7.50	−6.87	−0.25	−0.50	−0.50	−0.75	−1.00	−1.25	−1.50	−1.50	−1.75	−2.00	−2.25	−2.50
−7.75	−7.00	−0.25	−0.50	−0.50	−0.75	−1.00	−1.25	−1.50	−1.50	−1.75	−2.00	−2.25	−2.50
−8.00	−7.25	−0.25	−0.50	−0.50	−0.75	−1.00	−1.25	−1.50	−1.50	−1.75	−2.00	−2.25	−2.50
−8.25	−7.50	−0.25	−0.50	−0.50	−0.75	−1.00	−1.25	−1.50	−1.50	−1.75	−2.00	−2.25	−2.25
−8.50	−7.62	−0.25	−0.50	−0.50	−0.75	−1.00	−1.25	−1.50	−1.50	−1.75	−2.00	−2.25	−2.25
−8.75	−7.87	−0.25	−0.50	−0.50	−0.75	−1.00	−1.25	−1.50	−1.50	−1.75	−2.00	−2.25	−2.25
−9.00	−8.00	−0.25	−0.50	−0.50	−0.75	−1.00	−1.25	−1.25	−1.50	−1.75	−2.00	−2.25	−2.25
−9.25	−8.25	−0.25	−0.50	−0.50	−0.75	−1.00	−1.25	−1.25	−1.50	−1.75	−2.00	−2.00	−2.25
−9.50	−8.50	−0.25	−0.50	−0.50	−0.75	−1.00	−1.25	−1.25	−1.50	−1.75	−2.00	−2.00	−2.25
−9.75	−8.62	−0.25	−0.50	−0.50	−0.75	−1.00	−1.25	−1.25	−1.50	−1.75	−2.00	−2.00	−2.25
−10.00	−8.87	−0.25	−0.50	−0.50	−0.75	−1.00	−1.25	−1.25	−1.50	−1.75	−2.00	−2.00	−2.25
−10.25	−9.00	−0.25	−0.50	−0.50	−0.75	−1.00	−1.25	−1.25	−1.50	−1.75	−2.00	−2.00	−2.25
−10.50	−9.25	−0.25	−0.50	−0.50	−0.75	−1.00	−1.25	−1.25	−1.50	−1.75	−2.00	−2.00	−2.25
−10.75	−9.37	−0.25	−0.50	−0.50	−0.75	−1.00	−1.25	−1.25	−1.50	−1.75	−2.25	−2.00	−2.25
+4.00	+4.25	−0.25	−0.50	−0.75	−1.00	−1.25	−1.75	−2.00	−2.25	−2.50	−2.75	−3.00	−3.25
+4.25	+4.50	−0.25	−0.50	−0.75	−1.00	−1.50	−1.75	−2.00	−2.25	−2.50	−2.75	−3.00	−3.25
+4.50	+4.75	−0.25	−0.50	−0.75	−1.00	−1.50	−1.75	−2.00	−2.25	−2.50	−2.75	−3.00	−3.25
+4.75	+5.12	−0.25	−0.50	−0.75	−1.00	−1.50	−1.75	−2.00	−2.25	−2.50	−2.75	−3.00	−3.25
+5.00	+5.37	−0.25	−0.50	−0.75	−1.00	−1.50	−1.75	−2.00	−2.25	−2.50	−2.75	−3.00	−3.25
+5.25	+5.62	−0.25	−0.50	−0.75	−1.00	−1.50	−1.75	−2.00	−2.25	−2.50	−2.75	−3.00	−3.25
+5.50	+5.87	−0.25	−0.50	−0.75	−1.00	−1.50	−1.75	−2.00	−2.25	−2.50	−2.75	−3.00	−3.25
+5.75	+6.25	−0.25	−0.50	−0.75	−1.00	−1.50	−1.75	−2.00	−2.25	−2.50	−2.75	−3.00	−3.25
+6.00	+6.50	−0.25	−0.50	−0.75	−1.00	−1.50	−1.75	−2.00	−2.25	−2.50	−2.75	−3.00	−3.50
+6.25	+6.75	−0.25	−0.50	−1.00	−1.00	−1.50	−1.75	−2.00	−2.25	−2.50	−2.75	−3.00	−3.50
+6.50	+7.12	−0.25	−0.50	−1.00	−1.00	−1.50	−1.75	−2.00	−2.25	−2.50	−3.00	−3.25	−3.50
+6.75	+7.37	−0.25	−0.50	−1.00	−1.00	−1.50	−1.75	−2.00	−2.25	−2.50	−3.00	−3.25	−3.50
+7.00	+7.75	−0.25	−0.50	−1.00	−1.00	−1.50	−1.75	−2.00	−2.25	−2.75	−3.00	−3.25	−3.50
+7.25	+8.00	−0.25	−0.50	−1.00	−1.00	−1.50	−1.75	−2.00	−2.25	−2.75	−3.00	−3.25	−3.50
+7.50	+8.25	−0.25	−0.50	−1.00	−1.00	−1.50	−1.75	−2.00	−2.50	−2.75	−3.00	−3.25	−3.50
+7.75	+8.62	−0.25	−0.50	−1.00	−1.00	−1.50	−1.75	−2.00	−2.50	−2.75	−3.00	−3.25	−3.50
+8.00	+8.87	−0.25	−0.50	−1.00	−1.00	−1.50	−1.75	−2.25	−2.50	−2.75	−3.00	−3.25	−3.50
+8.25	+9.25	−0.25	−0.50	−1.00	−1.00	−1.50	−1.75	−2.25	−2.50	−2.75	−3.00	−3.25	−3.50
+8.50	+9.25	−0.25	−0.75	−1.00	−1.25	−1.50	−1.75	−2.25	−2.50	−2.75	−3.00	−3.25	−3.75
+8.75	+9.87	−0.25	−0.75	−1.00	−1.25	−1.50	−1.75	−2.25	−2.50	−2.75	−3.00	−3.25	−3.75
+9.00	+10.25	−0.25	−0.75	−1.00	−1.25	−1.50	−2.00	−2.25	−2.50	−2.75	−3.00	−3.50	−3.75
+9.25	+10.50	−0.25	−0.75	−1.00	−1.25	−1.50	−2.00	−2.25	−2.50	−2.75	−3.00	−3.50	−3.75
+9.50	+10.87	−0.25	−0.75	−1.00	−1.25	−1.50	−2.00	−2.25	−2.50	−2.75	−3.25	−3.50	−3.75
+9.75	+11.12	−0.25	−0.75	−1.00	−1.25	−1.50	−2.00	−2.25	−2.50	−2.75	−3.25	−3.50	−3.75
+10.00	+11.50	−0.25	−0.75	−1.00	−1.25	−1.50	−2.00	−2.25	−2.50	−3.00	−3.25	−3.50	−3.75
+10.25	+11.87	−0.25	−0.75	−1.00	−1.25	−1.75	−2.00	−2.25	−2.50	−3.00	−3.25	−3.50	−3.75
+10.50	+12.12	−0.25	−0.75	−1.00	−1.25	−1.75	−2.00	−2.25	−2.50	−3.00	−3.25	−3.50	−3.75
+10.75	+12.50	−0.25	−0.75	−1.00	−1.25	−1.75	−2.00	−2.25	−2.50	−3.00	−3.25	−3.50	−4.00
+11.00	+12.87	−0.25	−0.75	−1.00	−1.25	−1.75	−2.00	−2.25	−2.75	−3.00	−3.25	−3.50	−4.00
+11.25	+13.12	−0.25	−0.75	−1.00	−1.25	−1.75	−2.00	−2.25	−2.75	−3.00	−3.25	−3.50	−4.00
+11.50	+13.50	−0.25	−0.75	−1.00	−1.25	−1.75	−2.00	−2.25	−2.75	−3.00	−3.25	−3.75	−4.00
+11.75	+13.87	−0.25	−0.75	−1.00	−1.25	−1.75	−2.00	−2.25	−2.75	−3.00	−3.25	−3.75	−4.00

Example: Spectacle refraction (SR) at 13 mm = −5.75 − 2.50 × 180.
Matching up −5.75 (see highlighted boxes) on the left, gives effective spherical power (SRV) of −5.37.
Following values to the right and reading in the −2.50 cylinder column gives a cylinder value of −2.00.

Corneal plane refraction = −5.37 − 2.00 3 180.

Legend: In this chart of spherocylindrical corneal plane refractions, the spherical value is calculated and rounded off to the nearest 0.125 diopter, while the cylinder value is rounded off to the nearest 0.25 diopter.

2. SOFT-CONTACT LENSES MANUFACTURER DIRECTORY

Below is a list of companies that manufacture soft-contact lenses and their contact information.

ACCU LENS, INC.
5353 West Colfax Avenue
Denver, CO 80214-1811
Phone: (303) 232-6244
Toll-free: (800) 525-2470
Fax: (303) 235-0472
Website: www.acculens.com

ACUITY ONE, LLC.
7642 East Gray Road, Suite 103
Scottsdale, AZ 85260
Phone: (480) 607-2998
Toll-free: (877) 228-4891
Toll-free Fax: (877) 607-2871
E-mail: info@acuityone.com
Website: acuityone.com

ALDEN OPTICAL LABORATORIES, INC.
13295 Broadway
Alden, NY 14004
Phone: (716) 937-9181
Toll-free: (800) 253-3669
Toll-free Fax: (800) 899-5612
E-mail: info@aldenoptical.com
Website: www.aldenoptical.com

BAUSCH & LOMB
1400 North Goodman Street
Rochester, NY 14609
Phone: (585) 338-6000
Toll-free: (800) 553-5340
Fax: (585) 338-6896
Website: www.bausch.com

BLANCHARD CONTACT LENS, INC.
8025 S. Willow Street
Manchester, NH 03103
Phone: (603) 625-1664
Toll-free: (800) 367-4009
Fax: (603) 625-1644
E-mail: blanchardlabs@blanchardlab.com
Website: www.blanchardlab.com

CIBA VISION CORPORATION
11440 Johns Creek Parkway
Duluth, GA 30097
Phone: (678) 415-4255
Toll-free: (800) 241-5999
Fax: (800) 845-8842
Website: www.cibavision.com

CONTINENTAL SOFT LENS, INC.
P.O. Box 621029
Littleton, CO 80162
Phone: (303) 795-2130
Toll-free: (800) 637-3845
Fax: (303) 795-6984

COOPERVISION, INC.
370 Woodcliff Drive, Suite 200
Fairport, NY 14450
Phone: (585) 385-6810
Toll-free: (800) 538-7850
Fax: (888) 385-3217
E-mail: info@coopervision.com
Website: www.coopervision.com

CUSTOM COLOR CONTACTS
55 West 49th Street
New York, NY 10020
Phone: (212) 765-4444
Toll-free: (800) 598-2020
Fax: (212) 765-4459
E-mail: info@customcontacts.com
Website: www.customcontacts.com

EXTREME H2O/ HYDROGEL VISION CORP.
7575 Commerce Court
Sarasota, FL 34243
Toll-free: (877) 336-2482
Toll-free Fax: (888) 612-6379
E-mail: customercare@extreme-h2o.com
Website: www.hydrogelvision.com

IDEAL OPTICS, INC.
2775 Premier Parkway
Suite 600
Deluth, GA 30097
Phone: (770) 434-8291
Toll-free: (800) 554-7353
Fax: (770) 434-8291
Website: www.ideal-optics.com

KONTUR KONTACT LENS CO.
642 Alfred Nobel Drive
Hercules, CA 94547
Phone: (510) 964-9760
Toll-free: (800) 227-1320
Fax: (800) 650-6525
E-mail: info@kontur55.com
Website: www.kontur55.com

LENS DYNAMICS, INC.
3901 "E" NE 33rd Terrace
Kansas City, MO 64117
Phone: (303) 237-6927
Toll-free: (800) 228-2691
Fax: (800) 661-6707
　　　(303) 274-6707
E-mail: vaske@lensdynamics.com
Website: www.lensdynamics.com

METRO OPTICS, INC.
P.O. Box 81189
Austin, TX 78708
Phone: (512) 251-2382
Toll-free: (800) 223-1858
Fax: (512) 251-6554
E-mail: info@metro-optics.com
Website: www.metro-optics.com

OCU-EASE OPTICAL PRODUCTS, INC.
920 San Pablo Avenue
Pinole, CA 94564
Toll-free: (800) 521-8984
Fax: (800) 628-3273
E-mail: sandy@ocuease.com
Website: www.ocuease.com

PC OPTICAL PRODUCTS, INC.
801 12th Ave North
Minneapolis, MN 55411-4230
Phone: (612) 520-6150
Toll-free: (800) 433-4885
Fax: (612) 520-6153

PURILENS, INC.
1800 Rt. 34 North
Wall, NJ 07719
Toll-free: (877) 787-5367
Fax: (732) 972-9205
E-mail: lenses@lifestylecompany.com
Website: www.purilens.com

PRECISION VISION, LTD.
1490 S. Yampa Way
Aurora, CO 80017
Phone: (303) 743-0494
Toll-free: (800) 843-5367
Fax: (303) 632-8216
E-mail: info@precisionvision.com
Website: www.precisionvision.com

SODERBERG OPHTHALMIC SERVICES
801 12th Ave North
Minneapolis, MN 55411
Toll-free: (866) 566-0387
Fax: (800) 838-2972
E-mail: info@soderberginc.com
Website: www.soseyes.com

TRU-FORM OPTICS
400 Harwood Road
Bedford, TX 76021
Toll-free: (800) 792-1095
Fax: (817) 354-8319
E-mail: info@tfoptics.com
Website: www.tfoptics.com

UNILENS VISION INC.
10431 72nd Street North
Largo, FL 33777
Phone: (727) 544-2531
Toll-free: (800) 446-2020
Fax: (727) 545-1883
　　　(800) 808-8264
E-mail: unilens@aol.com *or* information@unilens.com
Website: www.unilens.com

UNITED CONTACT LENS, INC.
19111 61st Ave NE # 5
Arlington, WA 98223-6305
Phone: (360) 474-9577
Toll-free: (800) 446-1666
Fax: (425) 743-8795
Toll-free Fax: (888) 523-3156
E-mail: neal@unitedcontactlens.com
Website: www.unitedcontactlens.com

VALLEY CONTAX
200 South Mill Street
Springfield, OR 97477
Phone: (541) 744-9393
Toll-free: (800) 547-8815
Fax: (541) 744-9399
E-mail: contax@valleycontax.com
Website: www.valleycontax.com

VISTAKON
Customer Relations
D-QA
7500 Centurion Parkway
Jacksonville, FL 32256
Toll-free: (800) 843-2020
Website: www.acuvue.com

WESTCON CONTACT LENS COMPANY, INC.
611 Eisenhauer Street
Grand Junction, CO 81505
Phone: (970) 245-3845
Toll-free: (800) 346-4303
Fax: (970) 245-4516
　　　(800) 715-3388
E-mail: westcon@westconlens.com
Website: www.westconlens.com

WALMAN OPTICAL
801 12th Avenue North
Minneapolis, MN 55411
(See website for more office locations.)
Phone: (770) 622-9235
Toll-free: (800) 241-9312
Fax: (770) 622-8989
Website: www.walman.com

SECTION 5

VISION STANDARDS AND LOW-VISION AIDS

1. VISION STANDARDS

TABLE 1

VISION STANDARDS FOR PILOTS

	WITHOUT RX[1]	REQUIRING RX[1] CORRECTED TO	NEAR VISION WITH/ WITHOUT RX	PHORIAS[2]	FIELDS	COLOR	PATHOLOGY
1st class	20/20	20/100 to 20/20	20/40 (J_3)	6 D eso/exo 1 Δ hyper	Normal	Normal	4
2nd class	20/20	20/100 to 20/20	20/40 (J_3)	6 D eso/exo 1 Δ hyper	Normal	3	5
3rd class	20/50	To 20/30	20/60 (J_6)	...	...	3	5

1. Each eye.
2. If exceeded, further evaluation required to determine bifoveal fixation and adequate vergence phoria relationship.
3. Able to distinguish aviation signal red, aviation signal green, and white.
4. No acute or chronic pathologic condition of either eye of adnexa that might interfere with its proper function, might progress to that degree, or be aggravated by flying.
5. No serious pathology.

Note: By amendment regulations (12/21/76) correction may be by spectacles or contact lenses.

TABLE 2

VISION STANDARDS FOR ADMISSION TO SERVICE ACADEMIES

US Coast Guard Academy	Minimum uncorrected 20/200 each eye; correctable to 20/20 each eye; refractive error not more than ±5.50 D any meridian; astigmatism not over 3.00 D; anisometropia not exceeding 3.50 D; full visual fields; normal color vision; no chronic, disfiguring, disabling, ocular pathology.
US Merchant Marine Academy	Minimum uncorrected 20/100 each eye; correctable to 20/20 each eye; refractive error as for Coast Guard Academy; color vision normal by Farnsworth lantern test or pseudoisochromatic plates; certain pathologies may disqualify.
US Naval Academy	Uncorrected vision 20/20 each eye; limited waivers if correctable to 20/20 each eye and to refraction standards, Coast Guard Academy; color vision normal–no waivers; no chronic, disfiguring, disabling ocular pathology.
US Military Academy	Distance vision correctable to 20/20 each eye; refractive error as for Coast Guard Academy; able to distinguish vivid red and green; ET less than 15 prism diopters; XT less than 10 prism diopters; hypertropia less than 2 prism diopters; certain pathologies may disqualify.
US Air Force Academy	*Pilot:* Uncorrected vision 20/20 or better each eye, far and near; refractive error hyperopia no greater than +1.75 D and nearsightedness less than plano in any one meridian; the astigmatic error must not exceed 0.75 D. *Navigator:* Uncorrected vision 20/70 or better correctable with ordinary glasses to 20/20 each eye; near acuity 20/20 or better each eye, uncorrected; hyperopia not greater than +3.00 D and myopia not greater than −1.50 D any meridian; astigmatism not to exceed 2.00 D. *Commission:* Distance acuity correctable 20/40 one eye and 20/70 other, or 20/30 one eye and 20/100 other; near acuity correctable to 20/20 (J_1) one eye and 20/30 (J_2) in other; refractive error of equivalent sphere not more than ±8.00 D; no chronic, disfiguring, disabling ocular pathology.

Based on information as of May 17, 1983, Medical Examination Review Board, Department of Defense.

TABLE 3

VISION STANDARDS FOR COMMERCIAL DRIVERS

	VISUAL ACUITY BINOC	VISUAL FIELD (degrees) MONOC	BINOC	COLOR	OTHER	RETEST
Alabama	20/40	No	No	ND	No	No
Alaska	20/40	No	No	No	No	Periodic
Arizona	20/40	70/35	No	PD	No	Periodic
Arkansas	20/50	105	NS	No	NS	NS
California	20/40	No	No	No	NS	Periodic
Colorado	20/40	No	No	No	ST	Periodic
Connecticut	20/40	100	140	No	ST	No
Delaware	20/40	No	No	No	No	Periodic
Florida	20/70	No	130	No	No	Periodic
Georgia	20/60	140, 140	140	No	No	Periodic
Hawaii	20/40	70, 70	140	No	ST, EC	Periodic
Idaho	20/40	NS	NS	NS	NS	Periodic
Illinois	20/40	105	140	NS	NS	Periodic
Indiana	20/40	70	120	No	NS	Periodic
Iowa	20/40	No	140	PD	NS	Periodic
Kansas	20/40	55	110	No	NS	Periodic
Kentucky	20/45, PV	80	120	No	No	No
Louisiana	20/40	No	No	No	No	Periodic
Maine	20/40	NS	140	No	NS	No
Maryland	20/40	NS	140	PD	No	Periodic
Massachusetts	20/40	90,90	120	Yes	No	Periodic
Michigan	20/40	70, 70	140	No	NS	Periodic
Minnesota	20/40	NS	105	No	NS	Periodic
Mississippi	20/40	70(T)/35(N)	140	No	ST	No
Missouri	20/40	55, 55	No	No	No	Periodic
Montana	20/40	No	No	No	ST	Periodic
Nebraska	20/40	No	140	PD	No	Periodic
Nevada	20/40	No	140	NS	No	Periodic
New Hampshire	20/40	No	No	No	NS	Periodic
New Jersey	20/50	70, 70	No	No	No	NS
New Mexico	20/40	NS	120(T)/30(N)	No	NS	Periodic
New York	20/40	NS	140	No	NS	Periodic
North Carolina	20/50	No	60	No	No	Periodic
North Dakota	20/40	70, 70	105	No	No	Periodic
Ohio	20/40	70, 70	No	Yes	No	Periodic
Oklahoma	20/60	No	70	No	No	No
Oregon	20/40	No	110	No	No	No
Pennsylvania	20/40	No	120	No	No	No
Rhode Island	20/40	NS	NS	Yes	No	Periodic
South Carolina	20/40	NS	140	NS	NS	Periodic
South Dakota	20/40	No	No	No	No	Periodic
Tennessee	20/40	No	No	PD	No	No
Texas	20/50	No	No	ND	No	Periodic
Utah	20/40	NS	120(H)/20(V)	No	ST	Periodic
Vermont	20/40	60,60	No	No	NS	No
Virginia	20/40	100, 100	100	No	NS	Periodic
Washington	20/40	No	110	ND,PD	No	Periodic
West Virginia	20/40	No	No	No	No	No
Wisconsin	20/40	70, 70	140	PD	No	Periodic
Wyoming	20/40	No	120	No	No	Periodic

Note: Visual acuity is expressed in Snellen notation; visual field is given in degrees along the horizontal meridian.
Key: EC = eye coordination; H = horizontal; N = nasal field; ND = new driver; No = no standard; NS = standard not specified; PD = professional driver; PV = default to private vehicle standard; ST = stereopsis (absence of); T = with telescope; V = vertical.

Sources: US Dept of Transportation. *Visual Disorders and Commercial Drivers*. Washington, DC: Federal Highway Administration, Office of Motor Carriers; Nov 1991. US Dept of Transportation publication FHWA-MC-92-003, HCS-10/1-92(200)E.

Wang CC, Kosinski CJ, Schwartzberg JG, et al. *Physician's Guide to Assessing and Counseling Older Drivers*. Washington, DC: National Highway Traffic Safety Administration; 2003.

2. LOW-VISION AIDS

Under federal regulation, a patient is considered legally blind when the best vision attained in the better eye is 20/200 or less, or when, whatever the acuity achieved, the field of vision of the better eye is 20° or less. While most states have adopted these standards, individual variations may exist at the local level.

Patients whose vision is reduced or inadequate for their visual tasks — those whose best corrected vision ranges from 20/50 downward toward the 20/200 level — can frequently be aided by the same techniques and devices used for the legally blind and visually rehabilitated. These modalities include rehabilitation training programs and optical and nonoptical aids. They often can help restore independence and mobility, allowing the patient to remain productive.

For those patients considered partially sighted rather than partially blind, increased vision is obtained by magnification or approximation. For distance, this may be accomplished by telescopic devices. Although difficult to use while moving about, these instruments may be quite effective for distinguishing a street sign or the number of a house or bus. They are also useful aids in the theater or classroom and at sporting events.

Telescopic devices can be obtained in magnifications of 2.2, 2.5, 3.0, 3.5, 4.0, 6.0, 8.0, and 103 from suppliers such as Designs for Vision, Keeler, Nikon, Selsi, Walters, and Zeiss. Some are fixed focus; others may be refocused for viewing closer material. Telescopes fitted with reading cap lenses permit reading at greater distances than high-plus aids. A familiar example of this system is the surgical loupe.

Because the field diminishes as the power increases, the magnification of telescopic devices should be kept to the minimum needed to secure desired acuity. Differences in design and construction of these devices may cause slight variations in the fields produced at a given magnification. A representative sample may be drawn from the devices produced by Designs for Vision:

MAGNIFICATION	FIELD AT 20 FEET
2.2 standard	12°
2.2 wide angle	17°
3.0 standard	8°
3.0 wide angle	12°
4.0 standard	6°

Near vision can be augmented by higher adds, high-plus "Micro" lenses (American Optical, Lucerne Optical), binocular loupes, and handheld or stand magnifiers. The higher plus values permit approximation to increase the angle subtended with little or no demand on accommodation. The add to obtain J5 can be estimated by the inverse of the best distance vision obtained. For example, if best distance vision is 20/200, the add is 200/20, or 10 D.

Greater detail can be obtained through increased add power or supplementary magnifiers. If the patient will not read at extremely close range, lower adds may be used in combination with magnifiers. Required magnification at desired working distance can also be provided by a telemicroscope system modified with a reading cap or objective lens, as in a surgical loupe.

When binocular function is present, prism base-in may be required in the near prescription (about 1 prism diopter per diopter of add). Plastic-lens, half-eye spectacles of 6, 8, or 10 D with incorporated prism are available from American Optical and Luzerne Optical. Handheld magnifiers ranging from 23 to 83 are available from Bausch & Lomb, Coil, Reizen, Schweizer, and Zeiss and others. Once again, the higher powers have reduced fields of view. Patients with physical infirmities can use stand magnifiers that rest on the material and remain in focus as they are moved across the page.

Nonoptical aids include reading masks, large-print publications, heavily ruled stationery, check-writing guides, large playing cards, and easy-to-thread needles. Also available are fixed-power opaque projection magnifiers and closed-circuit television devices with variable magnification.

Television permits a greater range of magnification and can, when polarity is reversed, provide a white-on-black image instead of the usual black-on-white. This effect, for many, is an additional aid. Products are available from Telesensory and Visualtek. Advances in electronics have also made possible talking clocks, calculators, computers, and word processors whose "voices" open the way to gainful employment for the visually impaired.

For those with clouded vision, absorptive lenses provide glare protection and can help improve acuity. Neutral gray lenses with 5–15% transmission are specifically recommended for achromatopes, who may also require the protection of wide side-shield frames. Albinotic patients are aided by brown tints with 75% transmission indoors and 25% outdoors. Retinitis pigmentosa patients generally require daytime outdoor protection with the darker sunglass tints. Many are aided in night vision by the Kalichrome lenses (Bausch & Lomb) and the Hazemaster line (American Optical).

For more information on optical aids and other resources for the visually impaired, contact:

American Council of the Blind
Phone: 800-424-8666, 202-467-5081
Website: www.acb.org

American Foundation for the Blind
Phone: 800-232-5463, 212-502-7600
Website: www.afb.org

Library of Congress, National Library Service for the Blind and Physically Handicapped
Phone: 888-657-7323, 202-707-5100
Website: www.loc.gov/nls

U.S. FOOD AND DRUG ADMINISTRATION

Medical Product Reporting Programs

MedWatch (24-hour service).. 800-332-1088
*Reporting of problems with drugs, devices, biologics (except vaccines), medical foods,
and dietary supplements.*

Vaccine Adverse Event Reporting System (24-hour service)................................. 800-822-7967
Reporting of vaccine-related problems.

Mandatory Medical Device Reporting... 800-332-1088
*Reporting required from user facilities regarding device-related deaths
and serious injuries.*

Veterinary Adverse Drug Reaction Program 888-332-8387
Reporting of adverse drug events in animals.

Division of Drug Marketing, Advertising, and Communication (DDMAC) 301-796-1200
Inquiries from health professionals regarding product promotion.

Information for Health Professionals

Center for Drug Evaluation and Research Drug Information Hotline 888-463-6332
Information on human drugs including hormones.

Center for Biologics Office of Communications 800-835-4709
Information on biological products including vaccines and blood.

Center for Devices and Radiological Health 800-638-2041
Automated request for information on medical devices and radiation-emitting products.

Emergency Operations 866-300-4374
*Emergencies involving FDA-regulated products, tampering reports,
and emergency Investigational New Drug requests.*

Office of Orphan Products Development 301-796-8660
Information on products for rare diseases.

General Information

General Consumer Inquiries 888-463-6332
Consumer information on regulated products/issues.

Freedom of Information.. 301-796-3900
Requests for publicly available FDA documents.

Office of Public Affairs 301-796-4540
Interviews/press inquiries on FDA activities.

Center for Food Safety and Applied Nutrition 888-723-3366
*Information on food safety, seafood, dietary supplements, women's nutrition,
and cosmetics.*

Consumer Information Service, Center for Devices and Radiological Health........... 800-638-2041
*Information on medical devices, mammography facilities, and
radiation-emitting products.*

MANUFACTURER'S INDEX

PRODUCT INDEX

PRODUCT IDENTIFICATION GUIDE

To aid in quick identification, manufacturers participating in this section have furnished full-color photographs of selected ophthalmic products. Capsules and tablets are shown in actual size. Tubes, bottles, boxes, and other types of packaging appear in reduced size to fit available space.

For more information on any of the products in this section, please turn to the Pharmaceutical and Equipment Product Information Section, or check directly with the manufacturer. The page number of each product's text entry appears above its photograph.

While every effort has been made to guarantee faithful reproduction of the products in this section, changes in size, color, and design are always a possibility. Be sure to confirm a product's identity with the manufacturer or your pharmacist.

ALLERGAN, INC.

RX   ALLERGAN, INC.   P. 214

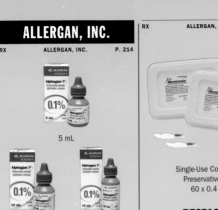

5 mL

10 mL   15 mL

0.1%

5 mL

10 mL   15 mL

0.15%

ALPHAGAN® P
(brimonidine tartrate ophthalmic solution)

RX   ALLERGAN, INC.   P. 216

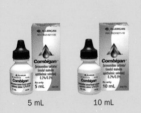

5 mL   10 mL

COMBIGAN®
(brimonidine tartrate/timolol maleate ophthalmic solution) 0.2%/0.5%

RX   ALLERGAN, INC.   P. 219

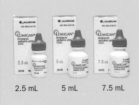

2.5 mL   5 mL   7.5 mL

LUMIGAN®
(bimatoprost ophthalmic solution) 0.03%

RX   ALLERGAN, INC.   P. 223

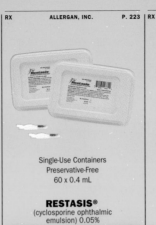

Single-Use Containers
Preservative-Free
60 x 0.4 mL

RESTASIS®
(cyclosporine ophthalmic emulsion) 0.05%

BAUSCH & LOMB

OTC   BAUSCH & LOMB INCORPORATED   P. 225

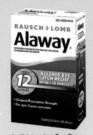

Antihistamine Eye Drops

Alaway®
(ketotifen fumarate ophthalmic solution) 0.025%

RX   BAUSCH & LOMB INCORPORATED   P. 226

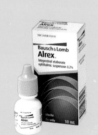

Available in 5 mL and 10 mL

Alrex®
(loteprednol etabonate ophthalmic suspension) 0.2%

RX   BAUSCH & LOMB INCORPORATED   P. 227

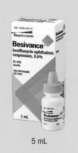

5 mL

Besivance®
(besifloxacin ophthalmic suspension) 0.6%

RX   BAUSCH & LOMB INCORPORATED   P. 229

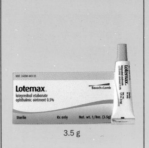

3.5 g

Lotemax®
(loteprednol etabonate ophthalmic ointment) 0.5%

RX   BAUSCH & LOMB INCORPORATED   P. 230

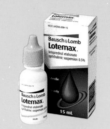

Available in 5 mL, 10 mL, and 15 mL

Lotemax®
(loteprednol etabonate ophthalmic suspension) 0.5%

DS   BAUSCH & LOMB INCORPORATED   P. 233

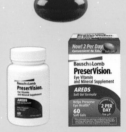

Adult 50+ Formula
Eye Vitamin and Mineral Supplement
Available in 30 ct and 50 ct

Ocuvite® Adult 50+ Formula

DS   BAUSCH & LOMB INCORPORATED   P. 233

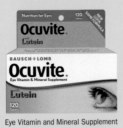

Eye Vitamin and Mineral Supplement
Available in 60 ct and 120 ct

Ocuvite® Lutein

DS   BAUSCH & LOMB INCORPORATED   P. 234

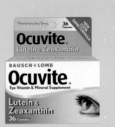

Eye Vitamin and Mineral Supplement
Available in 36 ct and 72 ct

Ocuvite® Lutein & Zeaxanthin

OTC   BAUSCH & LOMB INCORPORATED   P. 234

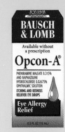

15 mL
Itching and Redness Reliever Eye Drops

Opcon-A®
(pheniramine maleate/naphazoline hydrochloride ophthalmic solution) 0.315%/0.02675%

DS   BAUSCH & LOMB INCORPORATED   P. 234

Eye Vitamin and Mineral Supplement
Available in 60 ct, 120 ct, and 150 ct

PreserVision® AREDS Soft Gels

DS   BAUSCH & LOMB INCORPORATED   P. 234

Eye Vitamin and Mineral Supplement
Available in 120 ct and 240 ct

PreserVision® AREDS Tablets

DS   BAUSCH & LOMB INCORPORATED   P. 235

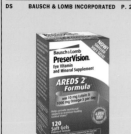

Eye Vitamin and Mineral Supplement
Available in 120 ct

PreserVision® Eye Vitamin AREDS 2 Formula Soft Gels

DS   BAUSCH & LOMB INCORPORATED   P. 235

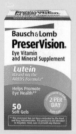

Eye Vitamin and Mineral Supplement
Available in 50 ct, 120 ct, and 180 ct

PreserVision® Lutein Soft Gels

OTC   BAUSCH & LOMB INCORPORATED   P. 236

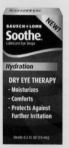

15 mL
Lubricant Eye Drops

Soothe® Hydration

OTC   BAUSCH & LOMB INCORPORATED   P. 236

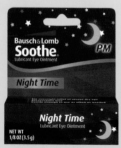

1/8 oz (3.5 g)
Lubricant Eye Ointment

Soothe® Night Time
(mineral oil/white petrolatum) 20%/80%

OTC   BAUSCH & LOMB INCORPORATED   P. 236

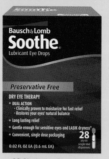

28 Single-Use Dispensers
Lubricant Eye Drops

Soothe® Preservative Free
(glycerin/propylene glycol) 0.6%/0.6%

RX   BAUSCH & LOMB INCORPORATED   P. 238

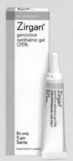

5 g

Zirgan®
(ganciclovir ophthalmic gel) 0.15%

RX   BAUSCH & LOMB INCORPORATED   P. 239

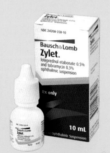

Available in 5 mL and 10 mL

Zylet®
(loteprednol etabonate/tobramycin
ophthalmic suspension) 0.5%/0.3%

FOCUS LABORATORIES

RX   FOCUS LABORATORIES   P. 240

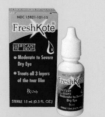

15 mL
Ophthalmic Solution

FreshKote®

RX   FOCUS LABORATORIES   P. 241

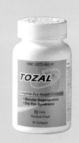

Tozal®
(lutein and zeaxanthin/omega-3 fatty
acids/antocyanosides)

MERCK

RX   MERCK   P. 241

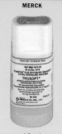

10 mL
3519* 2%

Trusopt®
Sterile Ophthalmic Solution
OCUMETER® PLUS Ophthalmic Dispenser
(dorzolamide HCl ophthalmic solution)

---

*Manufacturer's Identification Code

PRODUCT INFORMATION ON PHARMACEUTICALS AND EQUIPMENT

This book is made possible through the courtesy of the manufacturers whose products appear in this section. The information concerning each pharmaceutical product has been prepared by the manufacturer, and edited and approved by the manufacturer's medical department, medical director, or medical counsel.

For those products that have official package circulars, the descriptions in *Physicians' Desk Reference for Ophthalmic Medicines* must be in full compliance with Food and Drug Administration regulations pertaining to the labeling of prescription drugs. For more information, please turn to the Foreword. In presenting the following material, the publisher is not necessarily advocating the use of any product listed.

Alcon Laboratories, Inc.
and its affiliates
CORPORATE HEADQUARTERS
6201 SOUTH FREEWAY
FORT WORTH, TX 76134

Address Inquiries to:
(800) 757-9195
Outside the U.S. call (817) 568-6725
medinfo@alconlabs.com

AZOPT® ℞
(brinzolamide ophthalmic suspension) 1%

Description: AZOPT® (brinzolamide ophthalmic suspension) 1% contains a carbonic anhydrase inhibitor formulated for multidose topical ophthalmic use. Brinzolamide is described chemically as: (R)-(+)-4-Ethylamino-2- (3-methoxypropyl)-3,4-dihydro-2H-thieno [3,2-e]-1,2-thiazine-6-sulfonamide-1,1-dioxide. Its empirical formula is $C_{12}H_{21}N_3O_5S_3$. Brinzolamide has a molecular weight of 383.5 and a melting point of about 131°C. It is a white powder, which is insoluble in water, very soluble in methanol and soluble in ethanol.

AZOPT® (brinzolamide ophthalmic suspension) 1% is supplied as a sterile, aqueous suspension of brinzolamide which has been formulated to be readily suspended and slow settling, following shaking. It has a pH of approximately 7.5 and an osmolality of 300 mOsm/kg. Each mL of AZOPT® (brinzolamide ophthalmic suspension) 1% contains 10 mg brinzolamide. Inactive ingredients are mannitol, carbomer 974P, tyloxapol, edetate disodium, sodium chloride, hydrochloric acid and/ or sodium hydroxide (to adjust pH), and purified water. Benzalkonium chloride 0.01% is added as a preservative.

Clinical Pharmacology: Carbonic anhydrase (CA) is an enzyme found in many tissues of the body including the eye. It catalyzes the reversible reaction involving the hydration of carbon dioxide and the dehydration of carbonic acid. In humans, carbonic anhydrase exists as a number of isoenzymes, the most active being carbonic anhydrase II (CA-II), found primarily in red blood cells (RBCs), but also in other tissues. Inhibition of carbonic anhydrase in the ciliary processes of the eye decreases aqueous humor secretion, presumably by slowing the formation of bicarbonate ions with subsequent reduction in sodium and fluid transport.

The result is a reduction in intraocular pressure (IOP).

AZOPT® (brinzolamide ophthalmic suspension) 1% contains brinzolamide, an inhibitor of carbonic anhydrase II (CA-II). Following topical ocular administration, brinzolamide inhibits aqueous humor formation and reduces elevated intraocular pressure. Elevated intraocular pressure is a major risk factor in the pathogenesis of optic nerve damage and glaucomatous visual field loss.

Following topical ocular administration, brinzolamide is absorbed into the systemic circulation. Due to its affinity for CA-II, brinzolamide distributes extensively into the RBCs and exhibits a long half-life in whole blood (approximately 111 days). In humans, the metabolite N-desethyl brinzolamide is formed, which also binds to CA and accumulates in RBCs. This metabolite binds mainly to CA-I in the presence of brinzolamide. In plasma, both parent brinzolamide and N-desethyl brinzolamide concentrations are low and generally below assay quantitation limits (<10 ng/mL). Binding to plasma proteins is approximately 60%. Brinzolamide is eliminated predominantly in the urine as unchanged drug. N-Desethyl brinzolamide is also found in the urine along with lower concentrations of the N-desmethoxypropyl and O-desmethyl metabolites.

An oral pharmacokinetic study was conducted in which healthy volunteers received 1 mg capsules of brinzolamide twice per day for up to 32 weeks. This regimen approximates the amount of drug delivered by topical ocular administration of AZOPT® (brinzolamide ophthalmic suspension) 1% dosed to both eyes three times per day and simulates systemic drug and metabolite concentrations similar to those achieved with long-term topical dosing. RBC CA activity was measured to assess the degree of systemic CA inhibition. Brinzolamide saturation of RBC CA-II was achieved within 4 weeks (RBC concentrations of approximately 20 µM). N-Desethyl brinzolamide accumulated in RBCs to steady-state within 20–28 weeks reaching concentrations ranging from 6–30 µM. The inhibition of CA-II activity at steady-state was approximately 70–75%, which is below the degree of inhibition expected to have a pharmacological effect on renal function or respiration in healthy subjects.

In two, three-month clinical studies, AZOPT® (brinzolamide ophthalmic suspension) 1% dosed three times per day (TID) in patients with elevated intraocular pressure (IOP), produced significant reductions in IOPs (4–5 mmHg). These IOP reductions are equivalent to the reductions observed with TRUSOPT[1] (dorzolamide hydrochloride ophthalmic solution) 2% dosed TID in the same studies.

In two clinical studies in patients with elevated intraocular pressure, AZOPT® (brinzolamide ophthalmic suspension) 1% was associated with less stinging and burning upon instillation than TRUSOPT[1] 2%.

[1]TRUSOPT is a registered trademark of Merck & Co., Inc.

Indications and Usage: AZOPT® (brinzolamide ophthalmic suspension) 1% is indicated in the treatment of elevated intraocular pressure in patients with ocular hypertension or open-angle glaucoma.

Contraindications: AZOPT® (brinzolamide ophthalmic suspension) 1% is contraindicated in patients who are hypersensitive to any component of this product.

Warnings: AZOPT® (brinzolamide ophthalmic suspension) 1% is a sulfonamide and although administered topically it is absorbed systemically. Therefore, the same types of adverse reactions that are attributable to sulfonamides may occur with topical administration of AZOPT® (brinzolamide ophthalmic suspension) 1%. Fatalities have occurred, although rarely, due to severe reactions to sulfonamides including Stevens-Johnson syndrome, toxic epidermal necrolysis, fulminant hepatic necrosis, agranulocytosis, aplastic anemia, and other blood dyscrasias. Sensitization may recur when a sulfonamide is re-administered irrespective of the route of administration. If signs of serious reactions or hypersensitivity occur, discontinue the use of this preparation.

Precautions
General:
Carbonic anhydrase activity has been observed in both the cytoplasm and around the plasma membranes of the corneal endothelium. The effect of continued administration of AZOPT® (brinzolamide ophthalmic suspension) 1% on the corneal endothelium has not been fully evaluated. The management of patients with acute angle-closure glaucoma requires therapeutic interventions in addition to ocular hypotensive agents. AZOPT® (brinzolamide ophthalmic suspension) 1% has not been studied in patients with acute angle-closure glaucoma.

AZOPT® (brinzolamide ophthalmic suspension) 1% has not been studied in patients with severe renal impairment (CrCl <30 mL/min). Because AZOPT® (brinzolamide ophthalmic suspension) 1% and its metabolite are excreted predominantly by the kidney, AZOPT® (brinzolamide ophthalmic suspension) 1% is not recommended in such patients.

AZOPT® (brinzolamide ophthalmic suspension) 1% has not been studied in patients with hepatic impairment and should be used with caution in such patients.

There is a potential for an additive effect on the known systemic effects of carbonic anhydrase inhibition in patients receiving an oral carbonic anhydrase inhibitor and AZOPT® (brinzolamide ophthalmic suspension) 1%. The concomitant administration of AZOPT® (brinzolamide ophthalmic suspension) 1% and oral carbonic anhydrase inhibitors is not recommended.

Information For Patients:
AZOPT® (brinzolamide ophthalmic suspension) 1% is a sulfonamide and although administered topically, it is absorbed systemically; therefore, the same types of adverse reactions attributable to sulfonamides may occur with topical administration. Patients should be advised that if serious or unusual ocular or systemic reactions or signs of hypersensitivity occur, they should discontinue the use of the product and consult their physician *(see Warnings)*.

Continued on next page

Azopt—Cont.

Vision may be temporarily blurred following dosing with AZOPT® (brinzolamide ophthalmic suspension) 1%. Care should be exercised in operating machinery or driving a motor vehicle.

Patients should be instructed to avoid allowing the tip of the dispensing container to contact the eye or surrounding structures or other surfaces, since the product can become contaminated by common bacteria known to cause ocular infections. Serious damage to the eye and subsequent loss of vision may result from using contaminated solutions.

Patients should also be advised that if they have ocular surgery or develop an intercurrent ocular condition (e.g., trauma or infection), they should immediately seek their physician's advice concerning the continued use of the present multidose container.

If more than one topical ophthalmic drug is being used, the drugs should be administered at least ten minutes apart. The preservative in AZOPT® (brinzolamide ophthalmic suspension) 1%, benzalkonium chloride, may be absorbed by soft contact lenses. Contact lenses should be removed during instillation of AZOPT® (brinzolamide ophthalmic suspension) 1%, but may be reinserted 15 minutes after instillation.

Drug Interactions:
AZOPT® (brinzolamide ophthalmic suspension) 1% contains a carbonic anhydrase inhibitor. Acid-base and electrolyte alterations were not reported in the clinical trials with brinzolamide. However, in patients treated with oral carbonic anhydrase inhibitors, rare instances of drug interactions have occurred with high-dose salicylate therapy. Therefore, the potential for such drug interactions should be considered in patients receiving AZOPT® (brinzolamide ophthalmic suspension) 1%.

Carcinogenesis, Mutagenesis, Impairment of Fertility:
Carcinogenicity data on brinzolamide are not available. The following tests for mutagenic potential were negative: (1) *in vivo* mouse micronucleus assay; (2) *in vivo* sister chromatid exchange assay; and (3) Ames *E. coli* test. The *in vitro* mouse lymphoma forward mutation assay was negative in the absence of activation, but positive in the presence of microsomal activation.

In reproduction studies of brinzolamide in rats, there were no adverse effects on the fertility or reproductive capacity of males or females at doses up to 18 mg/kg/day (375 times the recommended human ophthalmic dose).

Pregnancy:
Teratogenic Effects: Pregnancy Category C. Developmental toxicity studies with brinzolamide in rabbits at oral doses of 1, 3, and 6 mg/kg/day (20, 62, and 125 times the recommended human ophthalmic dose) produced maternal toxicity at 6 mg/kg/day and a significant increase in the number of fetal variations, such as accessory skull bones, which was only slightly higher than the historic value at 1 and 6 mg/kg. In rats, statistically decreased body weights of fetuses from dams receiving oral doses of 18 mg/kg/day (375 times the recommended human ophthalmic dose) during gestation were proportional to the reduced maternal weight gain, with no statistically significant effects on organ or tissue development. Increases in unossified sternebrae, reduced ossification of the skull, and unossified hyoid that occurred at 6 and 18 mg/kg were not statistically significant. No treatment-related malformations were seen. Following oral administration of 14C-brinzolamide to pregnant rats, radioactivity was found to cross the placenta and was present in the fetal tissues and blood.

There are no adequate and well-controlled studies in pregnant women. AZOPT® (brinzolamide ophthalmic suspension) 1% should be used during pregnancy only if the potential benefit justifies the potential risk to the fetus.

Nursing Mothers:
In a study of brinzolamide in lactating rats, decreases in body weight gain in offspring at an oral dose of 15 mg/kg/day (312 times the recommended human ophthalmic dose) were seen during lactation. No other effects were observed. However, following oral administration of 14C-brinzolamide to lactating rats, radioactivity was found in milk at concentrations below those in the blood and plasma.

It is not known whether this drug is excreted in human milk. Because many drugs are excreted in human milk and because of the potential for serious adverse reactions in nursing infants from AZOPT® (brinzolamide ophthalmic suspension) 1%, a decision should be made whether to discontinue nursing or to discontinue the drug, taking into account the importance of the drug to the mother.

Pediatric Use:
A three-month controlled clinical study was conducted in which AZOPT® (brinzolamide ophthalmic suspension) 1% was dosed only twice a day in pediatric patients 4 weeks to 5 years of age. Patients were not required to discontinue their IOP-lowering medication(s) until initiation of monotherapy with AZOPT®. IOP-lowering efficacy was not demonstrated in this study in which the mean decrease in elevated IOP was between 0 and 2 mmHg. Five out of 32 patients demonstrated an increase in corneal diameter of one millimeter.

Geriatric Use: No overall differences in safety or effectiveness have been observed between elderly and younger patients.

Adverse Reactions:
In clinical studies of AZOPT® (brinzolamide ophthalmic suspension) 1%, the most frequently reported adverse events associated with AZOPT® (brinzolamide ophthalmic suspension) 1% were blurred vision and bitter, sour or unusual taste. These events occurred in approximately 5–10% of patients. Blepharitis, dermatitis, dry eye, foreign body sensation, headache, hyperemia, ocular discharge, ocular discomfort, ocular keratitis, ocular pain, ocular pruritus and rhinitis were reported at an incidence of 1–5%.

The following adverse reactions were reported at an incidence below 1%: allergic reactions, alopecia, chest pain, conjunctivitis, diarrhea, diplopia, dizziness, dry mouth, dyspnea, dyspepsia, eye fatigue, hypertonia, keratoconjunctivitis, keratopathy, kidney pain, lid margin crusting or sticky sensation, nausea, pharyngitis, tearing and urticaria.

Overdosage: Although no human data are available, electrolyte imbalance, development of an acidotic state, and possible nervous system effects may occur following oral administration of an overdose. Serum electrolyte levels (particularly potassium) and blood pH levels should be monitored.

Dosage and Administration: Shake well before use. The recommended dose is 1 drop of AZOPT® (brinzolamide ophthalmic suspension) 1% in the affected eye(s) three times daily.

AZOPT® (brinzolamide ophthalmic suspension) 1% may be used concomitantly with other topical ophthalmic drug products to lower intraocular pressure.

If more than one topical ophthalmic drug is being used, the drugs should be administered at least ten minutes apart.

How Supplied:
AZOPT® (brinzolamide ophthalmic suspension) 1% is supplied in plastic DROP-TAINER® dispensers with a controlled dispensing-tip as follows:

NDC 0065-0275-05	5 mL
NDC 0065-0275-10	10 mL
NDC 0065-0275-15	15 mL

Storage: Store AZOPT® (brinzolamide ophthalmic suspension) 1% at 4–30°C (39–86°F).

℞ Only
U.S. Patent Nos: 5,378,703; 5,461,081; 6,071,904.

*TRUSOPT is a registered trademark of Merk & Co., Inc.

DUREZOL® 0.05%
(difluprednate ophthalmic emulsion) 0.05%

HIGHLIGHTS OF PRESCRIBING INFORMATION
These highlights do not include all of the information needed to use Durezol® safely and effectively. See full prescribing information for Durezol.
DUREZOL®
(difluprednate ophthalmic emulsion) 0.05%
Initial U.S. approval: 2008

——————— INDICATIONS AND USAGE ———————

Durezol is a topical corticosteroid that is indicated for the treatment of inflammation and pain associated with ocular surgery. (1)

——————— DOSAGE AND ADMINISTRATION ———————

Instill one drop into the conjunctival sac of the affected eye(s) 4 times daily beginning 24 hours after surgery and continuing throughout the first weeks of the postoperative period, followed by times daily for a week and then a taper based on the response. (2)

——————— DOSAGE FORMS AND STRENGTHS ———————

Durezol contains 0.05% difluprednate, as a sterile preserved ophthalmic emulsion for topical ophthalmic use only. (3)

——————— CONTRAINDICATIONS ———————

Durezol, as with other ophthalmic corticosteroids is contraindicated in most active viral diseases of the cornea and conjunctiva including epithelial herpes simplex keratitis (dendritic keratitis), vaccinia and varicella, and also in mycobacterial infection of the eye and fungal diseases of ocular structures. (4)

——————— WARNINGS AND PRECAUTIONS ———————

- Intraocular pressure (IOP) increase—Prolonged use of corticosteroids may result in glaucoma with damage to the optic nerve, defects in visual acuity and fields of vision. If this product is used for 10 days or longer, IOP should be monitored. (5.1)
- Cataracts—Use of corticosteroids may result in posterior subcapsular cataract formation. (5.2)
- Delayed healing—The use of steroids after cataract surgery may delay healing and increase the incidence of bleb formation. In those diseases causing thinning of the cornea or sclera, perforations have been known to occur with the use of topical steroids. The initial prescription and renewal of the medication order beyond 28 days should be made by a physician only after examination of the patient with the aid of magnification such as slit lamp biomicroscopy and, where appropriate, fluorescein staining. (5.3)
- Bacterial infections—Prolonged use of corticosteroids may suppress the host response and thus increase the hazard of secondary ocular infections. In acute purulent conditions, steroids may mask infection or enhance existing infection. If signs and symptoms fail to improve after 2 days, the patient should be re-evaluated. (5.4)
- Viral infections—Employment of a corticosteroid medication in the treatment of patients with a history of herpes simplex requires great caution. Use of ocular steroids may prolong the course and may exacerbate the severity of many viral infections of the eye (including herpes simplex). (5.5)
- Fungal infections—Fungal infections of the cornea are particularly prone to develop coincidentally with long-term local steroid application. Fungus invasion must be considered in any persistent corneal ulceration where a steroid has been used or is in use. (5.6)

To report SUSPECTED ADVERSE REACTIONS contact Alcon Laboratories, Inc. at 1-800-757-9195 or FDA at 1-800-FDA-1088 or www.fda.gov/medwatch.
See 17 for PATIENT COUNSELING INFORMATION

Revised: 08/201

FULL PRESCRIBING INFORMATION: CONTENTS*

ULL PRESCRIBING INFORMATION

INDICATIONS AND USAGE

urezol (difluprednate ophthalmic emulsion) .05%, a topical corticosteroid, is indicated for the reatment of inflammation and pain associated ith ocular surgery.

DOSAGE AND ADMINISTRATION

nstill one drop into the conjunctival sac of the af- ected eye(s) 4 times daily beginning 24 hours after urgery and continuing throughout the first 2 veeks of the postoperative period, followed by 2 imes daily for a week and then a taper based on he response.

DOSAGE STRENGTHS

urezol contains 0.05% difluprednate as a sterile reserved emulsion for topical ophthalmic adminis- ration.

CONTRAINDICATIONS

he use of Durezol, as with other ophthalmic corti- osteroids, is contraindicated in most active viral iseases of the cornea and conjunctiva including ep- helial herpes simplex keratitis (dendritic kerati- s), vaccinia, and varicella, and also in mycobacte- ial infection of the eye and fungal disease of ocular tructures.

WARNINGS AND PRECAUTIONS

.1   IOP Increase

rolonged use of corticosteroids may result in glau- oma with damage to the optic nerve, defects in vi- ual acuity and fields of vision. Steroids should be sed with caution in the presence of glaucoma. If his product is used for 10 days or longer, intraocu- ar pressure should be monitored.

.2   Cataracts

Jse of corticosteroids may result in posterior sub- apsular cataract formation.

.3   Delayed Healing

he use of steroids after cataract surgery may delay ealing and increase the incidence of bleb forma- ion. In those diseases causing thinning of the cor- ea or sclera, perforations have been known to oc- ur with the use of topical steroids. The initial rescription and renewal of the medication order eyond 28 days should be made by a physician only fter examination of the patient with the aid of nagnification such as slit lamp biomicroscopy and, here appropriate, fluorescein staining.

.4   Bacterial Infections

rolonged use of corticosteroids may suppress the ost response and thus increase the hazard of econdary ocular infections. In acute purulent con- itions, steroids may mask infection or enhance ex- ting infection. If signs and symptoms fail to im- rove after 2 days, the patient should be re- valuated.

5.5   Viral Infections

Employment of a corticosteroid medication in the treatment of patients with a history of herpes sim- plex requires great caution. Use of ocular steroids may prolong the course and may exacerbate the se- verity of many viral infections of the eye (including herpes simplex).

5.6   Fungal Infections

Fungal infections of the cornea are particularly prone to develop coincidentally with long-term local steroid application. Fungus invasion must be con- sidered in any persistent corneal ulceration where a steroid has been used or is in use. Fungal culture should be taken when appropriate.

5.7   Topical Ophthalmic Use Only

Durezol is not indicated for intraocular administra- tion.

6   ADVERSE REACTIONS

Adverse reactions associated with ophthalmic ster- oids include elevated intraocular pressure, which may be associated with optic nerve damage, visual acuity and field defects, posterior subcapsular cata- ract formation, secondary ocular infection from pathogens including herpes simplex, and perfora- tion of the globe where there is thinning of the cor- nea or sclera.

Ocular adverse reactions occurring in 5–15% of sub- jects in clinical studies with Durezol included cor- neal edema, ciliary and conjunctival hyperemia, eye pain, photophobia, posterior capsule opacification, anterior chamber cells, anterior chamber flare, con- junctival edema, and blepharitis. Other ocular ad- verse reactions occurring in 1–5% of subjects in- cluded reduced visual acuity, punctate keratitis, eye inflammation, and iritis. Ocular adverse events oc- curring in <1% of subjects included application site discomfort or irritation, corneal pigmentation and striae, episcleritis, eye pruritis, eyelid irritation and crusting, foreign body sensation, increased lac- rimation, macular edema, scleral hyperemia, and uveitis. Most of these events may have been the consequence of the surgical procedure.

8   USE IN SPECIFIC POPULATIONS

8.1   Pregnancy

Teratogenic Effects

Pregnancy Category C. Difluprednate has been shown to be embryotoxic (decrease in embryonic body weight and a delay in embryonic ossification) and teratogenic (cleft palate and skeletal) anoma- lies when administered subcutaneously to rabbits during organogenesis at a dose of 1–10 μg/kg/day. The no-observed-effect-level (NOEL) for these ef- fects was 1 μg/kg/day, and 10 μg/kg/day was consid- ered to be a teratogenic dose that was concurrently found in the toxic dose range for fetuses and preg- nant females. Treatment of rats with 10 μg/kg/day subcutaneously during organogenesis did not result in any reproductive toxicity, nor was it maternally toxic. At 100 μg/kg/day after subcutaneous admin- istration in rats, there was a decrease in fetal weights and delay in ossification, and effects on weight gain in the pregnant females. It is difficult to extrapolate these doses of difluprednate to maxi- mum daily human doses of Durezol, since Durezol is administered topically with minimal systemic ab- sorption, and difluprednate blood levels were not measured in the reproductive animal studies. How- ever, since use of difluprednate during human preg- nancy has not been evaluated and cannot rule out the possibility of harm, Durezol should be used dur- ing pregnancy only if the potential benefit justifies the potential risk to the embryo or fetus.

8.3   Nursing Mothers

It is not known whether topical ophthalmic admin- istration of corticosteroids could result in sufficient systemic absorption to produce detectable quanti- ties in breast milk. Systemically administered cor- ticosteroids appear in human milk and could sup- press growth, interfere with endogenous

corticosteroid production, or cause other untoward effects. Caution should be exercised when Durezol is administered to a nursing woman.

8.4   Pediatric Use

Safety and effectiveness in pediatric patients has not been established.

8.5   Geriatric Use

No overall differences in safety or effectiveness have been observed between elderly and younger patients.

11   DESCRIPTION

Durezol (difluprednate ophthalmic emulsion) 0.05% is a sterile, topical anti-inflammatory corticosteroid for ophthalmic use. The chemical name is 6α,9difluoro-11β,17,21-trihydroxypregna-1,4-diene- 3,20-dione 21-acetate 17-butyrate (CAS number 23674-86-4). Difluprednate is represented by the following structural formula:

Difluprednate has a molecular weight of 508.56, and the empirical formula is $C_{27}H_{34}F_2O_7$.

Each mL contains: ACTIVE: difluprednate 0.5 mg (0.05%); INACTIVE: boric acid, castor oil, glycerin, polysorbate 80, water for injection, sodium acetate, sodium EDTA, sodium hydroxide(to adjust the pH to 5.2 to 5.8). The emulsion is essentially isotonic with a tonicity of 304 to 411 mOsm/kg. PRESERVATIVE: sorbic acid 0.1%.

12   CLINICAL PHARMACOLOGY

12.1   Mechanism of Action

Corticosteroids inhibit the inflammatory response to a variety of inciting agents that may delay or slow healing. They inhibit edema, fibrin deposition, capillary dilation, leukocyte migration, capillary proliferation, fibroblast proliferation, deposition of collagen, and scar formation associated with in- flammation. There is no generally accepted expla- nation for the mechanism of action of ocular corti- costeroids. However, corticosteroids are thought to act by the induction of phospholipase A_2 inhibitory proteins, collectively called lipocortins. It is postu- lated that these proteins control the biosynthesis of potent mediators of inflammation such as prostag- landins and leukotreines by inhibiting the release of their common precursor arachidonic acid. Arach- idonic acid is released from membrane phospholip- ids by phospholipase A_2.

Difluprednate is structurally similar to other corti- costeroids.

12.3   Pharmacokinetics

Difluprednate undergoes deacetylation in vivo to 6α,9-difluoroprednisolone 17-butyrate (DFB), an ac- tive metabolite of difluprednate.

Clinical pharmacokinetic studies of difluprednate after repeat ocular instillation of 2 drops of difluprednate (0.01% or 0.05%) QID for 7days showed that DFB levels in blood were below the quantification limit (50 ng/mL) at all time points for all subjects, indicating the systemic absorption of difluprednate after ocular instillation of Durezol is limited.

13   NONCLINICAL TOXICOLOGY

13.1   Carcinogenesis, Mutagenesis, and Impair- ment of Fertility

Difluprednate was not genotoxic in vitro in the Ames test, and in cultured mammalian cells CHL/IU (a fibroblastic cell line derived from the lungs of newborn female Chinese hamsters). An in vivo micronucleus test of difluprednate in mice was also negative. Treatment of male and female rats

Continued on next page

Ocular Inflammation and Pain Endpoints (Studies Pooled)

Day	Durezol QID (n=107)		Vehicle (n=220)	
	8	15	8	15
Anterior Chamber cell clearing (% subjects)	24 (22%)*	44 (41%)*	17 (7%)	25 (11%)
Pain free (% subjects)	62 (58%)*	67 (63%)*	59 (27%)	76 (35%)

* Statistically significantly better than vehicle, P<0.01

Durezol—Cont.

with subcutaneous difluprednate up to 10 μg/kg/day prior to and during mating did not impair fertility in either gender. Long term studies have not been conducted to evaluate the carcinogenic potential of difluprednate.

13.2   Animal Toxicology and/or Pharmacology

In multiple studies performed in rodents and non-rodents, subchronic and chronic toxicity tests of difluprednate showed systemic effects such as suppression of body weight gain; a decrease in lymphocyte count; atrophy of the lymphatic glands and adrenal gland; and for local effects, thinning of the skin; all of which were due to the pharmacologic action of the molecule and are well known glucocorticosteroid effects. Most, if not all of these effects were reversible after drug withdrawal. The NOEL for the subchronic and chronic toxicity tests were consistent between species and ranged from 1–1.25 μg/kg per day.

14   CLINICAL STUDIES

14.1   Postoperative Ocular Inflammation and Pain

Clinical efficacy was evaluated in 2 randomized, double-masked, placebo-controlled trials in which subjects with an anterior chamber cell grade ≥"2" (a cell count of 11 or higher) after cataract surgery were assigned to Durezol or placebo (vehicle) following surgery. One drop of Durezol or vehicle was self instilled either 2 (BID) or 4 (QID) times per day for 14 days, beginning the day after surgery. The presence of complete clearing (a cell count of 0) was assessed 8 and 15 days post-surgery using a slit lamp binocular microscope. In the intent-to-treat analyses of both studies, a significant benefit was seen in the QID Durezol-treated group in ocular inflammation and reduction of pain when compared with placebo. The consolidated clinical trial results are provided below.

[See table above]

16   HOW SUPPLIED/STORAGE AND HANDLING

Durezol (difluprednate ophthalmic emulsion) 0.05% is a sterile, aqueous topical ophthalmic emulsion supplied in an opaque plastic bottle with a controlled drop tip and a pink cap in the following size: 5 mL in a 5 mL bottle (NDC 0065-9240-05)

Storage

Store at 15–25°C (59–77°F). Do not freeze. Protect from light. When not in use keep the bottles in the protective carton.

17   PATIENT COUNSELING INFORMATION

This product is sterile when packaged. Patients should be advised not to allow the dropper tip to touch any surface, as this may contaminate the emulsion. If pain develops or if redness, itching, or inflammation becomes aggravated, the patient should be advised to consult a physician. As with all ophthalmic preparations containing a preservative, patients should be advised not to wear contact lenses when using Durezol.

Revised: August 2010

Manufactured for: Alcon Laboratories, Inc. 6201 South Freeway, Fort Worth, Texas 76134 USA 1-800-757-9195

MedInfo@AlconLabs.com

Manufactured by: Catalent Pharma Solutions Woodstock, IL 60098

© 2010 Alcon, Inc.

MOXEZA™   ℞

moxifloxacin hydrochloride solution

Sterile topical ophthalmic solution

HIGHLIGHTS OF PRESCRIBING INFORMATION

These highlights do not include all the information needed to use MOXEZA™ solution safely and effectively. See full prescribing information for MOXEZA™.

MOXEZA™ (moxifloxacin hydrochloride ophthalmic solution) 0.5% as base

Sterile topical ophthalmic solution

Initial U.S. Approval: 1999

——————— **INDICATIONS AND USAGE** ———————

MOXEZA™ solution is a topical fluoroquinolone anti-infective indicated for the treatment of bacterial conjunctivitis caused by susceptible strains of the following organisms:

Aerococcus viridans, *Corynebacterium macginleyi*, *Enterococcus faecalis*, *Micrococcus luteus*, *Staphylococcus arlettae*, *Staphylococcus aureus*, *Staphylococcus capitis*, *Staphylococcus epidermidis*, *Staphylococcus haemolyticus*, *Staphylococcus hominis*, *Staphylococcus saprophyticus*, *Staphylococcus warneri*, *Streptococcus mitis*, *Streptococcus pneumoniae*, *Streptococcus parasanguinis*, *Escherichia coli*, *Haemophilus influenzae*, *Klebsiella pneumoniae*, *Propionibacterium acnes*, *Chlamydia trachomatis*

*Efficacy for this organism was studied in fewer than 10 infections. (1)

——— **DOSAGE AND ADMINISTRATION** ———

Instill 1 drop in the affected eye(s) 2 times daily for 7 days. (2)

——— **DOSAGE FORMS AND STRENGTHS** ———

4 mL bottle filled with 3 mL sterile ophthalmic solution of moxifloxacin hydrochloride, 0.5% as base. (3)

——————— **CONTRAINDICATIONS** ———————

None. (4)

——— **WARNINGS AND PRECAUTIONS** ———

• Topical ophthalmic use only. (5.1)
• Hypersensitivity and anaphylaxis have been reported with systemic use of moxifloxacin. (5.2)
• Prolonged use may result in overgrowth of non-susceptible organisms, including fungi. (5.3)
• Patients should not wear contact lenses if they have signs or symptoms of bacterial conjunctivitis. (5.4)

——————— **ADVERSE REACTIONS** ———————

The most common adverse reactions reported in 1-2% of patients were eye irritation, pyrexia, and conjunctivitis. (6)

To report SUSPECTED ADVERSE REACTIONS, contact Alcon Laboratories, Inc. or FDA at 1-800-FDA-1088 or www.fda.gov/medwatch.

See 17 for PATIENT COUNSELING INFORMATION

Revised: 11/2010

FULL PRESCRIBING INFORMATION

1   INDICATIONS AND USAGE

MOXEZA™ solution is indicated for the treatmen of bacterial conjunctivitis caused by susceptibl strains of the following organisms:

Aerococcus viridans
Corynebacterium macginleyi
Enterococcus faecalis
Micrococcus luteus
Staphylococcus arlettae
Staphylococcus aureus
Staphylococcus capitis
Staphylococcus epidermidis
Staphylococcus haemolyticus
Staphylococcus hominis
Staphylococcus saprophyticus
Staphylococcus warneri
Streptococcus mitis
Streptococcus pneumoniae
Streptococcus parasanguinis
Escherichia coli
Haemophilus influenzae
Klebsiella pneumoniae
Propionibacterium acnes
Chlamydia trachomatis

*Efficacy for this organism was studied in fewe than 10 infections.

2   DOSAGE AND ADMINISTRATION

Instill 1 drop in the affected eye(s) 2 times daily fo 7 days.

3   DOSAGE FORMS AND STRENGTHS

4 mL bottle filled with 3 mL of sterile ophthalmi solution of moxifloxacin hydrochloride, 0.5% a base.

4   CONTRAINDICATIONS

None.

5   WARNINGS AND PRECAUTIONS

5.1   Topical Ophthalmic Use Only

NOT FOR INJECTION. MOXEZA™ solution is fo topical ophthalmic use only and should not be in jected subconjunctivally or introduced directly int the anterior chamber of the eye.

5.2   Hypersensitivity Reactions

In patients receiving systemically administere quinolones, including moxifloxacin, serious and oc casionally fatal hypersensitivity (anaphylactic) re actions have been reported, some following the firs ose. Some reactions were accompanied by cardio-ascular collapse, loss of consciousness, angio-dema (including laryngeal, pharyngeal or facial dema), airway obstruction, dyspnea, urticaria, and ching. If an allergic reaction to moxifloxacin oc-urs, discontinue use of the drug. Serious acute hy-ersensitivity reactions may require immediate mergency treatment. Oxygen and airway manage-ent should be administered as clinically indi-ated.

.3   Growth of Resistant Organisms with Pro-nged Use
s with other anti-infectives, prolonged use may re-lt in overgrowth of non-susceptible organisms, in-luding fungi. If superinfection occurs, discontinue se and institute alternative therapy. Whenever inical judgment dictates, the patient should be ex-mined with the aid of magnification, such as slit-mp biomicroscopy, and, where appropriate, fluo-escein staining.

.4   Avoidance of Contact Lens Wear
atients should be advised not to wear contact nses if they have signs or symptoms of bacterial onjunctivitis.

ADVERSE REACTIONS
ecause clinical trials are conducted under widely arying conditions, adverse reaction rates observed the clinical trials of a drug cannot be directly ompared to the rates in the clinical trials of an-ther drug and may not reflect the rates observed in ractice.
he data described below reflect exposure to IOXEZA™ solution in 1263 patients, between months and 92 years of age, with signs and symp-oms of bacterial conjunctivitis. The most fre-uently reported adverse reactions were eye irrita-on, pyrexia and conjunctivitis, reported in 1-2% of atients.

USE IN SPECIFIC POPULATIONS
1   Pregnancy
regnancy Category C. Moxifloxacin was not tera-ogenic when administered to pregnant rats during rganogenesis at oral doses as high as 500 mg/kg/ay (approximately 25,000 times the highest recom-ended total daily human ophthalmic dose); how-ver, decreased fetal body weights and slightly elayed fetal skeletal development were observed. here was no evidence of teratogenicity when preg-ant Cynomolgus monkeys were given oral doses as igh as 100 mg/kg/day (approximately 5,000 times he highest recommended total daily human oph-halmic dose). An increased incidence of smaller fe-uses was observed at 100 mg/kg/day.
ince there are no adequate and well-controlled tudies in pregnant women, MOXEZA™ solution hould be used during pregnancy only if the poten-al benefit justifies the potential risk to the fetus.

.3   Nursing Mothers
Ioxifloxacin has not been measured in human ilk, although it can be presumed to be excreted in uman milk. Caution should be exercised when IOXEZA™ solution is administered to a nursing other.

.4   Pediatric Use
he safety and effectiveness of MOXEZA™ solution infants below 4 months of age have not been es-ablished.
here is no evidence that the ophthalmic adminis-ration of moxifloxacin has any effect on weight earing joints, even though oral administration of ome quinolones has been shown to cause arthrop-thy in immature animals.

5   Geriatric Use
o overall differences in safety and effectiveness ave been observed between elderly and younger atients.

1   DESCRIPTION
IOXEZA™ is a sterile solution for topical ophthal-ic use.
Ioxifloxacin hydrochloride is an 8-methoxy fluoro-uinolone anti-infective, with a diazabicyclononyl ng at the C7 position.

$C_{21}H_{24}FN_3O_4 \bullet HCl$ Mol Wt 437.9
Chemical Name: 1-Cyclopropyl-6-fluoro-1,4-dihydro-8-methoxy-7-[(4aS,7aS)-octahydro-6H-pyrrolo[3,4-b]pyridin-6-yl]-4-oxo-3-quinolinecar-boxylic acid, monohydrochloride.
Each mL of MOXEZA™ solution contains 5.45 mg moxifloxacin hydrochloride, equivalent to 5 mg moxifloxacin base.
Inactives: Sodium chloride, xanthan gum, boric acid, sorbitol, tyloxapol, purified water, and hydro-chloric acid and/or sodium hydroxide to adjust pH. MOXEZA™ is a greenish-yellow, isotonic solution with an osmolality of 300-370 mOsm/kg and a pH of approximately 7.4. Moxifloxacin hydrochloride is a slightly yellow to yellow crystalline powder.

12   CLINICAL PHARMACOLOGY
12.1   Mechanism of Action
Moxifloxacin is a member of the fluoroquinolone class of anti-infective drugs. (See 12.4 Microbiol-ogy.)

12.3   Pharmacokinetics
Moxifloxacin steady-state plasma pharmacokinetics were evaluated in healthy adult male and female subjects who were administered multiple, bilateral, topical ocular doses of MOXEZA™ solution two times daily for four days with a final dose on day 5. The average steady-state AUC_{0-12} was 8.17 ± 5.31 ng*h/mL. Moxifloxacin C_{max} following twice-daily bilateral ophthalmic administration of moxifloxacin 0.5% for 5 days is approximately 0.02% of that achieved with the oral formulation of moxifloxacin hydrochloride (C_{max} following oral dos-ing of 400 mg AVELOX*, 4.5 ± 0.5 mcg/mL).

12.4   Microbiology
The antibacterial action of moxifloxacin results from inhibition of the topoisomerase II (DNA gy-rase) and topoisomerase IV. DNA gyrase is an es-sential enzyme that is involved in the replication, transcription and repair of bacterial DNA. Topo-isomerase IV is an enzyme known to play a key role in the partitioning of the chromosomal DNA during bacterial cell division.
The mechanism of action for quinolones, including moxifloxacin, is different from that of macrolides, aminoglycosides, or tetracyclines. Therefore, moxifloxacin may be active against pathogens that are resistant to these antibiotics and these antibi-otics may be active against pathogens that are re-sistant to moxifloxacin. There is no cross-resistance between moxifloxacin and the aforementioned clas-ses of antibiotics. Cross-resistance has been ob-served between systemic moxifloxacin and some other quinolones.
In vitro resistance to moxifloxacin develops via multiple-step mutations. Resistance to moxifloxacin occurs in vitro at a general frequency of between 1.8 × 10^{-9} to < 1 × 10^{-11} for Gram-positive bacteria.
Moxifloxacin has been shown to be active against most strains of the following microorganisms, both in vitro and in clinical infections as described in the INDICATIONS AND USAGE section:
Aerococcus viridans*
Corynebacterium macginleyi*
Enterococcus faecalis*
Micrococcus luteus*
Staphylococcus arlettae*
Staphylococcus aureus
Staphylococcus capitis
Staphylococcus epidermidis
Staphylococcus haemolyticus
Staphylococcus hominis
Staphylococcus saprophyticus*
Staphylococcus warneri*
Streptococcus mitis*

Streptococcus pneumoniae
Streptococcus parasanguinis*
Escherichia coli*
Haemophilus influenzae
Klebsiella pneumoniae*
Propionibacterium acnes
Chlamydia trachomatis*
*Efficacy for this organism was studied in fewer than 10 infections.
The following in vitro data are available, but their clinical significance in ophthalmic infections is un-known. The safety and effectiveness of MOXEZA™ solution in treating ophthalmic infections due to these organisms have not been established in ade-quate and well-controlled trials.
Moxifloxacin has been shown to be active in vitro against most strains of the microorganisms listed below. These organisms are considered susceptible when evaluated using systemic breakpoints; how-ever, a correlation between the in vitro systemic breakpoint and ophthalmologic efficacy has not been established. The list of organisms is provided as guidance only in assessing the potential treat-ment of conjunctival infections. Moxifloxacin exhib-its in vitro minimal inhibitory concentrations (MICs) of 2 mcg/mL or less (systemic susceptible breakpoint) against most (≥ 90%) strains of the fol-lowing ocular pathogens:
Aerobic Gram-positive microorganisms:
Staphylococcus caprae
Staphylococcus cohnii
Staphylococcus lugdunensis
Staphylococcus pasteuri
Streptococcus agalactiae
Streptococcus milleri group
Streptococcus oralis
Streptococcus pyogenes
Streptococcus salivarius
Streptococcussanguis
Aerobic Gram-negative microorganisms:
Acinetobacter baumannii
Acinetobacter calcoaceticus
Acinetobacter junii
Enterobacter aerogenes
Enterobacter cloacae
Haemophilus parainfluenzae
Klebsiella oxytoca
Moraxella catarrhalis
Moraxella osloensis
Morganella morganii
Neisseria gonorrhoeae
Neisseria meningitidis
Pantoea agglomerans
Proteus vulgaris
Pseudomonas stutzeri
Serratia liquefaciens
Serratia marcescens
Stenotrophomonas maltophilia
Anaerobic microorganisms:
Clostridium perfringens
Peptostreptococcus anaerobius
Peptostreptococcus magnus
Peptostreptococcus micros
Peptostreptococcus prevotii
Other microorganisms:
Mycobacterium tuberculosis
Mycobacterium avium
Mycobacterium kansasii
Mycobacterium marinum

13   NONCLINICAL TOXICOLOGY
13.1   Carcinogenesis, Mutagenesis, Impairment of Fertility
Long-term studies in animals to determine the car-cinogenic potential of moxifloxacin have not been performed.
Moxifloxacin was not mutagenic in four bacterial strains used in the Ames Salmonella reversion as-say. As with other quinolones, the positive response observed with moxifloxacin in strain TA 102 using the same assay may be due to the inhibition of DNA gyrase. Moxifloxacin was not mutagenic in the CHO/HGPRT mammalian cell gene mutation assay. An equivocal result was obtained in the same assay when v79 cells were used. Moxifloxacin was clasto-genic in the v79 chromosome aberration assay, but it did not induce unscheduled DNA synthesis in cul-tured rat hepatocytes. There was no evidence of genotoxicity in vivo in a micronucleus test or a dom-inant lethal test in mice.

Continued on next page

Moxeza—Cont.

Moxifloxacin had no effect on fertility in male and female rats at oral doses as high as 500 mg/kg/day, approximately 25,000 times the highest recommended total daily human ophthalmic dose. At 500 mg/kg orally there were slight effects on sperm morphology (head-tail separation) in male rats and on the estrous cycle in female rats.

14 CLINICAL STUDIES

In one randomized, double-masked, multicenter, vehicle-controlled clinical trial in which patients with bacterial conjunctivitis were dosed with MOXEZA™ solution 2 times a day, MOXEZA™ was superior to its vehicle for both clinical and microbiological outcomes. Clinical cure achieved on Day 4 was 63% (265/424) in MOXEZA™ solution treated patients, versus 51% (214/423) in vehicle treated patients. Microbiologic success (eradication of baseline pathogens) was achieved on Day 4 in 75% (316/424) of MOXEZA™ solution treated patients versus 56% (237/423) of vehicle treated patients. Microbiologic eradication does not always correlate with clinical outcome in anti-infective trials.

16 HOW SUPPLIED/STORAGE AND HANDLING

MOXEZA™ solution is supplied as a sterile ophthalmic solution in the Alcon DROP-TAINER® dispensing system consisting of a natural low density polyethylene bottle and dispensing plug and tan polypropylene closure. Tamper evidence is provided with a shrink band around the closure and neck area of the package.

3 mL in a 4 mL bottle - NDC 0065-0006-03
Storage: Store at 2°C- 25°C (36°F - 77°F).

17 PATIENT COUNSELING INFORMATION

Patients should be advised not to touch the dropper tip to any surface to avoid contaminating the contents.

Patients should be advised not to wear contact lenses if they have signs and symptoms of bacterial conjunctivitis.

Systemically administered quinolones, including moxifloxacin, have been associated with hypersensitivity reactions, even following a single dose. Patients should be told to discontinue use immediately and contact their physician at the first sign of a rash or allergic reaction.

Licensed to Alcon, Inc. by Bayer Schering Pharma AG.
U.S. PAT. NO. 4,990,517; 5,607,942; 6,716,830; 7,671,070
Alcon ®
Alcon Laboratories, Inc.
6201 South Freeway
Fort Worth, Texas 76134 USA
MedInfo@AlconLabs.com
©2010 Alcon, Inc.
*Avelox is a registered trademark of Bayer AG.

NEVANAC®   ℞

(nepafenac ophthalmic suspension)
0.1%, topical ophthalmic

HIGHLIGHTS OF PRESCRIBING INFORMATION
These highlights do not include all the information needed to use NEVANAC® safely and effectively. See full prescribing information for NEVANAC®.
NEVANAC® (nepafenac ophthalmic suspension) 0.1%, topical ophthalmic
Initial U.S. Approval: 2005

INDICATIONS AND USAGE

NEVANAC ophthalmic suspension is a nonsteroidal, anti-inflammatory prodrug indicated for the treatment of pain and inflammation associated with cataract surgery (1).

DOSAGE AND ADMINISTRATION

One drop of NEVANAC ophthalmic suspension should be applied to the affected eye(s) three-times-daily beginning 1 day prior to cataract surgery, continued on the day of surgery and through the first 2 weeks of the postoperative period. (2)

DOSAGE FORMS AND STRENGTHS

Sterile ophthalmic suspension: 0.1% (3)
3 mL in a 4 mL bottle

CONTRAINDICATIONS

Hypersensitivity to any of the ingredients in the formula or to other NSAIDS. (4)

WARNINGS AND PRECAUTIONS

Increased bleeding time due to increased thrombocyte aggregation (5.1)
Delayed healing (5.2)
Corneal effects including keratitis (5.3)

ADVERSE REACTIONS

Most common adverse reactions (5 to 10%) are capsular opacity, decreased visual acuity, foreign body sensation, increased intraocular pressure, and sticky sensation. (6.1)
To report SUSPECTED ADVERSE REACTIONS, contact Alcon Laboratories, Inc. at 1-800-757-9195 or FDA at 1-800-FDA-1088 or www.fda.gov/medwatch.

INFORMATION FOR PATIENTS

See 17 for PATIENT COUNSELING INFORMATION and FDA-approved patient labeling
Revised: 09/2007

FULL PRESCRIBING INFORMATION: CONTENTS*

FULL PRESCRIBING INFORMATION

1   Indications and Usage

NEVANAC® ophthalmic suspension is indicated for the treatment of pain and inflammation associated with cataract surgery.

2   Dosage and Administration

2.1   Recommended Dosing

One drop of NEVANAC® should be applied to the affected eye(s) three-times-daily beginning 1 day prior to cataract surgery, continued on the day surgery and through the first 2 weeks of the pos operative period.

2.2   Use with Other Topical Ophthalmic Medications

NEVANAC® may be administered in conjunctio with other topical ophthalmic medications such beta-blockers, carbonic anhydrase inhibitor alpha-agonists, cycloplegics, and mydriatics.

3   Dosage Forms and Strengths

Sterile ophthalmic suspension: 0.1%
3 mL in a 4 mL bottle

4   Contraindications

NEVANAC® is contraindicated in patients wi previously demonstrated hypersensitivity to any the ingredients in the formula or to other NSAI

5   Warnings and Precautions

5.1   Increased Bleeding Time

With some nonsteroidal anti-inflammatory dru including NEVANAC®, there exists the potenti for increased bleeding time due to interference wi thrombocyte aggregation. There have been repor that ocularly applied nonsteroidal an inflammatory drugs may cause increased bleedi of ocular tissues (including hyphemas) in conjun tion with ocular surgery. It is recommended th NEVANAC® ophthalmic suspension be used wi caution in patients with known bleeding tendenci or who are receiving other medications which ma prolong bleeding time.

5.2   Delayed Healing

Topical nonsteroidal anti-inflammatory dru (NSAIDs) including NEVANAC®, may slow or d lay healing. Topical corticosteroids are also know to slow or delay healing. Concomitant use of topic NSAIDs and topical steroids may increase the p tential for healing problems.

5.3   Corneal Effects

Use of topical NSAIDs may result in keratitis. some susceptible patients, continued use of topic NSAIDs may result in epithelial breakdown, co neal thinning, corneal erosion, corneal ulceration corneal perforation. These events may be sigh threatening. Patients with evidence of corneal ep thelial breakdown should immediately discontinu use of topical NSAIDs including NEVANAC® an should be closely monitored for corneal health.

Postmarketing experience with topical NSAID suggests that patients with complicated ocular su geries, corneal denervation, corneal epithelial de fects, diabetes mellitus, ocular surface disease (e.g., dry eye syndrome), rheumatoid arthritis, repeat ocular surgeries within a short period time may be at increased risk for corneal advers events which may become sight threatening. Top cal NSAIDs should be used with caution in thes patients.

Postmarketing experience with topical NSAID also suggests that use more than 1 day prior to su gery or use beyond 14 days post surgery may in crease patient risk and severity of corneal advers events.

5.4   Contact Lens Wear

NEVANAC® should not be administered while u ing contact lenses.

6   Adverse Reactions

Because clinical studies are conducted under wide varying conditions, adverse reaction rates observe in the clinical studies of a drug cannot be direct compared to the rates in the clinical studies of an other drug and may not reflect the rates observed practice.

6.1   Ocular Adverse Reactions

The most frequently reported ocular adverse rea tions following cataract surgery were capsula opacity, decreased visual acuity, foreign body sens tion, increased intraocular pressure, and sticky se sation. These events occurred in approximately 5 10% of patients.

Other ocular adverse reactions occurring at an in cidence of approximately 1 to 5% included conjun tival edema, corneal edema, dry eye, lid margi crusting, ocular discomfort, ocular hyperemia, oc lar pain, ocular pruritus, photophobia, tearing an itreous detachment. Some of these events may be he consequence of the cataract surgical procedure.

2 Non-Ocular Adverse Reactions

on-ocular adverse reactions reported at an incidence of 1 to 4% included headache, hypertension, ausea/vomiting, and sinusitis.

Use in Specific Populations

1 Pregnancy

eratogenic Effects.

Pregnancy Category C: Reproduction studies performed with nepafenac in rabbits and rats at oral oses up to 10 mg/kg/day have revealed no evidence f teratogenicity due to nepafenac, despite the induction of maternal toxicity. At this dose, the animal plasma exposure to nepafenac and amfenac was approximately 260 and 2400 times human plasma exposure at the recommended human topical ophthalmic dose for rats and 80 and 680 times uman plasma exposure for rabbits, respectively. In ats, maternally toxic doses ≥10 mg/kg were associated with dystocia, increased postimplantation oss, reduced fetal weights and growth, and reduced etal survival.

Nepafenac has been shown to cross the placental arrier in rats. There are no adequate and well-ontrolled studies in pregnant women. Because animal reproduction studies are not always predictive f human response, NEVANAC® should be used uring pregnancy only if the potential benefit justies the potential risk to the fetus.

Non-teratogenic Effects.

Because of the known effects of prostaglandin biosynthesis inhibiting drugs on the fetal cardiovascular system (closure of the ductus arteriosus), the use of NEVANAC® during late pregnancy should be avoided.

3 Nursing Mothers

NEVANAC® is excreted in the milk of lactating ats. It is not known whether this drug is excreted n human milk. Because many drugs are excreted n human milk, caution should be exercised when NEVANAC® ophthalmic suspension is administered to a nursing woman.

4 Pediatric Use

The safety and effectiveness of NEVANAC® in pediatric patients below the age of 10 years have not been established.

5 Geriatric Use

No overall differences in safety and effectiveness ave been observed between elderly and younger patients.

1 Description

NEVANAC® (nepafenac ophthalmic suspension) .1% is a sterile, topical, nonsteroidal anti-nflammatory (NSAID) prodrug for ophthalmic use. Each mL of NEVANAC® suspension contains 1 mg f nepafenac. Nepafenac is designated chemically as 2-amino-3-benzoylbenzeneacetamide with an empirical formula of $C_{15}H_{14}N_2O_2$. The structural ormula of nepafenac is:

Nepafenac is a yellow crystalline powder. The molecular weight of nepafenac is 254.28. NEVANAC® ophthalmic suspension is supplied as a sterile, aqueous 0.1% suspension with a pH approximately of 7.4.

The osmolality of NEVANAC® ophthalmic suspension is approximately 305 mOsmol/kg. Each mL of NEVANAC® contains: Active: nepafenac .1% Inactives: mannitol, carbomer 974P, sodium chloride, tyloxapol, edetate disodium, benzalkonium chloride 0.005% (preservative), sodium hydroxide and/or hydrochloric acid to adjust pH and purified water, USP.

2 Clinical Pharmacology

2.1 Mechanism of Action

After topical ocular dosing, nepafenac penetrates the cornea and is converted by ocular tissue hydroases to amfenac, a nonsteroidal anti-inflammatory drug. Amfenac is thought to inhibit the action of prostaglandin H synthase (cyclooxygenase), an enzyme required for prostaglandin production.

2.3 Pharmacokinetics

Low but quantifiable plasma concentrations of nepafenac and amfenac were observed in the majority of subjects 2 and 3 hours post dose, respectively,

following bilateral topical ocular three-times-daily dosing of nepafenac ophthalmic suspension, 0.1%. The mean steady-state C_{max} for nepafenac and for amfenac were 0.310 ± 0.104 ng/ml and 0.422 ± 0.121 ng/ml, respectively, following ocular administration.

Nepafenac at concentrations up to 300 ng/mL did not inhibit the in vitro metabolism of 6 specific marker substrates of cytochrome P450 (CYP) isozymes (CYP1A2, CYP2C9, CYP2C19, CYP2D6, CYP2E1, and CYP3A4). Therefore, drug-drug interactions involving CYP mediated metabolism of concomitantly administered drugs are unlikely. Drug-drug interactions mediated by protein binding are also unlikely.

13 Nonclinical Toxicology

13.1 Carcinogenesis, Mutagenesis, Impairment of Fertility

Nepafenac has not been evaluated in long-term carcinogenicity studies. Increased chromosomal aberrations were observed in Chinese hamster ovary cells exposed in vitro to nepafenac suspension. Nepafenac was not mutagenic in the Ames assay or in the mouse lymphoma forward mutation assay. Oral doses up to 5,000 mg/kg did not result in an increase in the formation of micronucleated polychromatic erythrocytes in vivo in the mouse micronucleus assay in the bone marrow of mice.

Nepafenac did not impair fertility when administered orally to male and female rats at 3 mg/kg (approximately 90 and 380 times the plasma exposure to the parent drug, nepafenac, and the active metabolite, amfenac, respectively, at the recommended human topical ophthalmic dose).

14 Clinical Studies

In two double-masked, randomized clinical trials in which patients were dosed three-times-daily beginning one day prior to cataract surgery, continued on the day of surgery and for the first two weeks of the postoperative period, NEVANAC® ophthalmic suspension demonstrated clinical efficacy, compared to its vehicle in treating postoperative inflammation.

Patients treated with NEVANAC® ophthalmic suspension were less likely to have ocular pain and measurable signs of inflammation (cells and flare) in the early postoperative period through the end of treatment than those treated with its vehicle.

For ocular pain in both studies a significantly higher percentage of patients (approximately 80%) in the nepafenac group reported no ocular pain on the day following cataract surgery (Day 1) compared to those in the vehicle group (approximately 50%).

Results from clinical studies indicated that NEVANAC® has no significant effect upon intraocular pressure; however, changes in intraocular pressure may occur following cataract surgery.

16 How Supplied/Storage and Handling

NEVANAC® (nepafenac ophthalmic suspension) is supplied in a natural, oval, low density polyethylene DROP-TAINER® dispenser with a natural low density polyethylene dispensing plug and gray polypropylene cap. Tamper evidence is provided with a shrink band around the closure and neck area of the package.

3 mL in 4 mL bottle NDC 0065-0002-03
Storage: Store at 2-25°C (36-77°F).

17 Patient Counseling Information

17.1 Slow or Delayed Healing

Patients should be informed of the possibility that slow or delayed healing may occur while using nonsteroidal anti-inflammatory drugs (NSAIDs).

17.2 Avoiding Contamination of the Product

Patients should be instructed to avoid allowing the tip of the dispensing container to contact the eye or surrounding structures because this could cause the tip to become contaminated by common bacteria known to cause ocular infections. Serious damage to the eye and subsequent loss of vision may result from using contaminated solutions.

17.3 Contact Lens Wear

NEVANAC® should not be administered while wearing contact lens.

17.4 Intercurrent Ocular Conditions

Patients should be advised that if they develop an intercurrent ocular condition (e.g., trauma, or infection) or have ocular surgery, they should immediately seek their physician's advice concerning the continued use of the multi-dose container.

17.5 Concomitant Topical Ocular Therapy

If more than one topical ophthalmic medication is being used, the medicines must be administered at least 5 minutes apart.

17.6 Shake Well Before Use

Patients should be advised to shake the bottle well.
U.S. Patent No; 5,475,034
ALCON LABORATORIES, INC.
Fort Worth, Texas 76134 USA
© 2007, 2008 Alcon, Inc.

PATADAY™   ℞
(olopatadine hydrochloride ophthalmic solution) 0.2%

DESCRIPTION

PATADAY™ (olopatadine hydrochloride ophthalmic solution) 0.2% is a sterile ophthalmic solution containing olopatadine for topical administration to the eyes. Olopatadine hydrochloride is a white, crystalline, water-soluble powder with a molecular weight of 373.88 and a molecular formula of $C_{21}H_{23}NO_3 \bullet HCl$.

Chemical Name: 11-[(Z)-3-(Dimethylamino) propylidene]-6-11-dihydrodibenz[b,e] oxepin-2-acetic acid, hydrochloride.

Each mL of PATADAY™ solution contains: Active: 2.22 mg olopatadine hydrochloride equivalent to 2 mg olopatadine.

Inactives: povidone; dibasic sodium phosphate; sodium chloride; edetate disodium; benzalkonium chloride 0.01% (preservative) hydrochloric acid / sodium hydroxide (adjust pH); and purified water.

It has a pH of approximately 7 and an osmolality of approximately 300 mOsm/kg.

CLINICAL PHARMACOLOGY

Olopatadine is a relatively selective histamine H_1 antagonist and an inhibitor of the release of histamine from the mast cells. Decreased chemotaxis and inhibition of eosinophil activation has also been demonstrated. Olopatadine is devoid of effects on alpha-adrenergic, dopaminergic, and muscarinic type 1 and 2 receptors.

Systemic bioavailability data upon topical ocular administration of PATADAY™ solution are not available. Following topical ocular administration of olopatadine 0.15% ophthalmic solution in man, olopatadine was shown to have a low systemic exposure. Two studies in normal volunteers (totaling 24 subjects) dosed bilaterally with olopatadine 0.15% ophthalmic solution once every 12 hours for 2 weeks demonstrated plasma concentrations to be generally below the quantitation limit of the assay (< 0.5 ng/mL). Samples in which olopatadine was quantifiable were typically found within 2 hours of dosing and ranged from 0.5 to 1.3 ng/mL. The elimination half-life in plasma following oral dosing was 8 to 12 hours, and elimination was predominantly through renal excretion. Approximately 60–70% of the dose was recovered in the urine as parent drug. Two metabolites, the mono-desmethyl and the N-oxide, were detected at low concentrations in the urine.

CLINICAL STUDIES

Results from clinical studies of up to 12 weeks duration demonstrate that PATADAY™ solution when dosed once a day is effective in the treatment of ocular itching associated with allergic conjunctivitis.

INDICATIONS AND USAGE

PATADAY™ solution is indicated for the treatment of ocular itching associated with allergic conjunctivitis.

CONTRAINDICATIONS

Hypersensitivity to any components of this product.

Continued on next page

Pataday—Cont.

WARNINGS
For topical ocular use only. Not for injection or oral use.

PRECAUTIONS
Information for Patients
As with any eye drop, to prevent contaminating the dropper tip and solution, care should be taken not to touch the eyelids or surrounding areas with the dropper tip of the bottle. Keep bottle tightly closed when not in use. Patients should be advised not to wear a contact lens if their eye is red.
PATADAY™ (olopatadine hydrochloride ophthalmic solution) 0.2% should not be used to treat contact lens related irritation. The preservative in PATADAY™ solution, benzalkonium chloride, may be absorbed by soft contact lenses. Patients who wear soft contact lenses and **whose eyes are not red**, should be instructed to wait at least ten minutes after instilling PATADAY™ (olopatadine hydrochloride ophthalmic solution) 0.2% before they insert their contact lenses.

Carcinogenesis, Mutagenesis, Impairment of Fertility
Olopatadine administered orally was not carcinogenic in mice and rats in doses up to 500 mg/kg/day and 200 mg/kg/day, respectively. Based on a 40 μL drop size and a 50 kg person, these doses were approximately 150,000 and 50,000 times higher than the maximum recommended ocular human dose (MROHD). No mutagenic potential was observed when olopatadine was tested in an *in vitro* bacterial reverse mutation (Ames) test, an *in vitro* mammalian chromosome aberration assay or an *in vivo* mouse micronucleus test.
Olopatadine administered to male and female rats at oral doses of approximately 100,000 times MROHD level resulted in a slight decrease in the fertility index and reduced implantation rate; no effects on reproductive function were observed at doses of approximately 15,000 times the MROHD level.

Pregnancy:
Teratogenic effects: Pregnancy Category C
Olopatadine was found not to be teratogenic in rats and rabbits. However, rats treated at 600 mg/kg/day, or 150,000 times the MROHD and rabbits treated at 400 mg/kg/day, or approximately 100,000 times the MROHD, during organogenesis showed a decrease in live fetuses. In addition, rats treated with 600 mg/kg/day of olopatadine during organogenesis showed a decrease in fetal weight. Further, rats treated with 600 mg/kg/day of olopatadine during late gestation through the lactation period showed a decrease in neonatal survival and body weight.
There are, however, no adequate and well-controlled studies in pregnant women. Because animal studies are not always predictive of human responses, this drug should be used in pregnant women only if the potential benefit to the mother justifies the potential risk to the embryo or fetus.

Nursing Mothers:
Olopatadine has been identified in the milk of nursing rats following oral administration. It is not known whether topical ocular administration could result in sufficient systemic absorption to produce detectable quantities in the human breast milk. Nevertheless, caution should be exercised when PATADAY™ (olopatadine hydrochloride ophthalmic solution) 0.2% is administered to a nursing mother.

Pediatric Use:
Safety and effectiveness in pediatric patients below the age of 3 years have not been established.

Geriatric Use:
No overall differences in safety and effectiveness have been observed between elderly and younger patients.

ADVERSE REACTIONS
Symptoms similar to cold syndrome and pharyngitis were reported at an incidence of approximately 10%.

The following adverse experiences have been reported in 5% or less of patients:
Ocular: blurred vision, burning or stinging, conjunctivitis, dry eye, foreign body sensation, hyperemia, hypersensitivity, keratitis, lid edema, pain and ocular pruritus.
Non-ocular: asthenia, back pain, flu syndrome, headache, increased cough, infection, nausea, rhinitis, sinusitis and taste perversion.
Some of these events were similar to the underlying disease being studied.

DOSAGE AND ADMINISTRATION
The recommended dose is one drop in each affected eye once a day.

HOW SUPPLIED
PATADAY™ (olopatadine hydrochloride ophthalmic solution) 0.2% is supplied in a white, oval, low density polyethylene DROP-TAINER® dispenser with a natural low density polyethylene dispensing plug and a white polypropylene cap. Tamper evidence is provided with a shrink band around the closure and neck area of the package.
NDC 0065-0272-25   2.5 mL fill in 4 mL oval bottle
Storage:
Store at 2°C to 25°C (36°F to 77°F)
U.S. Patents Nos. 5,116,863; 5,641,805; 6,995,186; 7,402,609
Rx Only
ALCON LABORATORIES, INC.
Fort Worth, Texas 76134 USA
© 2006-2008, 2010 Alcon, Inc.

SYSTANE® BALANCE LUBRICANT   OTC
EYE DROPS

Drug Facts

Active Ingredients	Purpose
Propylene Glycol 0.6%	Lubricant

Uses
• For the temporary relief of burning and irritation due to dryness of the eye

Warnings
For external use only.
Do not use
• if this product changes color
• if you are sensitive to any ingredient in this product
When using this product
• do not touch tip of container to any surface to avoid contamination
• replace cap after each use
Stop use and ask a doctor if
• you feel eye pain
• changes in vision occur
• redness or irritation of the eye(s) gets worse, persists or lasts more than 72 hours
Keep out of reach of children.
If swallowed, get medical help or contact a Poison Control Center right away.

Directions
• Shake well before using.
• Instill 1 or 2 drops in the affected eye(s) as needed.
Other Information
• Store at room temperature.
Inactive Ingredients:
Boric acid, dimyristoyl phosphatidylglycerol, edetate disodium, hydroxypropyl guar, mineral oil, polyoxyl 40 stearate, POLYQUAD® (polyquaternium-1) 0.001% preservative, sorbitan tristearate, sorbitol and purified water. May contain hydrochloric acid and/or sodium hydroxide to adjust pH.
Questions:
In the U.S. call **1-800-757-9195**
www.systane.com
MedInfo@AlconLabs.com
SYSTANE®BALANCE Lubricant Eye Drops has the proven power to restore the natural tear's lipid layer to treat dryness and provide long lasting relief.
U.S. Patent Nos. 5,278,151; 5,294,607; 5,578,586; 6,583,124; 6,838,449; 6,849,253

©2010 Alcon, Inc.
Alcon Laboratories, Inc.
Fort Worth, TX 76134 USA

SYSTANE® ULTRA LUBRICANT   OT
EYE DROPS

Drug Facts

Active Ingredients	Purpos
Polyethylene Glycol 400 0.4%	Lubrica
Propylene Glycol 0.3%	Lubrica

Uses:
• For the temporary relief of burning and irritatio due to dryness of the eye
Warnings: For external use only.
Do not use
• if this product changes color or becomes cloudy
• if you are sensitive to any ingredient in this product
When using this product
• do not touch tip of container to any surface avoid contamination
• replace cap after each use
Stop use and ask a doctor if
• you feel eye pain
• changes in vision occur
• redness or irritation of the eye(s) gets worse, persists or lasts more than 72 hours
Keep out of reach of children.
If swallowed, get medical help or contact a Poison Control Center right away.

Directions:
• Shake well before using.
• Instill 1 or 2 drops in the affected eye(s) a needed.
Other Information
• Store at room temperature.
Inactive Ingredients:
Aminomethylpropanol, boric acid, hydroxypropy guar, POLYQUAD® (polyquaternium-1) 0.001° preservative, potassium chloride, purified water, sodium chloride, sorbitol. May contain hydrochloric acid and/or sodium hydroxide to adjust pH.
Questions:
In the U.S. call **1-800-757-9195**
www.systane.com
MedInfo@AlconLabs.com
TAMPER EVIDENT: For your protection, this bottl has an imprinted seal around the neck. Do not us if seal is damaged or missing at time of purchase Open your eyes to a breakthrough in comfort wit SYSTANE® ULTRA Lubricant Eye Drop SYSTANE® ULTRA elevates the science of dry ey therapy to a new level. From first blink, eyes fee lubricated and refreshed. Feel the difference in dr eye relief with SYSTANE® ULTRA.
U.S. Patent Nos. 6,403,609, 6,583,124 an 6,838,449.
©2008-2011 Alcon, Inc.

Alcon Laboratories, In
Fort Worth, TX 76134 US

TRAVATAN Z®   I
[*tra-va-tan*]
(travoprost ophthalmic solution) 0.004%
OPHTHALMIC SOLUTION

HIGHLIGHTS OF PRESCRIBING INFORMATION
These highlights do not include all the informatio needed to use TRAVATAN Z® (travopros ophthalmic solution) 0.004% safely and effectively See full prescribing information for TRAVATAN Z® TRAVATAN Z® (travoprost ophthalmic solutior 0.004%
Initial U.S. Approval: 2001

--------- INDICATIONS AND USAGE ---------

TRAVATAN Z® is a prostaglandin analog indicate for the reduction of elevated intraocular pressure i patients with open-angle glaucoma or ocular hyper tension. (1)

DOSAGE AND ADMINISTRATION

One drop in the affected eye(s) once daily in the evening. (2)

DOSAGE FORMS AND STRENGTHS

Solution containing 0.04 mg/mL travoprost ophthalmic solution. (3)

WARNINGS AND PRECAUTIONS

- Pigmentation.
Pigmentation of the iris, periorbital tissue (eyelid) and eyelashes can occur. Iris pigmentation likely to be permanent. (5.1)
- Eyelash Changes.
Gradual change to eyelashes including increased length, thickness and number of lashes. Usually reversible. (5.2)

ADVERSE REACTIONS

Most common adverse reaction (30% to 50%) is conjunctival hyperemia. (6.1)

To report SUSPECTED ADVERSE REACTIONS, contact Alcon Laboratories Inc. at 1-800-757-9195 or FDA at 1-800-FDA-1088 or www.fda.gov/medwatch.

USE IN SPECIFIC POPULATIONS

Use in pediatric patients below the age of 16 years is not recommended because of potential safety concerns related to increased pigmentation following long-term chronic use. (8.4)

See 17 for PATIENT COUNSELING INFORMATION

Revised: 09/2010

FULL PRESCRIBING INFORMATION

1 INDICATIONS AND USAGE

TRAVATAN Z® (travoprost ophthalmic solution) 0.004% is indicated for the reduction of elevated intraocular pressure in patients with open-angle glaucoma or ocular hypertension.

2 DOSAGE AND ADMINISTRATION

The recommended dosage is one drop in the affected eye(s) once daily in the evening. TRAVATAN Z® (travoprost ophthalmic solution) should not be administered more than once daily since it has been shown that more frequent administration of prostaglandin analogs may decrease the intraocular pressure lowering effect.

Reduction of the intraocular pressure starts approximately 2 hours after the first administration with maximum effect reached after 12 hours.

TRAVATAN Z® may be used concomitantly with other topical ophthalmic drug products to lower intraocular pressure. If more than one topical ophthalmic drug is being used, the drugs should be administered at least five (5) minutes apart.

3 DOSAGE FORMS AND STRENGTHS

Ophthalmic solution containing travoprost 0.04 mg/mL.

4 CONTRAINDICATIONS

None

5 WARNINGS AND PRECAUTIONS

5.1 Pigmentation

Travoprost ophthalmic solution has been reported to cause changes to pigmented tissues. The most frequently reported changes have been increased pigmentation of the iris, periorbital tissue (eyelid) and eyelashes. Pigmentation is expected to increase as long as travoprost is administered. The pigmentation change is due to increased melanin content in the melanocytes rather than to an increase in the number of melanocytes. After discontinuation of travoprost, pigmentation of the iris is likely to be permanent, while pigmentation of the periorbital tissue and eyelash changes have been reported to be reversible in some patients. Patients who receive treatment should be informed of the possibility of increased pigmentation. The long term effects of increased pigmentation are not known.

Iris color change may not be noticeable for several months to years. Typically, the brown pigmentation around the pupil spreads concentrically towards the periphery of the iris and the entire iris or parts of the iris become more brownish. Neither nevi nor freckles of the iris appear to be affected by treatment. While treatment with TRAVATAN Z® (travoprost ophthalmic solution) 0.004% can be continued in patients who develop noticeably increased iris pigmentation, these patients should be examined regularly. (see PATIENT COUNSELING INFORMATION, 17.1).

5.2 Eyelash Changes

TRAVATAN Z® may gradually change eyelashes and vellus hair in the treated eye. These changes include increased length, thickness, and number of lashes. Eyelash changes are usually reversible upon discontinuation of treatment.

5.3 Intraocular Inflammation

TRAVATAN Z® should be used with caution in patients with active intraocular inflammation (e.g., uveitis) because the inflammation may be exacerbated.

5.4 Macular Edema

Macular edema, including cystoid macular edema, has been reported during treatment with travoprost ophthalmic solution. TRAVATAN Z® should be used with caution in aphakic patients, in pseudophakic patients with a torn posterior lens capsule, or in patients with known risk factors for macular edema.

5.5 Angle-closure, Inflammatory or Neovascular Glaucoma

TRAVATAN Z® has not been evaluated for the treatment of angle-closure, inflammatory or neovascular glaucoma.

5.6 Bacterial Keratitis

There have been reports of bacterial keratitis associated with the use of multiple-dose containers of topical ophthalmic products. These containers had been inadvertently contaminated by patients who, in most cases, had a concurrent corneal disease or a disruption of the ocular epithelial surface (see PATIENT COUNSELING INFORMATION, 17.3).

5.7 Use with Contact Lenses

Contact lenses should be removed prior to instillation of TRAVATAN Z® and may be reinserted 15 minutes following its administration.

6 ADVERSE REACTIONS

6.1 Clinical Studies Experience

Because clinical studies are conducted under widely varying conditions, adverse reaction rates observed in the clinical studies of a drug cannot be directly compared to rates in the clinical studies of another drug and may not reflect the rates observed in practice.

The most common adverse reaction observed in controlled clinical studies with TRAVATAN® (travoprost ophthalmic solution) 0.004% and TRAVATAN Z® (travoprost ophthalmic solution) 0.004% was ocular hyperemia which was reported in 30 to 50% of patients. Up to 3% of patients discontinued therapy due to conjunctival hyperemia.

Ocular adverse reactions reported at an incidence of 5 to 10% in these clinical studies included decreased visual acuity, eye discomfort, foreign body sensation, pain and pruritus.

Ocular adverse reactions reported at an incidence of 1 to 4% in clinical studies with TRAVATAN® or TRAVATAN Z® included abnormal vision, blepharitis, blurred vision, cataract, conjunctivitis, corneal staining, dry eye, iris discoloration, keratitis, lid margin crusting, ocular inflammation, photophobia, subconjunctival hemorrhage and tearing.

Nonocular adverse reactions reported at an incidence of 1 to 5% in these clinical studies were allergy, angina pectoris, anxiety, arthritis, back pain, bradycardia, bronchitis, chest pain, cold/flu syndrome, depression, dyspepsia, gastrointestinal disorder, headache, hypercholesterolemia, hypertension, hypotension, infection, pain, prostate disorder, sinusitis, urinary incontinence and urinary tract infections.

8 USE IN SPECIFIC POPULATIONS

8.1 Pregnancy

Pregnancy Category C

Teratogenic effects: Travoprost was teratogenic in rats, at an intravenous (IV) dose up to 10 mcg/kg/day (250 times the maximal recommended human ocular dose (MRHOD), evidenced by an increase in the incidence of skeletal malformations as well as external and visceral malformations, such as fused sternebrae, domed head and hydrocephaly. Travoprost was not teratogenic in rats at IV doses up to 3 mcg/kg/day (75 times the MRHOD), or in mice at subcutaneous doses up to 1 mcg/kg/day (25 times the MRHOD). Travoprost produced an increase in post-implantation losses and a decrease in fetal viability in rats at IV doses > 3 mcg/kg/day (75 times the MRHOD) and in mice at subcutaneous doses > 0.3 mcg/kg/day (7.5 times the MRHOD).

In the offspring of female rats that received travoprost subcutaneously from Day 7 of pregnancy to lactation Day 21 at doses of ≥ 0.12 mcg/kg/day (3 times the MRHOD), the incidence of postnatal mortality was increased, and neonatal body weight gain was decreased. Neonatal development was also affected, evidenced by delayed eye opening, pinna detachment and preputial separation, and by decreased motor activity.

There are no adequate and well-controlled studies of TRAVATAN Z® (travoprost ophthalmic solution) 0.004% administration in pregnant women. Because animal reproductive studies are not always predictive of human response, TRAVATAN Z® should be administered during pregnancy only if the potential benefit justifies the potential risk to the fetus.

8.3 Nursing Mothers

A study in lactating rats demonstrated that radiolabeled travoprost and/or its metabolites were excreted in milk. It is not known whether this drug or its metabolites are excreted in human milk. Because many drugs are excreted in human milk, caution should be exercised when TRAVATAN Z® is administered to a nursing woman.

Continued on next page

Travatan Z—Cont.

8.4 Pediatric Use
Use in pediatric patients below the age of 16 years is not recommended because of potential safety concerns related to increased pigmentation following long-term chronic use.

8.5 Geriatric Use
No overall clinical differences in safety or effectiveness have been observed between elderly and other adult patients.

8.6 Hepatic and Renal Impairment
Travoprost ophthalmic solution 0.004% has been studied in patients with hepatic impairment and also in patients with renal impairment. No clinically relevant changes in hematology, blood chemistry, or urinalysis laboratory data were observed in these patients.

11 DESCRIPTION
Travoprost is a synthetic prostaglandin F analogue. Its chemical name is [1R-[1α(Z),2β(1E,3R*),3α,5α]]-7-[3,5-Dihydroxy-2-[3-hydroxy-4-[3-(trifluoromethyl) phenoxy]-1-butenyl]cyclopentyl]-5-heptenoic acid, 1-methylethylester. It has a molecular formula of $C_{26}H_{35}F_3O_6$ and a molecular weight of 500.55. The chemical structure of travoprost is:

Travoprost is a clear, colorless to slightly yellow oil that is very soluble in acetonitrile, methanol, octanol, and chloroform. It is practically insoluble in water.

TRAVATAN Z® (travoprost ophthalmic solution) 0.004% is supplied as sterile, buffered aqueous solution of travoprost with a pH of approximately 5.7 and an osmolality of approximately 290 mOsmol/kg.

TRAVATAN Z® contains Active: travoprost 0.04 mg/mL; Inactives: polyoxyl 40 hydrogenated castor oil, sofZia® (boric acid, propylene glycol, sorbitol, zinc chloride), sodium hydroxide and/or hydrochloric acid (to adjust pH) and purified water, USP. Preserved in the bottle with an ionic buffered system, sofZia®.

12 CLINICAL PHARMACOLOGY
12.1 Mechanism of Action
Travoprost free acid, a prostaglandin analog is a selective FP prostanoid receptor agonist which is believed to reduce intraocular pressure by increasing uveoscleral outflow. The exact mechanism of action is unknown at this time.

12.3 Pharmacokinetics
Travoprost is absorbed through the cornea and is hydrolyzed to the active free acid. Data from four multiple dose pharmacokinetic studies (totaling 107 subjects) have shown that plasma concentrations of the free acid are below 0.01 ng/ml (the quantitation limit of the assay) in two-thirds of the subjects. In those individuals with quantifiable plasma concentrations (N=38), the mean plasma C_{max} was 0.018 ± 0.007 ng/ml (ranged 0.01 to 0.052 ng/mL) and was reached within 30 minutes. From these studies, travoprost is estimated to have a plasma half-life of 45 minutes. There was no difference in plasma concentrations between Days 1 and 7, indicating steady-state was reached early and that there was no significant accumulation.

Travoprost, an isopropyl ester prodrug, is hydrolyzed by esterases in the cornea to its biologically active free acid. Systemically, travoprost free acid is metabolized to inactive metabolites via beta-oxidation of the α(carboxylic acid) chain to give the

1,2-dinor and 1,2,3,4-tetranor analogs, via oxidation of the 15-hydroxyl moiety, as well as via reduction of the 13,14 double bond.

The elimination of travoprost free acid from plasma was rapid and levels were generally below the limit of quantification within one hour after dosing. The terminal elimination half-life of travoprost free acid was estimated from fourteen subjects and ranged from 17 minutes to 86 minutes with the mean half-life of 45 minutes. Less than 2% of the topical ocular dose of travoprost was excreted in the urine within 4 hours as the travoprost free acid.

13 NONCLINICAL TOXICOLOGY
13.1 Carcinogenesis, Mutagenesis, Impairment of Fertility
Two-year carcinogenicity studies in mice and rats at subcutaneous doses of 10, 30, or 100 mcg/kg/day did not show any evidence of carcinogenic potential. However, at 100 mcg/kg/day, male rats were only treated for 82 weeks, and the maximum tolerated dose (MTD) was not reached in the mouse study. The high dose (100 mcg/kg) corresponds to exposure levels over 400 times the human exposure at the maximum recommended human ocular dose (MRHOD) of 0.04 mcg/kg, based on plasma active drug levels.

Travoprost was not mutagenic in the Ames test, mouse micronucleus test or rat chromosome aberration assay. A slight increase in the mutant frequency was observed in one of two mouse lymphoma assays in the presence of rat S-9 activation enzymes.

Travoprost did not affect mating or fertility indices in male or female rats at subcutaneous doses up to 10 mcg/kg/day [250 times the maximum recommended human ocular dose of 0.04 mcg/kg/day on a mcg/kg basis (MRHOD)]. At 10 mcg/kg/day, the mean number of corpora lutea was reduced, and the post-implantation losses were increased. These effects were not observed at 3 mcg/kg/day (75 times the MRHOD).

14 CLINICAL STUDIES
In clinical studies, patients with open-angle glaucoma or ocular hypertension and baseline pressure of 25-27 mmHg who were treated with TRAVATAN® (travoprost ophthalmic solution) 0.004% or TRAVATAN Z® (travoprost ophthalmic solution) 0.004% dosed once-daily in the evening demonstrated 7-8 mmHg reductions in intraocular pressure. In subgroup analyses of these studies, mean IOP reduction in black patients was up to 1.8 mmHg greater than in non-black patients. It is not known at this time whether this difference is attributed to race or to heavily pigmented irides.

In a multi-center, randomized, controlled trial, patients with mean baseline intraocular pressure of 24-26 mmHg on TIMOPTIC[1] 0.5% BID who were treated with TRAVATAN® (travoprost ophthalmic solution) 0.004% dosed QD adjunctively to TIMOPTIC[1] 0.5% BID demonstrated 6-7 mmHg reductions in intraocular pressure.

[1]TIMOPTIC is a registered trademark of Merck & Co., Inc.

16 HOW SUPPLIED/STORAGE AND HANDLING
TRAVATAN Z® (travoprost ophthalmic solution) 0.004% is a sterile, isotonic, buffered, preserved, aqueous solution of travoprost (0.04 mg/mL) supplied in Alcon's oval DROP-TAINER® package system.

TRAVATAN Z® is supplied as a 2.5 mL solution in a 4 mL and a 5 mL solution in a 7.5 mL natural polypropylene dispenser bottle with a natural polypropylene dropper tip and a turquoise polypropylene or high density polyethylene overcap. Tamper evidence is provided with a shrink band around the closure and neck area of the package.

2.5 mL fill	NDC 0065-0260-25
5 mL fill	NDC 0065-0260-05

Storage: Store at 2° - 25°C (36° - 77°F).

17 PATIENT COUNSELING INFORMATION
17.1 Potential for Pigmentation
Patients should be advised about the potential for increased brown pigmentation of the iris, which

may be permanent. Patients should also be informed about the possibility of eyelid skin darkening, which may be reversible after discontinuati of TRAVATAN Z® (travoprost ophthalmic solutio 0.004%.

17.2 Potential for Eyelash Changes
Patients should also be informed of the possibili of eyelash and vellus hair changes in the treate eye during treatment with TRAVATAN Z®. The changes may result in a disparity between eyes length, thickness, pigmentation, number of ey lashes or vellus hairs, and/or direction of eyelas growth. Eyelash changes are usually reversib upon discontinuation of treatment.

17.3 Handling the Container
Patients should be instructed to avoid allowing th tip of the dispensing container to contact the ey surrounding structures, fingers, or any other su face in order to avoid contamination of the solutic by common bacteria known to cause ocular infe tions. Serious damage to the eye and subseque loss of vision may result from using contaminate solutions.

17.4 When to Seek Physician Advice
Patients should also be advised that if they develo an intercurrent ocular condition (e.g., trauma or in fection), have ocular surgery, or develop any ocula reactions, particularly conjunctivitis and eyelid re actions, they should immediately seek their phys cian's advice concerning the continued use TRAVATAN Z®.

17.5 Use with Contact Lenses
Contact lenses should be removed prior to instilla tion of TRAVATAN® and may be reinserted 15 mi utes following its administration.

17.6 Use with Other Ophthalmic Drugs
If more than one topical ophthalmic drug is bein used, the drugs should be administered at least fiv (5) minutes between applications.

Rx Only
U.S. Patent Nos. 5,631,287; 5,889,052; 6,011,06 6,235,781; 6,503,497; and 6,849,253

Alcon®
ALCON LABORATORIES, INC.
Fort Worth, Texas 76134 USA
© 2006, 2010 Alcon, Inc.
9006070-0910

TRIESENCE® SUSPENSION
(triamcinolone acetonide injectable suspension

HIGHLIGHTS OF PRESCRIBING INFORMATION
These highlights do not include all the informatio needed to use TRIESENCE® (triamcinolon acetonide injectable suspension) 40 mg/mL safel and effectively. See full prescribing information fo TRIESENCE® suspension.
TRIESENCE® (triamcinolone acetonide injectabl suspension) 40 mg/mL
Initial U.S. Approval: 1957

INDICATIONS AND USAGE
TRIESENCE® suspension is a synthetic corticoste roid indicated for:
• Treatment of the following ophthalmic diseases
   sympathetic ophthalmia, temporal arteritis
   uveitis, and ocular inflammatory conditions unre
   sponsive to topical corticosteroids. (1.1)
• Visualization during vitrectomy. (1.2)

DOSAGE AND ADMINISTRATION
• Initial recommended dose for all indications ex
   cept visualization: 4 mg (100 microliters o
   40 mg/mL suspension) with subsequent dosage a
   needed over the course of treatment. (2.1)
• Recommended dose for visualization: 1 to 4 mg
   (25 to 100 microliters of 40 mg/mL suspension
   administered intravitreally. (2.2)

DOSAGE FORMS AND STRENGTHS
Single use 1 mL vial containing 40 mg/mL o triamcinolone acetonide suspension. (3)

CONTRAINDICATIONS
• Patients with systemic fungal infections. (4)

Hypersensitivity to triamcinolone or any component of this product. (4)

WARNINGS AND PRECAUTIONS

TRIESENCE® suspension should not be administered intravenously. (5.1)

Ophthalmic effects: May include cataracts, infections, and glaucoma. Monitor intraocular pressure. (5.1)

Hypothalamic-pituitary-adrenal (HPA) axis suppression, Cushing's syndrome and hyperglycemia: Monitor patients for these conditions and taper doses gradually. (5.2)

Infections: Increased susceptibility to new infection and increased risk of exacerbation, dissemination, or reactivation of latent infection.(5.3)

Elevated blood pressure, salt and water retention, and hypokalemia: Monitor blood pressure and sodium, potassium serum levels. (5.4)

GI perforation: Increased risk in patients with certain GI disorders. (5.5)

Behavioral and mood disturbances: May include euphoria, insomnia, mood swings, personality changes, severe depression, and psychosis. (5.6)

Decreases in bone density: Monitor bone density in patients receiving long term corticosteroid therapy. (5.7)

• Live or live attenuated vaccines: Do not administer to patients receiving immunosuppressive doses of corticosteroids. (5.8)

• Negative effects on growth and development: Monitor pediatric patients on long-term corticosteroid therapy. (5.9)

• Use in pregnancy: Fetal harm can occur with first trimester use. (5.10)

• Weight gain: May cause increased appetite. (5.11)

To report SUSPECTED ADVERSE REACTIONS, contact Alcon Laboratories, Inc. at 1-800-757-9195 or FDA at 1-800-FDA-1088 or www.fda.gov/medwatch.

DRUG INTERACTIONS

• Anticoagulant agents: May enhance or diminish anticoagulant effects. Monitor coagulationindices. (7)

• Antidiabetic agents: May increase blood glucose concentrations. Dose adjustments of antidiabetic agents may be required. (7)

• CYP 3A4 inducers and inhibitors: May respectively increase or decrease clearance of corticosteroids necessitating dose adjustment. (7)

• NSAIDS including aspirin and salicylates: Increased risk of gastrointestinal side effects. (7)

See 17 for PATIENT COUNSELING INFORMATION

Revised: 11/2007

FULL PRESCRIBING INFORMATION

1   INDICATIONS AND USAGE

1.1   Ophthalmic Diseases

TRIESENCE® (triamcinolone acetonide injectable suspension) 40 mg/mL is indicated for:
• sympathetic ophthalmia,
• temporal arteritis,
• uveitis, and
• ocular inflammatory conditions unresponsive to topical corticosteroids.

1.2   Visualization during Vitrectomy

TRIESENCE® suspension is indicated for visualization during vitrectomy.

2   DOSAGE AND ADMINISTRATION

2.1   Dosage for Treatment of Ophthalmic Diseases

The initial recommended dose of TRIESENCE® suspension is 4 mg (100 microliters of 40 mg/mL suspension) with subsequent dosage as needed over the course of treatment.

2.2   Dosage for Visualization during Vitrectomy

The recommended dose of TRIESENCE® suspension is 1 to 4 mg (25 to 100 microliters of 40 mg/mL suspension) administered intravitreally.

2.3   Preparation for Administration

STRICT ASEPTIC TECHNIQUE IS MANDATORY. The vial should be vigorously shaken for 10 seconds before use to ensure a uniform suspension. Prior to withdrawal, the suspension should be inspected for clumping or granular appearance (agglomeration). An agglomerated product results from exposure to freezing temperatures and should not be used. After withdrawal, TRIESENCE® suspension should be injected without delay to prevent settling in the syringe. Careful technique should be employed to avoid the possibility of entering a blood vessel or introducing organisms that can cause infection.

2.4   Administration

The injection procedure should be carried out under controlled aseptic conditions, which include the use of sterile gloves, a sterile drape, and a sterile eyelid speculum (or equivalent). Adequate anesthesia and a broad-spectrum microbicide should be given prior to the injection. Following the injection, patients should be monitored for elevation in intraocular pressure and for endophthalmitis. Monitoring may consist of a check for perfusion of the optic nerve head immediately after the injection, tonometry within 30 minutes following the injection, and biomicroscopy between two and seven days following the injection. Patients should be instructed to report any symptoms suggestive of endophthalmitis without delay.

Each vial should only be used for the treatment of a single eye. If the contralateral eye requires treatment, a new vial should be used and the sterile field, syringe, gloves, drapes, eyelid speculum, and injection needles should be changed before TRIESENCE® suspension is administered to the other eye.

3   DOSAGE FORMS AND STRENGTHS

Single use 1 mL vial containing 40 mg/mL of sterile triamcinolone acetonide suspension.

4   CONTRAINDICATIONS

Corticosteroids are contraindicated in patients with systemic fungal infections.

Triamcinolone is contraindicated in patients who are hypersensitive to corticosteroids or any components of this product. Rare instances of anaphylactoid reactions have occurred in patients receiving corticosteroid therapy. [See Adverse Reactions (6)].

5   WARNINGS AND PRECAUTIONS

5.1   Ophthalmic Effects

TRIESENCE® suspension should not be administered intravenously. Strict aseptic technique is mandatory.

Risk of infection

Corticosteroids may mask some signs of infection, and new infections may appear during their use. There may be decreased resistance and inability to localize infection when corticosteroids are used. Corticosteroids may enhance the establishment of secondary ocular infections due to fungi or viruses. If an infection occurs during corticosteroid therapy, it should be promptly controlled by suitable antimicrobial therapy.

See also Increased Risks Related to Infection (5.3).

Elevated Intraocular Pressure

Increases in intraocular pressure associated with triamcinolone acetonide injection have been observed in 20-60% of patients. This may lead to glaucoma with possible damage to the optic nerve. Effects on intraocular pressure may last up to 6 months following injection and are usually managed by topical glaucoma therapy. A small percentage of patients may require aggressive non-topical treatment. Intraocular pressure as well as perfusion of the optic nerve head should be monitored and managed appropriately.

Endophthalmitis

The rate of infectious culture positive endophthalmitis is 0.5%. Proper aseptic techniques should always be used when administering triamcinolone acetonide. In addition, patients should be monitored following the injection to permit early treatment should an infection occur.

Cataracts

Use of corticosteroids may produce cataracts, particularly posterior subcapsular cataracts.

Patients with Ocular Herpes Simplex

Corticosteroids should be used cautiously in patients with ocular herpes simplex because of possible corneal perforation. Corticosteroids **should not be used in active** ocular herpes simplex.

5.2   Alterations in Endocrine Function

Hypothalamic-pituitary-adrenal (HPA) axis suppression, Cushing's syndrome, and hyperglycemia. Monitor patients for these conditions with chronic use.

Corticosteroids can produce reversible HPA axis suppression with the potential for glucocorticosteroid insufficiency after withdrawal of treatment. Drug induced secondary adrenocortical insufficiency may be minimized by gradual reduction of dosage. This type of relative insufficiency may persist for months after discontinuation of therapy; therefore, in any situation of stress occurring during that period, hormone therapy should be reinstituted.

Metabolic clearance of corticosteroids is decreased in hypothyroid patients and increased in hyperthyroid patients. Changes in thyroid status of the patient may necessitate adjustment in dosage.

5.3   Increased Risks Related to Infections

Corticosteroids may increase the risks related to infections with any pathogen, including viral, bacterial, fungal, protozoan, or helminthic infections. The degree to which the dose, route and duration of corticosteroid administration correlates with the specific risks of infection is not well characterized; however, with increasing doses of corticosteroids, the rate of occurrence of infectious complications increases.

Continued on next page

Triesence—Cont.

Corticosteroids may mask some signs of infection and may reduce resistance to new infections.

Corticosteroids may exacerbate infections and increase risk of disseminated infection. The use of corticosteroids in active tuberculosis should be restricted to those cases of fulminating or disseminated tuberculosis in which the corticosteroid is used for the management of the disease in conjunction with an appropriate antituberculous regimen. Chickenpox and measles can have a more serious or even fatal course in non-immune children or adults on corticosteroids. In children or adults who have not had these diseases, particular care should be taken to avoid exposure. If a patient is exposed to chickenpox, prophylaxis with varicella zoster immune globulin (VZIG) may be indicated. If patient is exposed to measles, prophylaxis with pooled intramuscular immunoglobulin (IG) may be indicated. If chickenpox develops, treatment with antiviral agents may be considered.

Corticosteroids should be used with great care in patients with known or suspected Strongyloides (threadworm) infestation. In such patients, corticosteroid-induced immunosuppression may lead to Strongyloides hyperinfection and dissemination with widespread larval migration, often accompanied by severe enterocolitis and potentially fatal gram-negative septicemia.

Corticosteroids may increase risk of reactivation or exacerbation of latent infection. If corticosteroids are indicated in patients with latent tuberculosis or tuberculin reactivity, close observation is necessary as reactivation of the disease may occur. During prolonged corticosteroid therapy, these patients should receive chemoprophylaxis.

Corticosteroids may activate latent amebiasis. Therefore, it is recommended that latent or active amebiasis be ruled out before initiating corticosteroid therapy in any patient who has spent time in the tropics or in any patient with unexplained diarrhea.

Corticosteroids should not be used in cerebral malaria.

5.4 Alterations in Cardiovascular/Renal Function

Corticosteroids can cause elevation of blood pressure, salt and water retention, and increased excretion of potassium and calcium. These effects are less likely to occur with the synthetic derivatives except when used in large doses. Dietary salt restriction and potassium supplementation may be necessary. These agents should be used with caution in patients with hypertension, congestive heart failure, or renal insufficiency.

Literature reports suggest an association between use of corticosteroids and left ventricular free wall rupture after a recent myocardial infarction; therefore, therapy with corticosteroids should be used with caution in these patients.

5.5 Use in Patients with Gastrointestinal Disorders

There is an increased risk of gastrointestinal perforation in patients with certain GI disorders. Signs of GI perforation, such as peritoneal irritation, may be masked in patients receiving corticosteroids. Corticosteroids should be used with caution if there is a probability of impending perforation, abscess or other pyogenic infections; diverticulitis; fresh intestinal anastomoses; and active or latent peptic ulcer.

5.6 Behavioral and Mood Disturbances

Corticosteroid use may be associated with central nervous system effects ranging from euphoria, insomnia, mood swings, personality changes, and severe depression, to frank psychotic manifestations. Also, existing emotional instability or psychotic tendencies may be aggravated by corticosteroids.

5.7 Decrease in Bone Density

Corticosteroids decrease bone formation and increase bone resorption both through their effect on calcium regulation (i.e., decreasing absorption and increasing excretion) and inhibition of osteoblast function. This, together with a decrease in the protein matrix of the bone secondary to an increase in

protein catabolism, and reduced sex hormone production, may lead to inhibition of bone growth in children and adolescents and the development of osteoporosis at any age. Special consideration should be given to patients at increased risk of osteoporosis (i.e., postmenopausal women) before initiating corticosteroid therapy and bone density should be monitored in patients on long term corticosteroid therapy.

5.8 Vaccination

Administration of live or live attenuated vaccines is contraindicated in patients receiving immunosuppressive doses of corticosteroids. Killed or inactivated vaccines may be administered; however, the response to such vaccines can not be predicted. Immunization procedures may be undertaken in patients who are receiving corticosteroids as replacement therapy, e.g., for Addison's disease.

While on corticosteroid therapy, patients should not be vaccinated against smallpox. Other immunization procedures should not be undertaken in patients who are on corticosteroids, especially on high dose, because of possible hazards of neurological complications and a lack of antibody response.

5.9 Effect on Growth and Development

Long-term use of corticosteroids can have negative effects on growth and development in children. Growth and development of pediatric patients on prolonged corticosteroid therapy should be carefully monitored.

5.10 Use in Pregnancy

Triamcinolone acetonide can cause fetal harm when administered to a pregnant woman. Human and animal studies suggest that use of corticosteroids during the first trimester of pregnancy is associated with an increased risk of orofacial clefts, intrauterine growth restriction and decreased birth weight. If this drug is used during pregnancy, or if the patient becomes pregnant while using this drug, the patient should be apprised of the potential hazard to the fetus. [See Use in Specific Populations (8.1)].

5.11 Weight Gain

Systemically administered corticosteroids may increase appetite and cause weight gain.

5.12 Neuromuscular Effects

Although controlled clinical trials have shown corticosteroids to be effective in speeding the resolution of acute exacerbations of multiple sclerosis, they do not show that they affect the ultimate outcome or natural history of the disease. The studies do show that relatively high doses of corticosteroids are necessary to demonstrate a significant effect.

An acute myopathy has been observed with the use of high doses of corticosteroids, most often occurring in patients with disorders of neuromuscular transmission (e.g., myasthenia gravis), or in patients receiving concomitant therapy with neuromuscular blocking drugs (e.g., pancuronium). This acute myopathy is generalized, may involve ocular and respiratory muscles, and may result in quadriparesis. Elevation of creatine kinase may occur. Clinical improvement or recovery after stopping corticosteroids may require weeks to years.

5.13 Kaposi's Sarcoma

Kaposi's sarcoma has been reported to occur in patients receiving corticosteroid therapy, most often for chronic conditions.

Discontinuation of corticosteroids may result in clinical improvement.

6 ADVERSE REACTIONS

Because clinical trials are conducted under widely varying conditions, adverse reaction rates observed in the clinical trials of a drug cannot be directly compared to rates in the clinical trials of another drug and may not reflect the rates observed in practice.

Adverse event data were collected from 300 published articles containing data from controlled and uncontrolled clinical trials which evaluated over 14,000 eyes treated with different concentrations of triamcinolone acetonide. The most common dose administered within these trials was triamcinolone acetonide 4 mg administered as primary or adjunctive therapy primarily as a single injection.

The most common reported adverse events following administration of triamcinolone acetonide were elevated intraocular pressure and cataract progression. These events have been reported to occur in 20-60% of patients.

Less common reactions occurring in up to 2% include endophthalmitis (infectious and non-infectious), hypopyon, injection site reactions (described as blurring and transient discomfort), glaucoma, vitreous floaters, and detachment of retinal pigment epithelium, optic disc vascular disorder, eye inflammation, conjunctival hemorrhage, and visual acuity reduced. Cases of exophthalmos have also been reported.

Common adverse reactions for systemically administered corticosteroids include fluid retention, alteration in glucose tolerance, elevation in blood pressure, behavioral and mood changes, increased appetite and weight gain.

Other reactions reported to have occurred with the administration of corticosteroids include:

Allergic Reactions: Anaphylactoid reaction, anaphylaxis, angioedema

Cardiovascular: Bradycardia, cardiac arrest, cardiac arrhythmias, cardiac enlargement, circulatory collapse, congestive heart failure, fat embolism, hypertrophic cardiomyopathy in premature infants, myocardial rupture following recent myocardial infarction, pulmonary edema, syncope, tachycardia, thromboembolism, thrombophlebitis, vasculitis

Dermatologic: Acne, allergic dermatitis, cutaneous and subcutaneous atrophy, dry scalp, edema, facial erythema, hyper or hypo-pigmentation, impaired wound healing, increased sweating, petechiae and ecchymoses, rash, sterile abscess, striae, suppressed reactions to skin tests, thin fragile skin, thinning scalp hair, urticaria

Endocrine: Abnormal fat deposits, decreased carbohydrate tolerance, development of Cushingoid state, hirsutism, manifestations of latent diabetes mellitus and increased requirements for insulin or oral hypoglycemic agents in diabetics, menstrual irregularities, moon facies, secondary adrenocortical and pituitary unresponsiveness (particularly in times of stress, as in trauma, surgery or illness) suppression of growth in children

Fluid and Electrolyte Disturbances: Potassium loss, hypokalemic alkalosis, sodium retention

Gastrointestinal: Abdominal distention, elevation in serum liver enzymes levels (usually reversible upon discontinuation), hepatomegaly, hiccups, malaise, nausea, pancreatitis, peptic ulcer with possible perforation and hemorrhage, ulcerative esophagitis

Metabolic: Negative nitrogen balance due to protein catabolism

Musculoskeletal: Aseptic necrosis of femoral and humeral heads, charcot-like arthropathy, loss of muscle mass, muscle weakness, osteoporosis, pathologic fracture of long bones, steroid myopathy, tendon rupture, vertebral compression fractures

Neurological: Arachnoiditis, convulsions, depression, emotional instability, euphoria, headache, increased intracranial pressure with papilledema (pseudo-tumor cerebri) usually following discontinuation of treatment, insomnia, meningitis, neuritis, neuropathy, paraparesis/paraplegia, paresthesia, sensory disturbances, vertigo

Reproductive: Alteration in motility and number of spermatozoa.

7 DRUG INTERACTIONS

- **Amphotericin B:** There have been cases reported in which concomitant use of Amphotericin B and hydrocortisone was followed by cardiac enlargement and congestive heart failure. See *Potassium depleting agents*.
- **Anticholinesterase agents:** Concomitant use of anticholinesterase agents and corticosteroids may produce severe weakness in patients with myasthenia gravis. If possible, anticholinesterase agents should be withdrawn at least 24 hours before initiating corticosteroid therapy.
- **Anticoagulant agents:** Co-administration of corticosteroids and warfarin usually results in inhibition of response to warfarin, although there

have been some conflicting reports. Therefore, coagulation indices should be monitored frequently to maintain the desired anticoagulant effect.

- **Antidiabetic agents:** Because corticosteroids may increase blood glucose concentrations, dosage adjustments of antidiabetic agents may be required.
- **Antitubercular drugs:** Serum concentrations of isoniazid may be decreased.
- **CYP 3A4 inducers (e.g., barbiturates, phenytoin, carbamazepine, and rifampin):** Drugs such as barbiturates, phenytoin, ephedrine, and rifampin, which induce hepatic microsomal drug metabolizing enzyme activity may enhance metabolism of corticosteroid and require that the dosage of corticosteroid be increased.
- **CYP 3A4 inhibitors (e.g., ketoconazole, macrolide antibiotics):** Ketoconazole has been reported to decrease the metabolism of certain corticosteroids by up to 60% leading to an increased risk of corticosteroid side effects.
- **Cholestyramine:** Cholestyramine may increase the clearance of corticosteroids.
- **Cyclosporine:** Increased activity of both cyclosporine and corticosteroids may occur when the two are used concurrently. Convulsions have been reported with concurrent use.
- **Digitalis:** Patients on digitalis glycosides may be at increased risk of arrhythmias due to hypokalemia.
- **Estrogens, including oral contraceptives:** Estrogens may decrease the hepatic metabolism of certain corticosteroids thereby increasing their effect.
- **NSAIDS including aspirin and salicylates:** Concomitant use of aspirin or other non-steroidal antiinflammatory agents and corticosteroids increases the risk of gastrointestinal side effects. Aspirin should be used cautiously in conjunction with corticosteroids in hypoprothrombinemia. The clearance of salicylates may be increased with concurrent use of corticosteroids.
- **Potassium depleting agents (e.g., diuretics, Amphotericin B):** When corticosteroids are administered concomitantly with potassium-depleting agents, patients should be observed closely for development of hypokalemia.
- **Skin tests:** Corticosteroids may suppress reactions to skin tests.
- **Toxoids and live or inactivated vaccines:** Due to inhibition of antibody response, patients on prolonged corticosteroid therapy may exhibit a diminished response to toxoids and live or inactivated vaccines. Corticosteroids may also potentiate the replication of some organisms contained in live attenuated vaccines.

8 USE IN SPECIFIC POPULATIONS
8.1 Pregnancy
Teratogenic Effects: Pregnancy Category D *[See Warnings and Precautions (5.10)]*
Multiple cohort and case controlled studies in humans suggest that maternal corticosteroid use during the first trimester increases the rate of cleft lip with or without cleft palate from about 1/1000 infants to 3- 5/1000 infants. Two prospective case control studies showed decreased birth weight in infants exposed to maternal corticosteroids in utero. Triamcinolone acetonide was teratogenic in rats, rabbits, and monkeys. In rats and rabbits, triamcinolone acetonide was teratogenic at inhalation doses of 0.02 mg/kg and above and in monkeys, triamcinolone acetonide was teratogenic at an inhalation dose of 0.5 mg/kg (1/4 and 7 times the recommended human dose). Dose-related teratogenic effects in rats and rabbits included cleft palate and/or internal hydrocephaly and axial skeletal defects, whereas the effects observed in monkeys were cranial malformations. These effects are similar to those noted with other corticosteroids.
Corticosteroids should be used during pregnancy only if the potential benefit justifies the potential risk to the fetus. Infants born to mothers who received corticosteroids during pregnancy should be carefully observed for signs of hypoadrenalism.

Cortisone, 25	Prednisone, 5	Paramethasone, 2
Hydrocortisone, 20	Methylprednisolone, 4	Betamethasone, 0.75
Prednisolone, 5	Triamcinolone, 4	Dexamethasone, 0.75

8.3 Nursing Mothers
Corticosteroids are secreted in human milk. Reports suggest that steroid concentrations in human milk are 5 to 25% of maternal serum levels, and that total infant daily doses are small, less than 0.2% of the maternal daily dose. The risk of infant exposure to steroids through breast milk should be weighed against the known benefits of breastfeeding for both the mother and baby.

8.4 Pediatric Use
The efficacy and safety of corticosteroids in the pediatric population are based on the well established course of effect of corticosteroids which is similar in pediatric and adult populations.
The adverse effects of corticosteroids in pediatric patients are similar to those in adults. *[See Adverse Reactions (6)]*.
Like adults, pediatric patients should be carefully observed with frequent measurements of blood pressure, weight, height, intraocular pressure, and clinical evaluation for the presence of infection, psychosocial disturbances, thromboembolism, peptic ulcers, cataracts, and osteoporosis. Children, who are treated with corticosteroids by any route, including systemically administered corticosteroids, may experience a decrease in their growth velocity. This negative impact of corticosteroids on growth has been observed at low systemic doses and in the absence of laboratory evidence of HPA axis suppression (i.e., cosyntropin stimulation and basal cortisol plasma levels). Growth velocity may therefore be a more sensitive indicator of systemic corticosteroid exposure in children than some commonly used tests of HPA axis function. The linear growth of children treated with corticosteroids by any route should be monitored, and the potential growth effects of prolonged treatment should be weighed against clinical benefits obtained and the availability of other treatment alternatives. In order to minimize the potential growth effects of corticosteroids, children should be titrated to the lowest effective dose.

8.5 Geriatric Use
No overall differences in safety or effectiveness were observed between elderly subjects and younger subjects, and other reported clinical experience with triamcinolone has not identified differences in responses between the elderly and younger patients. However, the incidence of corticosteroid-induced side effects may be increased in geriatric patients and are dose-related. Osteoporosis is the most frequently encountered complication, which occurs at a higher incidence rate in corticosteroid-treated geriatric patients as compared to younger populations and in age-matched controls. Losses of bone mineral density appear to be greatest early on in the course of treatment and may recover over time after steroid withdrawal or use of lower doses.

11 DESCRIPTION
TRIESENCE® (triamcinolone acetonide injectable suspension) 40 mg/mL is a synthetic corticosteroid with anti-inflammatory action. Each mL of the sterile, aqueous suspension provides 40 mg of triamcinolone acetonide, with sodium chloride for isotonicity, 0.5% (w/v) carboxymethylcellulose sodium and 0.015% polysorbate 80. It also contains potassium chloride, calcium chloride (dihydrate), magnesium chloride (hexahydrate), sodium acetate (trihydrate), sodium citrate (dihydrate) and water for injection. Sodium hydroxide and hydrochloric acid may be present to adjust pH to a target value 6 – 7.5.
The chemical name for triamcinolone acetonide is 9-Fluro- 11β, 16α, 17,21-tetrahydroxypregna-1,4-diene-3,20-dione cyclic 16,17- acetal with acetone. Its structural formula of $C_{24}H_{31}FO_6$ is:

434.50 MW

Triamcinolone acetonide occurs as a white to cream-colored, crystalline powder having not more than a slight odor and is practically insoluble in water and very soluble in alcohol.

12 CLINICAL PHARMACOLOGY
12.1 Mechanism Of Action
Naturally occurring glucocorticoids (hydrocortisone and cortisone), which also have salt-retaining properties, are used as replacement therapy in adrenocortical deficiency states. Their synthetic analogs such as prednisolone and triamcinolone are primarily used for their anti-inflammatory effects in disorders of many organ systems.
Triamcinolone acetonide possesses glucocorticoid activity typical of this class of drug, but with little or no mineralocorticoid activity. For the purposes of comparison, the following is the equivalent milligram dosage of the various glucocorticoids:
[See table above]
Corticosteroids have been demonstrated to depress the production of eosinophils and lymphocytes, but erythropoiesis and production of polymorphonuclear leukocytes are stimulated. Inflammatory processes (edema, fibrin deposition, capillary dilatation, migration of leukocytes and phagocytosis) and the later stages of wound healing (capillary proliferation, deposition of collagen, cicatrization) are inhibited.

12.3 Pharmacokinetics
Aqueous humor pharmacokinetics of triamcinolone have been assessed in 5 patients following a single intravitreal administration (4 mg) of triamcinolone acetonide. Aqueous humor samples were obtained from 5 patients (5 eyes) via an anterior chamber paracentesis on Days 1, 3, 10, 17 and 31 post injection. Peak aqueous humor concentrations of triamcinolone ranged from 2151 to 7202 ng/mL, half-life 76 to 635 hours, and the area under the concentration-time curve (AUC0-t) from 231 to 1911 ng.h/mL following the single intravitreal administration. The mean elimination half-life was 18.7 ± 5.7 days in 4 nonvitrectomized eyes (4 patients). In a patient who had undergone vitrectomy (1 eye), the elimination half-life of triamcinolone from the vitreous was much faster (3.2 days) relative to patients that had not undergone vitrectomy.

13 NONCLINICAL TOXICOLOGY
13.1 Carcinogenesis, Mutagenesis, Impairment of Fertility
No evidence of mutagenicity was detected from invitro tests conducted with triamcinolone acetonide including a reverse mutation test in Salmonella bacteria and a forward mutation test in Chinese hamster ovary cells. With regard to carcinogenicity, in a two-year study in rats, triamcinolone acetonide caused no treatment-related carcinogenicity at oral doses up to 0.001mg/kg and in a two-year study in mice, triamcinolone acetonide caused no treatment-related carcinogenicity at oral doses up to 0.003 mg/kg (less than 1/25th of the recommended human dose). In male and female rats, triamcinolone acetonide caused no change in pregnancy rate at oral doses up to 0.015 mg/kg, but caused increased fetal resorptions and stillbirths

Continued on next page

Triesence—Cont.

and decreases in pup weight and survival at doses of 0.005 mg/kg (less than 1/10th of the recommended human dose).

13.2   Animal Toxicology and/or Pharmacology
Studies were conducted with triamcinolone acetonide, including those employing the proposed dosage form, i.e., 4.0% triamcinolone acetonide injectable suspension formulation containing 0.5% carboxymethylcellulose and 0.015% polysorbate-80 in a balanced salt solution.

Triamcinolone acetonide was demonstrated to be non-inflammatory when injected intravitreally in NZW rabbits, non-cytotoxic to mouse L-929 cells in an in-vitro assay and non-sensitizing in a guinea-pig maximization assay. Furthermore, the results of single-dose intravitreal injection studies with triamcinolone acetonide in both rabbits and monkeys demonstrate that the drug is well tolerated for up to one month with only minor findings of slight decrease in body weight gain and slight corneal thinning.

16   HOW SUPPLIED/STORAGE AND HANDLING
TRIESENCE® (triamcinolone acetonide injectable suspension) 40 mg/mL is supplied as 1 mL of a 40 mg/mL sterile triamcinolone acetonide suspension in a flint Type 1 single use glass vial with a gray rubber stopper and an open target aluminum seal. Each labeled vial is sealed in a polycarbonate blister with a backing material which provides tamper evidence and is stored in a carton.
• 1 mL single use vial (NDC 0065-0543-01)
Storage
Store at 4°-25°C (39°-77°F). Do Not Freeze. Protect from light by storing in carton.

17   PATIENT COUNSELING INFORMATION
Patients should discuss with their physician if they have had recent or ongoing infections or if they have recently received a vaccine.
There are a number of medicines that can interact with corticosteroids such as triamcinolone. Patients should inform their health-care provider of all the medicines they are taking, including over-the-counter and prescription medicines (such as phenytoin, diuretics, digitalis or digoxin, rifampin, amphotericin B, cyclosporine, insulin or diabetes medicines, ketoconazole, estrogens including birth control pills and hormone replacement therapy, blood thinners such as warfarin, aspirin or other NSAIDS, barbiturates), dietary supplements, and herbal products. If patients are taking any of these drugs, alternate therapy, dosage adjustment, and/or special test may be needed during the treatment.
Patients should be advised of common adverse reactions that could occur with corticosteroid use to include elevated intraocular pressure, cataracts, fluid retention, alteration in glucose tolerance, elevation in blood pressure, behavioral and mood changes, increased appetite and weight gain.
U.S. Patent No. 6,395,294
© 2007, 2008 Alcon, Inc.
Alcon®
ALCON LABORATORIES, INC.
Fort Worth, Texas 76134 USA

Allergan, Inc.
**2525 DUPONT DRIVE
P.O. BOX 19534
IRVINE, CA 92623-9534**

Direct Inquiries to:
(714) 246-4500

ALPHAGAN® P   ℞
(brimonidine tartrate ophthalmic solution) 0.1% and 0.15%
HIGHLIGHTS OF PRESCRIBING INFORMATION
These highlights do not include all the information needed to use ALPHAGAN® P safely and effectively. See full prescribing information for ALPHAGAN® P.
ALPHAGAN® P (brimonidine tartrate ophthalmic solution) 0.1% and 0.15%
Initial U.S. Approval: 1996

———— **INDICATIONS AND USAGE** ————
ALPHAGAN® P is an alpha adrenergic receptor agonist indicated for the reduction of elevated intraocular pressure (IOP) in patients with open-angle glaucoma or ocular hypertension. (1)

—— **DOSAGE AND ADMINISTRATION** ——
One drop in the affected eye(s), three times daily, approximately 8 hours apart. (2)

—— **DOSAGE FORMS AND STRENGTHS** ——
Solution containing 1 or 1.5 mg/mL brimonidine tartrate. (3)

———— **CONTRAINDICATIONS** ————
Neonates and infants (under the age of 2 years). (4.1)

—— **WARNINGS AND PRECAUTIONS** ——
Potentiation of vascular insufficiency. (5.1)

———— **ADVERSE REACTIONS** ————
Most common adverse reactions occurring in approximately 5% to 20% of patients receiving brimonidine ophthalmic solution (0.1%-0.2%) included allergic conjunctivitis, burning sensation, conjunctival folliculosis, conjunctival hyperemia, eye pruritus, hypertension, ocular allergic reaction, oral dryness, and visual disturbance. (6.1)

To report **SUSPECTED ADVERSE REACTIONS**, contact Allergan at 1-800-433-8871 or the FDA at 1-800-FDA-1088 or www.fda.gov/medwatch.

———— **DRUG INTERACTIONS** ————
• Antihypertensives/cardiac glycosides may lower blood pressure. (7.1)
• Use with CNS depressants may result in an additive or potentiating effect. (7.2)
• Tricyclic antidepressants may potentially blunt the hypotensive effect of systemic clonidine. (7.3)
• Monoamine oxidase inhibitors may result in increased hypotension. (7.4)

—— **USE IN SPECIFIC POPULATIONS** ——
Use with caution in children ≥ 2 years of age. (8.4)

See 17 for PATIENT COUNSELING INFORMATION

                                    Revised: 06/2011

————————————————————————————
FULL PRESCRIBING INFORMATION: CONTENTS*

FULL PRESCRIBING INFORMATION
1   INDICATIONS AND USAGE
ALPHAGAN® P (brimonidine tartrate ophthalmic solution) 0.1% or 0.15% is an alpha adrenergic receptor agonist indicated for the reduction of elevated intraocular pressure (IOP) in patients with open-angle glaucoma or ocular hypertension.

2   DOSAGE AND ADMINISTRATION
The recommended dose is one drop of ALPHAGAN® P in the affected eye(s) three times daily, approximately 8 hours apart. ALPHAGAN® P ophthalmic solution may be used concomitantly with other topical ophthalmic drug products to lower intraocular pressure. If more than one topical ophthalmic product is to be used, the different products should be instilled at least 5 minutes apart.

3   DOSAGE FORMS AND STRENGTHS
Solution containing 1 mg/mL or 1.5 mg/mL brimonidine tartrate.

4   CONTRAINDICATIONS
4.1   Neonates and Infants (under the age of 2 years)
ALPHAGAN® P is contraindicated in neonates and infants (under the age of 2 years).
4.2   Hypersensitivity Reactions
ALPHAGAN® P is contraindicated in patients who have exhibited a hypersensitivity reaction to any component of this medication in the past.

5   WARNINGS AND PRECAUTIONS
5.1   Potentiation of Vascular Insufficiency
ALPHAGAN® P may potentiate syndromes associated with vascular insufficiency. ALPHAGAN® P should be used with caution in patients with depression, cerebral or coronary insufficiency, Raynaud's phenomenon, orthostatic hypotension, or thromboangiitis obliterans.
5.2   Severe Cardiovascular Disease
Although brimonidine tartrate ophthalmic solution had minimal effect on the blood pressure of patients in clinical studies, caution should be exercised in treating patients with severe cardiovascular disease.
5.3   Contamination of Topical Ophthalmic Products After Use
There have been reports of bacterial keratitis associated with the use of multiple-dose containers of topical ophthalmic products. These containers had been inadvertently contaminated by patients who, in most cases, had a concurrent corneal

...disease or a disruption of the ocular epithelial surface (see **PATIENT COUNSELING INFORMATION**, 17).

6 ADVERSE REACTIONS
6.1 Clinical Studies Experience
Because clinical studies are conducted under widely varying conditions, adverse reaction rates observed in the clinical studies of a drug cannot be directly compared to rates in the clinical studies of another drug and may not reflect the rates observed in practice.

Adverse reactions occurring in approximately 10-20% of the subjects receiving brimonidine ophthalmic solution (0.1-0.2%) included: allergic conjunctivitis, conjunctival hyperemia, and eye pruritus. Adverse reactions occurring in approximately 5-9% included: burning sensation, conjunctival folliculosis, hypertension, ocular allergic reaction, oral dryness, and visual disturbance.

Adverse reactions occurring in approximately 1-4% of the subjects receiving brimonidine ophthalmic solution (0.1-0.2%) included: abnormal taste, allergic reaction, asthenia, blepharitis, blepharoconjunctivitis, blurred vision, bronchitis, cataract, conjunctival edema, conjunctival hemorrhage, conjunctivitis, cough, dizziness, dyspepsia, dyspnea, epiphora, eye discharge, eye dryness, eye irritation, eye pain, eyelid edema, eyelid erythema, fatigue, flu syndrome, follicular conjunctivitis, foreign body sensation, gastrointestinal disorder, headache, hypercholesterolemia, hypotension, infection (primarily colds and respiratory infections), insomnia, keratitis, lid disorder, pharyngitis, photophobia, rash, rhinitis, sinus infection, sinusitis, somnolence, stinging, superficial punctate keratopathy, tearing, visual field defect, vitreous detachment, vitreous disorder, vitreous floaters, and worsened visual acuity.

The following reactions were reported in less than 1% of subjects: corneal erosion, hordeolum, nasal dryness, and taste perversion.

6.2 Postmarketing Experience
The following reactions have been identified during postmarketing use of brimonidine tartrate ophthalmic solutions in clinical practice. Because they are reported voluntarily from a population of unknown size, estimates of frequency cannot be made. The reactions, which have been chosen for inclusion due to either their seriousness, frequency of reporting, possible causal connection to brimonidine tartrate ophthalmic solutions, or a combination of these factors, include: bradycardia, depression, hypersensitivity, iritis, keratoconjunctivitis sicca, miosis, nausea, skin reactions (including erythema, eyelid pruritus, rash, and vasodilation), syncope, and tachycardia. Apnea, bradycardia, coma, hypotension, hypothermia, hypotonia, lethargy, pallor, respiratory depression, and somnolence have been reported in infants receiving brimonidine tartrate ophthalmic solutions.

7 DRUG INTERACTIONS
7.1 Antihypertensives/Cardiac Glycosides
Because **ALPHAGAN® P** may reduce blood pressure, caution in using drugs such as antihypertensives and/or cardiac glycosides with **ALPHAGAN® P** is advised.

7.2 CNS Depressants
Although specific drug interaction studies have not been conducted with **ALPHAGAN® P**, the possibility of an additive or potentiating effect with CNS depressants (alcohol, barbiturates, opiates, sedatives, or anesthetics) should be considered.

7.3 Tricyclic Antidepressants
Tricyclic antidepressants have been reported to blunt the hypotensive effect of systemic clonidine. It is not known whether the concurrent use of these agents with **ALPHAGAN® P** in humans can lead to resulting interference with the IOP lowering effect. Caution is advised in patients taking tricyclic antidepressants which can affect the metabolism and uptake of circulating amines.

7.4 Monoamine Oxidase Inhibitors
Monoamine oxidase (MAO) inhibitors may theoretically interfere with the metabolism of brimonidine and potentially result in an increased systemic side-effect such as hypotension. Caution is advised in patients taking MAO inhibitors which can affect the metabolism and uptake of circulating amines.

8 USE IN SPECIFIC POPULATIONS
8.1 Pregnancy
Pregnancy Category B: Teratogenicity studies have been performed in animals.

Brimonidine tartrate was not teratogenic when given orally during gestation days 6 through 15 in rats and days 6 through 18 in rabbits. The highest doses of brimonidine tartrate in rats (2.5 mg/kg/day) and rabbits (5.0 mg/kg/day) achieved AUC exposure values 360- and 20-fold higher, or 260- and 15-fold higher, respectively, than similar values estimated in humans treated with **ALPHAGAN® P** 0.1% or 0.15%, 1 drop in both eyes three times daily. There are no adequate and well-controlled studies in pregnant women; however, in animal studies, brimonidine crossed the placenta and entered into the fetal circulation to a limited extent. Because animal reproduction studies are not always predictive of human response, **ALPHAGAN® P** should be used during pregnancy only if the potential benefit to the mother justifies the potential risk to the fetus.

8.3 Nursing Mothers
It is not known whether brimonidine tartrate is excreted in human milk, although in animal studies, brimonidine tartrate has been shown to be excreted in breast milk. Because of the potential for serious adverse reactions from **ALPHAGAN® P** in nursing infants, a decision should be made whether to discontinue nursing or to discontinue the drug, taking into account the importance of the drug to the mother.

8.4 Pediatric Use
ALPHAGAN® P is contraindicated in children under the age of 2 years (see **CONTRAINDICATIONS**, 4.1). During postmarketing surveillance, apnea, bradycardia, coma, hypotension, hypothermia, hypotonia, lethargy, pallor, respiratory depression, and somnolence have been reported in infants receiving brimonidine. The safety and effectiveness of brimonidine tartrate have not been studied in children below the age of 2 years.

In a well-controlled clinical study conducted in pediatric glaucoma patients (ages 2 to 7 years) the most commonly observed adverse reactions with brimonidine tartrate ophthalmic solution 0.2% dosed three times daily were somnolence (50-83% in patients ages 2 to 6 years) and decreased alertness. In pediatric patients 7 years of age (>20 kg), somnolence appears to occur less frequently (25%). Approximately 16% of patients on brimonidine tartrate ophthalmic solution discontinued from the study due to somnolence.

8.5 Geriatric Use
No overall differences in safety or effectiveness have been observed between elderly and other adult patients.

8.6 Special Populations
ALPHAGAN® P has not been studied in patients with hepatic impairment.
ALPHAGAN® P has not been studied in patients with renal impairment. The effect of dialysis on brimonidine pharmacokinetics in patients with renal failure is not known.

10 OVERDOSAGE
Very limited information exists on accidental ingestion of brimonidine in adults; the only adverse reaction reported to date has been hypotension. Symptoms of brimonidine overdose have been reported in neonates, infants, and children receiving **ALPHAGAN® P** as part of medical treatment of congenital glaucoma or by accidental oral ingestion (see **USE IN SPECIFIC POPULATIONS**, 8.4). Treatment of an oral overdose includes supportive and symptomatic therapy; a patent airway should be maintained.

11 DESCRIPTION
ALPHAGAN® P (brimonidine tartrate ophthalmic solution) 0.1% or 0.15%, sterile, is a relatively selective alpha-2 adrenergic receptor agonist (topical intraocular pressure lowering agent). The structural formula of brimonidine tartrate is:

5-Bromo-6-(2-imidazolidinylideneamino) quinoxaline L-tartrate; MW= 442.24

In solution, **ALPHAGAN® P** (brimonidine tartrate ophthalmic solution) has a clear, greenish-yellow color. It has an osmolality of 250-350 mOsmol/kg and a pH of 7.4-8.0 (0.1%) or 6.9-7.4 (0.15%).

Brimonidine tartrate appears as an off-white to pale-yellow powder and is soluble in both water (0.6 mg/mL) and in the product vehicle (1.4 mg/mL) at pH 7.7.

Each mL of **ALPHAGAN® P** contains the active ingredient brimonidine tartrate 0.1% (1 mg/mL) or 0.15% (1.5 mg/mL) with the inactive ingredients sodium carboxymethylcellulose; sodium borate; boric acid; sodium chloride; potassium chloride; calcium chloride; magnesium chloride; PURITE® 0.005% (0.05 mg/mL) as a preservative; purified water; and hydrochloric acid and/or sodium hydroxide to adjust pH.

12 CLINICAL PHARMACOLOGY
12.1 Mechanism of Action
ALPHAGAN® P is a relatively selective alpha-2 adrenergic receptor agonist with a peak ocular hypotensive effect occurring at two hours post-dosing.

Fluorophotometric studies in animals and humans suggest that brimonidine tartrate has a dual mechanism of action by reducing aqueous humor production and increasing uveoscleral outflow.

12.3 Pharmacokinetics
Absorption
After ocular administration of either a 0.1% or 0.2% solution, plasma concentrations peaked within 0.5 to 2.5 hours and declined with a systemic half-life of approximately 2 hours.

Distribution
The protein binding of brimonidine has not been studied.

Metabolism
In humans, brimonidine is extensively metabolized by the liver.

Excretion
Urinary excretion is the major route of elimination of brimonidine and its metabolites. Approximately 87% of an orally-administered radioactive dose of brimonidine was eliminated within 120 hours, with 74% found in the urine.

13 NONCLINICAL TOXICOLOGY
13.1 Carcinogenesis, Mutagenesis, Impairment of Fertility
No compound-related carcinogenic effects were observed in either mice or rats following a 21-month and 24-month study, respectively. In these studies, dietary administration of brimonidine tartrate at doses up to 2.5 mg/kg/day in mice and 1 mg/kg/day in rats achieved 150 and 120 times or 90 and 80 times, respectively, the plasma C_{max} drug concentration in humans treated with one drop of **ALPHAGAN® P** 0.1% or 0.15% into both eyes 3 times per day, the recommended daily human dose.

Brimonidine tartrate was not mutagenic or clastogenic in a series of in vitro and in vivo studies including the Ames bacterial reversion test, chromosomal aberration assay in Chinese Hamster Ovary (CHO) cells, and three in vivo studies in CD-1 mice: a host-mediated assay, cytogenetic study, and dominant lethal assay.

Reproduction and fertility studies in rats with brimonidine tartrate demonstrated no adverse

Continued on next page

Alphagan P—Cont.

effect on male or female fertility at doses which achieve up to approximately 125 and 90 times the systemic exposure following the maximum recommended human ophthalmic dose of **ALPHAGAN**® P 0.1% or 0.15%, respectively.

14 CLINICAL STUDIES
Elevated IOP presents a major risk factor in glaucomatous field loss. The higher the level of IOP, the greater the likelihood of optic nerve damage and visual field loss. Brimonidine tartrate has the action of lowering intraocular pressure with minimal effect on cardiovascular and pulmonary parameters.

Clinical studies were conducted to evaluate the safety, efficacy, and acceptability of **ALPHAGAN**® P (brimonidine tartrate ophthalmic solution) 0.15% compared with **ALPHAGAN**® administered three-times-daily in patients with open-angle glaucoma or ocular hypertension. Those results indicated that **ALPHAGAN**® P (brimonidine tartrate ophthalmic solution) 0.15% is comparable in IOP lowering effect to **ALPHAGAN**® (brimonidine tartrate ophthalmic solution) 0.2%, and effectively lowers IOP in patients with open-angle glaucoma or ocular hypertension by approximately 2-6 mmHg.

A clinical study was conducted to evaluate the safety, efficacy, and acceptability of **ALPHAGAN**® P (brimonidine tartrate ophthalmic solution) 0.1% compared with **ALPHAGAN**® administered three-times-daily in patients with open-angle glaucoma or ocular hypertension. Those results indicated that **ALPHAGAN**® P (brimonidine tartrate ophthalmic solution) 0.1% is equivalent in IOP lowering effect to **ALPHAGAN**® (brimonidine tartrate ophthalmic solution) 0.2%, and effectively lowers IOP in patients with open-angle glaucoma or ocular hypertension by approximately 2-6 mmHg.

16 HOW SUPPLIED/STORAGE AND HANDLING
ALPHAGAN® P is supplied sterile, in teal opaque plastic LDPE bottles and tips, with purple high impact polystyrene (HIPS) caps as follows:
0.1%
5 mL in 10 mL bottle	NDC 0023-9321-05
10 mL in 10 mL bottle	NDC 0023-9321-10
15 mL in 15 mL bottle	NDC 0023-9321-15

0.15%
5 mL in 10 mL bottle	NDC 0023-9177-05
10 mL in 10 mL bottle	NDC 0023-9177-10
15 mL in 15 mL bottle	NDC 0023-9177-15

Storage: Store at 15°-25°C (59°-77°F).

17 PATIENT COUNSELING INFORMATION
Patients should be instructed that ocular solutions, if handled improperly or if the tip of the dispensing container contacts the eye or surrounding structures, can become contaminated by common bacteria known to cause ocular infections. Serious damage to the eye and subsequent loss of vision may result from using contaminated solutions (see **WARNINGS AND PRECAUTIONS**, 5.3). Always replace the cap after using. If solution changes color or becomes cloudy, do not use. Do not use the product after the expiration date marked on the bottle.

Patients also should be advised that if they have ocular surgery or develop an intercurrent ocular condition (e.g., trauma or infection), they should immediately seek their physician's advice concerning the continued use of the present multidose container.

If more than one topical ophthalmic drug is being used, the drugs should be administered at least five minutes apart.

As with other similar medications, **ALPHAGAN**® P may cause fatigue and/or drowsiness in some patients. Patients who engage in hazardous activities should be cautioned of the potential for a decrease in mental alertness.

© 2011 Allergan, Inc.
Irvine, CA 92612, U.S.A.

® marks owned by Allergan, Inc.
U.S. Patents 5,424,078; 6,562,873; 6,627,210; 6,641,834; and 6,673,337
71816US14C

Shown in Product Identification Guide, page 103

COMBIGAN® ℞
(brimonidine tartrate/timolol maleate ophthalmic solution) 0.2%/0.5%

HIGHLIGHTS OF PRESCRIBING INFORMATION
These highlights do not include all the information needed to use COMBIGAN® safely and effectively. See full prescribing information for COMBIGAN®.
COMBIGAN® (brimonidine tartrate/timolol maleate ophthalmic solution) 0.2%/0.5%
Initial U.S. Approval: 2007

INDICATIONS AND USAGE
COMBIGAN® is an alpha adrenergic receptor agonist with a beta adrenergic receptor inhibitor indicated for the reduction of elevated intraocular pressure (IOP) in patients with glaucoma or ocular hypertension who require adjunctive or replacement therapy due to inadequately controlled IOP; the IOP-lowering of **COMBIGAN**® dosed twice a day was slightly less than that seen with the concomitant administration of timolol maleate ophthalmic solution, 0.5% dosed twice a day and brimonidine tartrate ophthalmic solution, 0.2% dosed three times per day. (1)

DOSAGE AND ADMINISTRATION
• One drop in the affected eye(s), twice daily approximately 12 hours apart. (2)

DOSAGE FORMS AND STRENGTHS
• Solution containing 2 mg/mL brimonidine tartrate and 5 mg/mL timolol. (3)

CONTRAINDICATIONS
• Bronchial asthma, a history of bronchial asthma, severe chronic obstructive pulmonary disease. (4, 5.1, 5.3)
• Sinus bradycardia, second or third degree atrioventricular block, overt cardiac failure, cardiogenic shock. (4, 5.2)
• Hypersensitivity to any component of this product. (4)

WARNINGS AND PRECAUTIONS
• Potentiation of Respiratory Reactions Including Asthma (5.1)
• Cardiac Failure (5.2)
• Obstructive Pulmonary Disease (5.3)
• Potentiation of Vascular Insufficiency (5.4)
• Increased Reactivity to Allergens (5.5)
• Potentiation of Muscle Weakness (5.6)
• Masking of Hypoglycemic Symptoms in Patients with Diabetes Mellitus (5.7)
• Masking of Thyrotoxicosis (5.8)

ADVERSE REACTIONS
Most common adverse reactions occurring in approximately 5 to 15% of patients included allergic conjunctivitis, conjunctival folliculosis, conjunctival hyperemia, eye pruritus, ocular burning, and stinging. (6.1)

To report SUSPECTED ADVERSE REACTIONS, contact Allergan at 1-800-433-8871 or the FDA at 1-800-FDA-1088 or www.fda.gov/medwatch.

DRUG INTERACTIONS
• Antihypertensives/cardiac glycosides may lower blood pressure. (7.1)
• Concomitant use with systemic beta-blockers may potentiate systemic beta-blockade. (7.2)
• Oral or intravenous calcium antagonists may cause atrioventricular conduction disturbances, left ventricular failure, and hypotension. (7.3)
• Catecholamine-depleting drugs may have additive effects and produce hypotension and/or marked bradycardia. (7.4)

• Use with CNS depressants may result in additive or potentiating effect. (7.5)
• Digitalis and calcium antagonists may have additive effects in prolonging atrioventricular conduction time. (7.6)
• CYP2D6 inhibitors may potentiate systemic beta-blockade. (7.7)
• Tricyclic antidepressants may potentially blunt the hypotensive effect of systemic clonidine. (7.8)
• Monoamine oxidase inhibitors may result in increased hypotension. (7.9)

USE IN SPECIFIC POPULATIONS
• Not for use in children below the age of 2 years. (8.4)

See 17 for PATIENT COUNSELING INFORMATION

Revised: 09/201_

FULL PRESCRIBING INFORMATION

1 INDICATIONS AND USAGE
COMBIGAN® (brimonidine tartrate/timolol maleate ophthalmic solution) 0.2%/0.5% is an alpha adrenergic receptor agonist with a beta adrenergic receptor inhibitor indicated for the reduction of elevated intraocular pressure (IOP) in patients with glaucoma or ocular hypertension who require adjunctive or replacement therapy due to inadequately controlled IOP; the IOP-lowering of **COMBIGAN**® dosed twice a day was slightly less

than that seen with the concomitant administration of 0.5% timolol maleate ophthalmic solution dosed twice a day and 0.2% brimonidine tartrate ophthalmic solution dosed three times per day.

2 DOSAGE AND ADMINISTRATION

The recommended dose is one drop of **COMBIGAN®** in the affected eye(s) twice daily approximately 12 hours apart. If more than one topical ophthalmic product is to be used, the different products should be instilled at least 5 minutes apart.

3 DOSAGE FORMS AND STRENGTHS

Solution containing 2 mg/mL brimonidine tartrate and 5 mg/mL timolol (6.8 mg/mL timolol maleate).

4 CONTRAINDICATIONS

Asthma, COPD
COMBIGAN® is contraindicated in patients with bronchial asthma; a history of bronchial asthma; severe chronic obstructive pulmonary disease (see **WARNINGS AND PRECAUTIONS**, 5.1, 5.3).

Sinus Bradycardia, AV Block, Cardiac Failure, Cardiogenic Shock
COMBIGAN® is contraindicated in patients with sinus bradycardia; second or third degree atrioventricular block; overt cardiac failure (see **WARNINGS AND PRECAUTIONS**, 5.2); cardiogenic shock.

Hypersensitivity Reactions
Local hypersensitivity reactions have occurred following the use of different components of **COMBIGAN®**. **COMBIGAN®** is contraindicated in patients who have exhibited a hypersensitivity reaction to any component of this medication in the past.

5 WARNINGS AND PRECAUTIONS

5.1 Potentiation of Respiratory Reactions Including Asthma

COMBIGAN® contains timolol maleate; and although administered topically can be absorbed systemically. Therefore, the same types of adverse reactions found with systemic administration of beta-adrenergic blocking agents may occur with topical administration. For example, severe respiratory reactions including death due to bronchospasm in patients with asthma have been reported following systemic or ophthalmic administration of timolol maleate (see **CONTRAINDICATIONS**, 4).

5.2 Cardiac Failure

Sympathetic stimulation may be essential for support of the circulation in individuals with diminished myocardial contractility, and its inhibition by beta-adrenergic receptor blockade may precipitate more severe failure.

In patients without a history of cardiac failure, continued depression of the myocardium with beta-blocking agents over a period of time can, in some cases, lead to cardiac failure. At the first sign or symptom of cardiac failure, **COMBIGAN®** should be discontinued (see also **CONTRAINDICATIONS**, 4).

5.3 Obstructive Pulmonary Disease

Patients with chronic obstructive pulmonary disease (e.g., chronic bronchitis, emphysema) of mild or moderate severity, bronchospastic disease, or a history of bronchospastic disease [other than bronchial asthma or a history of bronchial asthma, in which **COMBIGAN®** is contraindicated (see **CONTRAINDICATIONS**, 4)] should, in general, not receive beta-blocking agents, including **COMBIGAN®**.

5.4 Potentiation of Vascular Insufficiency

COMBIGAN® may potentiate syndromes associated with vascular insufficiency. **COMBIGAN®** should be used with caution in patients with depression, cerebral or coronary insufficiency, Raynaud's phenomenon, orthostatic hypotension, or thromboangiitis obliterans.

5.5 Increased Reactivity to Allergens

While taking beta-blockers, patients with a history of atopy or a history of severe anaphylactic reactions to a variety of allergens may be more reactive to repeated accidental, diagnostic, or therapeutic challenge with such allergens. Such patients may be unresponsive to the usual doses of epinephrine used to treat anaphylactic reactions.

5.6 Potentiation of Muscle Weakness

Beta-adrenergic blockade has been reported to potentiate muscle weakness consistent with certain myasthenic symptoms (e.g., diplopia, ptosis, and generalized weakness). Timolol has been reported rarely to increase muscle weakness in some patients with myasthenia gravis or myasthenic symptoms.

5.7 Masking of Hypoglycemic Symptoms in Patients with Diabetes Mellitus

Beta-adrenergic blocking agents should be administered with caution in patients subject to spontaneous hypoglycemia or to diabetic patients (especially those with labile diabetes) who are receiving insulin or oral hypoglycemic agents. Beta-adrenergic receptor blocking agents may mask the signs and symptoms of acute hypoglycemia.

5.8 Masking of Thyrotoxicosis

Beta-adrenergic blocking agents may mask certain clinical signs (e.g., tachycardia) of hyperthyroidism. Patients suspected of developing thyrotoxicosis should be managed carefully to avoid abrupt withdrawal of beta-adrenergic blocking agents that might precipitate a thyroid storm.

5.9 Contamination of Topical Ophthalmic Products After Use

There have been reports of bacterial keratitis associated with the use of multiple-dose containers of topical ophthalmic products. These containers had been inadvertently contaminated by patients who, in most cases, had a concurrent corneal disease or a disruption of the ocular epithelial surface (see **PATIENT COUNSELING INFORMATION**, 17).

5.10 Impairment of Beta-adrenergically Mediated Reflexes During Surgery

The necessity or desirability of withdrawal of beta-adrenergic blocking agents prior to major surgery is controversial. Beta-adrenergic receptor blockade impairs the ability of the heart to respond to beta-adrenergically mediated reflex stimuli. This may augment the risk of general anesthesia in surgical procedures. Some patients receiving beta-adrenergic receptor blocking agents have experienced protracted severe hypotension during anesthesia. Difficulty in restarting and maintaining the heartbeat has also been reported. For these reasons, in patients undergoing elective surgery, some authorities recommend gradual withdrawal of beta-adrenergic receptor blocking agents.

If necessary during surgery, the effects of beta-adrenergic blocking agents may be reversed by sufficient doses of adrenergic agonists.

6 ADVERSE REACTIONS

6.1 Clinical Studies Experience

Because clinical studies are conducted under widely varying conditions, adverse reaction rates observed in the clinical studies of a drug cannot be directly compared to rates in the clinical studies of another drug and may not reflect the rates observed in practice.

COMBIGAN®
In clinical trials of 12 months duration with **COMBIGAN®**, the most frequent reactions associated with its use occurring in approximately 5% to 15% of the patients included: allergic conjunctivitis, conjunctival folliculosis, conjunctival hyperemia, eye pruritus, ocular burning, and stinging. The following adverse reactions were reported in 1% to 5% of patients: asthenia, blepharitis, corneal erosion, depression, epiphora, eye discharge, eye dryness, eye irritation, eye pain, eyelid edema, eyelid erythema, eyelid pruritus, foreign body sensation, headache, hypertension, oral dryness, somnolence, superficial punctate keratitis, and visual disturbance.

Other adverse reactions that have been reported with the individual components are listed below.

Brimonidine Tartrate (0.1%-0.2%)
Abnormal taste, allergic reaction, blepharoconjunctivitis, blurred vision, bronchitis, cataract, conjunctival edema, conjunctival hemorrhage, conjunctivitis, cough, dizziness, dyspepsia, dyspnea, fatigue, flu syndrome, follicu-

lar conjunctivitis, gastrointestinal disorder, hypercholesterolemia, hypotension, infection (primarily colds and respiratory infections), hordeolum, insomnia, keratitis, lid disorder, nasal dryness, ocular allergic reaction, pharyngitis, photophobia, rash, rhinitis, sinus infection, sinusitis, taste perversion, tearing, visual field defect, vitreous detachment, vitreous disorder, vitreous floaters, and worsened visual acuity.

Timolol (Ocular Administration)
Body as a whole: chest pain; *Cardiovascular*: Arrhythmia, bradycardia, cardiac arrest, cardiac failure, cerebral ischemia, cerebral vascular accident, claudication, cold hands and feet, edema, heart block, palpitation, pulmonary edema, Raynaud's phenomenon, syncope, and worsening of angina pectoris; *Digestive*: Anorexia, diarrhea, nausea; *Immunologic*: Systemic lupus erythematosus; *Nervous System / Psychiatric*: Increase in signs and symptoms of myasthenia gravis, insomnia, nightmares, paresthesia, behavioral changes and psychic disturbances including confusion, hallucinations, anxiety, disorientation, nervousness, and memory loss; *Skin*: Alopecia, psoriasiform rash or exacerbation of psoriasis; *Hypersensitivity*: Signs and symptoms of systemic allergic reactions, including anaphylaxis, angioedema, urticaria, and generalized and localized rash; *Respiratory*: Bronchospasm (predominantly in patients with pre-existing bronchospastic disease), dyspnea, nasal congestion, respiratory failure; *Endocrine*: Masked symptoms of hypoglycemia in diabetes patients (see **WARNINGS AND PRECAUTIONS**, 5.7); *Special Senses*: diplopia, choroidal detachment following filtration surgery, cystoid macular edema, decreased corneal sensitivity, pseudopemphigoid, ptosis, refractive changes, tinnitus; *Urogenital*: Decreased libido, impotence, Peyronie's disease, retroperitoneal fibrosis.

6.2 Postmarketing Experience

Brimonidine
The following reactions have been identified during post-marketing use of brimonidine tartrate ophthalmic solutions in clinical practice. Because they are reported voluntarily from a population of unknown size, estimates of frequency cannot be made. The reactions, which have been chosen for inclusion due to either their seriousness, frequency of reporting, possible causal connection to brimonidine tartrate ophthalmic solutions, or a combination of these factors, include: bradycardia, depression, iritis, keratoconjunctivitis sicca, miosis, nausea, skin reactions (including erythema, eyelid pruritus, rash, and vasodilation), and tachycardia. Apnea, bradycardia, hypotension, hypothermia, hypotonia, and somnolence have been reported in infants receiving brimonidine tartrate ophthalmic solutions.

Oral Timolol/Oral Beta-blockers
The following additional adverse reactions have been reported in clinical experience with ORAL timolol maleate or other ORAL beta-blocking agents and may be considered potential effects of ophthalmic timolol maleate: *Allergic*: Erythematous rash, fever combined with aching and sore throat, laryngospasm with respiratory distress; *Body as a whole*: Decreased exercise tolerance, extremity pain, weight loss; *Cardiovascular*: Vasodilatation, worsening of arterial insufficiency; *Digestive*: Gastrointestinal pain, hepatomegaly, ischemic colitis, mesenteric arterial thrombosis, vomiting; *Hematologic*: Agranulocytosis, nonthrombocytopenic purpura, thrombocytopenic purpura; *Endocrine*: Hyperglycemia, hypoglycemia; *Skin*: Increased pigmentation, pruritus, skin irritation, sweating; *Musculoskeletal*: Arthralgia; *Nervous System / Psychiatric*: An acute reversible syndrome characterized by disorientation for time and place, decreased performance on neuropsychometrics, diminished concentration, emotional lability, local weakness, reversible mental depression progressing to catatonia, slightly

Continued on next page

Combigan—Cont.

clouded sensorium, vertigo; *Respiratory*: Bronchial obstruction, rales; *Urogenital*: Urination difficulties.

7 DRUG INTERACTIONS
7.1 Antihypertensives/Cardiac Glycosides
Because **COMBIGAN®** may reduce blood pressure, caution in using drugs such as antihypertensives and/or cardiac glycosides with **COMBIGAN®** is advised.

7.2 Beta-adrenergic Blocking Agents
Patients who are receiving a beta-adrenergic blocking agent orally and **COMBIGAN®** should be observed for potential additive effects of beta-blockade, both systemic and on intraocular pressure. The concomitant use of two topical beta-adrenergic blocking agents is not recommended.

7.3 Calcium Antagonists
Caution should be used in the co-administration of beta-adrenergic blocking agents, such as **COMBIGAN®**, and oral or intravenous calcium antagonists because of possible atrioventricular conduction disturbances, left ventricular failure, and hypotension. In patients with impaired cardiac function, co-administration should be avoided.

7.4 Catecholamine-depleting Drugs
Close observation of the patient is recommended when a beta blocker is administered to patients receiving catecholamine-depleting drugs such as reserpine, because of possible additive effects and the production of hypotension and/or marked bradycardia, which may result in vertigo, syncope, or postural hypotension.

7.5 CNS Depressants
Although specific drug interaction studies have not been conducted with **COMBIGAN®**, the possibility of an additive or potentiating effect with CNS depressants (alcohol, barbiturates, opiates, sedatives, or anesthetics) should be considered.

7.6 Digitalis and Calcium Antagonists
The concomitant use of beta-adrenergic blocking agents with digitalis and calcium antagonists may have additive effects in prolonging atrioventricular conduction time.

7.7 CYP2D6 Inhibitors
Potentiated systemic beta-blockade (e.g., decreased heart rate, depression) has been reported during combined treatment with CYP2D6 inhibitors (e.g., quinidine, SSRIs) and timolol.

7.8 Tricyclic Antidepressants
Tricyclic antidepressants have been reported to blunt the hypotensive effect of systemic clonidine. It is not known whether the concurrent use of these agents with **COMBIGAN®** in humans can lead to resulting interference with the IOP-lowering effect. Caution, however, is advised in patients taking tricyclic antidepressants which can affect the metabolism and uptake of circulating amines.

7.9 Monoamine Oxidase Inhibitors
Monoamine oxidase (MAO) inhibitors may theoretically interfere with the metabolism of brimonidine and potentially result in an increased systemic side-effect such as hypotension. Caution is advised in patients taking MAO inhibitors which can affect the metabolism and uptake of circulating amines.

8 USE IN SPECIFIC POPULATIONS
8.1 Pregnancy
Pregnancy Category C: Teratogenicity studies have been performed in animals.
Brimonidine tartrate was not teratogenic when given orally during gestation days 6 through 15 in rats and days 6 through 18 in rabbits. The highest doses of brimonidine tartrate in rats (1.65 mg/kg/day) and rabbits (3.33 mg/kg/day) achieved AUC exposure values 580 and 37-fold higher, respectively, than similar values estimated in humans treated with **COMBIGAN®**, 1 drop in both eyes twice daily.
Teratogenicity studies with timolol in mice, rats, and rabbits at oral doses up to 50 mg/kg/day [4,200 times the maximum recommended human ocular

dose of 0.012 mg/kg/day on a mg/kg basis (MRHOD)] demonstrated no evidence of fetal malformations. Although delayed fetal ossification was observed at this dose in rats, there were no adverse effects on postnatal development of offspring. Doses of 1,000 mg/kg/day (83,000 times the MRHOD) were maternotoxic in mice and resulted in an increased number of fetal resorptions. Increased fetal resorptions were also seen in rabbits at doses 8,300 times the MRHOD without apparent maternotoxicity.
There are no adequate and well-controlled studies in pregnant women; however, in animal studies, brimonidine crossed the placenta and entered into the fetal circulation to a limited extent. Because animal reproduction studies are not always predictive of human response, **COMBIGAN®** should be used during pregnancy only if the potential benefit to the mother justifies the potential risk to the fetus.

8.3 Nursing Mothers
Timolol has been detected in human milk following oral and ophthalmic drug administration. It is not known whether brimonidine tartrate is excreted in human milk, although in animal studies, brimonidine tartrate has been shown to be excreted in breast milk. Because of the potential for serious adverse reactions from **COMBIGAN®** in nursing infants, a decision should be made whether to discontinue nursing or to discontinue the drug, taking into account the importance of the drug to the mother.

8.4 Pediatric Use
COMBIGAN® is not recommended for use in children under the age of 2 years. During post-marketing surveillance, apnea, bradycardia, hypotension, hypothermia, hypotonia, and somnolence have been reported in infants receiving brimonidine. The safety and effectiveness of brimonidine tartrate and timolol maleate have not been studied in children below the age of 2 years. The safety and effectiveness of **COMBIGAN®** have been established in the age group 2 – 16 years of age. Use of **COMBIGAN®** in this age group is supported by evidence from adequate and well-controlled studies of **COMBIGAN®** in adults with additional data from a study of the concomitant use of brimonidine tartrate ophthalmic solution 0.2% and timolol maleate ophthalmic solution 0.5% in pediatric glaucoma patients (ages 2 to 7 years). In this study, brimonidine tartrate ophthalmic solution 0.2% was dosed three times a day as adjunctive therapy to beta-blockers. The most commonly observed adverse reactions were somnolence (50%-83% in patients 2 to 6 years) and decreased alertness. In pediatric patients 7 years of age or older (>20 kg), somnolence appears to occur less frequently (25%). Approximately 16% of patients on brimonidine tartrate ophthalmic solution discontinued from the study due to somnolence.

8.5 Geriatric Use
No overall differences in safety or effectiveness have been observed between elderly and other adult patients.

10 OVERDOSAGE
No information is available on overdosage with **COMBIGAN®** in humans. There have been reports of inadvertent overdosage with timolol ophthalmic solution resulting in systemic effects similar to those seen with systemic beta-adrenergic blocking agents such as dizziness, headache, shortness of breath, bradycardia, bronchospasm, and cardiac arrest. Treatment of an oral overdose includes supportive and symptomatic therapy; a patent airway should be maintained.

11 DESCRIPTION
COMBIGAN® (brimonidine tartrate/timolol maleate ophthalmic solution) 0.2%/0.5%, sterile, is a relatively selective alpha-2 adrenergic receptor agonist with a non-selective beta-adrenergic receptor inhibitor (topical intraocular pressure lowering agent).

The structural formulae are:
Brimonidine tartrate:

5-bromo-6-(2-imidazolidinylideneamino) quinoxaline L-tartrate; MW= 442.24
Timolol maleate:

(-)-1-(*tert*-butylamino)-3-[(4-morpholino-1,2,5-thiadiazol-3-yl)-oxy]-2-propanol maleate (1:1) (salt), MW= 432.50 as the maleate salt
In solution, **COMBIGAN®** (brimonidine tartrate/timolol maleate ophthalmic solution 0.2%/0.5% has a clear, greenish-yellow color. It has an osmolality of 260-330 mOsmol/kg and a pH during its shelf life of 6.5-7.3.
Brimonidine tartrate appears as an off-white, or white to pale-yellow powder and is soluble in both water (1.5 mg/mL) and in the product vehicle (3.0 mg/mL) at pH 7.2. Timolol maleate appears as a white, odorless, crystalline powder and is soluble in water, methanol, and alcohol.
Each mL of **COMBIGAN®** contains the active ingredients brimonidine tartrate 0.2% and timolol 0.5% with the inactive ingredients benzalkonium chloride 0.005%; sodium phosphate, monobasic; sodium phosphate, dibasic; purified water; and hydrochloric acid and/or sodium hydroxide to adjust pH.

12 CLINICAL PHARMACOLOGY
12.1 Mechanism of Action
COMBIGAN® is comprised of two components: brimonidine tartrate and timolol. Each of these two components decreases elevated intraocular pressure, whether or not associated with glaucoma. Elevated intraocular pressure is a major risk factor in the pathogenesis of optic nerve damage and glaucomatous visual field loss. The higher the level of intraocular pressure, the greater the likelihood of glaucomatous field loss and optic nerve damage.
COMBIGAN® is a selective alpha-2 adrenergic receptor agonist with a non-selective beta-adrenergic receptor inhibitor. Both brimonidine and timolol have a rapid onset of action, with peak ocular hypotensive effect seen at two hours post-dosing for brimonidine and one to two hours for timolol.
Fluorophotometric studies in animals and humans suggest that brimonidine tartrate has a dual mechanism of action by reducing aqueous humor production and increasing nonpressure dependent uveoscleral outflow.
Timolol maleate is a beta$_1$ and beta$_2$ adrenergic receptor inhibitor that does not have significant intrinsic sympathomimetic, direct myocardial depressant, or local anesthetic (membrane stabilizing) activity.

12.3 Pharmacokinetics
Absorption
Systemic absorption of brimonidine and timolol was assessed in healthy volunteers and patients following topical dosing with **COMBIGAN®**. Normal volunteers dosed with one drop of **COMBIGAN®** twice daily in both eyes for seven days showed peak plasma brimonidine and timolol concentrations of 30 pg/mL and 400 pg/mL, respectively. Plasma concentrations of brimonidine peaked at 1 to 4 hours after ocular dosing. Peak plasma concentrations of timolol occurred approximately 1 to 3 hours post-dose.
In a crossover study of **COMBIGAN®**, brimonidine tartrate 0.2%, and timolol 0.5% administered twice daily for 7 days in healthy volunteers, the mean brimonidine area-under-the-plasma-concentration-

time curve (AUC) for **COMBIGAN®** was 128 ± 61 pg•hr/mL versus 141 ± 106 pg•hr/mL for the respective monotherapy treatments; mean C_{max} values of brimonidine were comparable following **COMBIGAN®** treatment versus monotherapy (32.7 ± 15.0 pg/mL versus 34.7 ± 22.6 pg/mL, respectively). Mean timolol AUC for **COMBIGAN®** was similar to that of the respective monotherapy treatment (2919 ± 1679 pg•hr/mL versus 2909 ± 1231 pg•hr/mL, respectively); mean C_{max} of timolol was approximately 20% lower following **COMBIGAN®** treatment versus monotherapy.

In a parallel study in patients dosed twice daily with **COMBIGAN®**, twice daily with timolol 0.5%, or three times daily with brimonidine tartrate 0.2%, one-hour post dose plasma concentrations of timolol and brimonidine were approximately 30-40% lower with **COMBIGAN®** than their respective monotherapy values. The lower plasma brimonidine concentrations with **COMBIGAN®** appears to be due to twice-daily dosing for **COMBIGAN®** versus three-times dosing with brimonidine tartrate 0.2%.

Distribution
The protein binding of timolol is approximately 60%. The protein binding of brimonidine has not been studied.

Metabolism
In humans, brimonidine is extensively metabolized by the liver. Timolol is partially metabolized by the liver.

Excretion
In the crossover study in healthy volunteers, the plasma concentration of brimonidine declined with a systemic half-life of approximately 3 hours. The apparent systemic half-life of timolol was about 7 hours after ocular administration.

Urinary excretion is the major route of elimination of brimonidine and its metabolites. Approximately 87% of an orally-administered radioactive dose of brimonidine was eliminated within 120 hours, with 74% found in the urine. Unchanged timolol and its metabolites are excreted by the kidney.

Special Populations
COMBIGAN® has not been studied in patients with hepatic impairment.
COMBIGAN® has not been studied in patients with renal impairment.
A study of patients with renal failure showed that timolol was not readily removed by dialysis. The effect of dialysis on brimonidine pharmacokinetics in patients with renal failure is not known.
Following oral administration of timolol maleate, the plasma half-life of timolol is essentially unchanged in patients with moderate renal insufficiency.

13   NONCLINICAL TOXICOLOGY
13.1   Carcinogenesis, Mutagenesis, Impairment of Fertility
With brimonidine tartrate, no compound-related carcinogenic effects were observed in either mice or rats following a 21-month and 24-month study, respectively. In these studies, dietary administration of brimonidine tartrate at doses up to 2.5 mg/kg/day in mice and 1 mg/kg/day in rats achieved 150 and 210 times, respectively, the plasma C_{max} drug concentration in humans treated with one drop of **COMBIGAN®** into both eyes twice daily, the recommended daily human dose.

In a two-year study of timolol maleate administered orally to rats, there was a statistically significant increase in the incidence of adrenal pheochromocytomas in male rats administered 300 mg/kg/day [approximately 25,000 times the maximum recommended human ocular dose of 0.012 mg/kg/day on a mg/kg basis (MRHOD)]. Similar differences were not observed in rats administered oral doses equivalent to approximately 8,300 times the daily dose of **COMBIGAN®** in humans.

In a lifetime oral study of timolol maleate in mice, there were statistically significant increases in the incidence of benign and malignant pulmonary tumors, benign uterine polyps and mammary adenocarcinomas in female mice at 500 mg/kg/day,

(approximately 42,000 times the MRHOD), but not at 5 or 50 mg/kg/day (approximately 420 to 4,200 times higher, respectively, than the MRHOD). In a subsequent study in female mice, in which post-mortem examinations were limited to the uterus and the lungs, a statistically significant increase in the incidence of pulmonary tumors was again observed at 500 mg/kg/day.

The increased occurrence of mammary adenocarcinomas was associated with elevations in serum prolactin which occurred in female mice administered oral timolol at 500 mg/kg/day, but not at doses of 5 or 50 mg/kg/day. An increased incidence of mammary adenocarcinomas in rodents has been associated with administration of several other therapeutic agents that elevate serum prolactin, but no correlation between serum prolactin levels and mammary tumors has been established in humans. Furthermore, in adult human female subjects who received oral dosages of up to 60 mg of timolol maleate (the maximum recommended human oral dosage), there were no clinically meaningful changes in serum prolactin.

Brimonidine tartrate was not mutagenic or clastogenic in a series of in vitro and in vivo studies including the Ames bacterial reversion test, chromosomal aberration assay in Chinese Hamster Ovary (CHO) cells, and three in vivo studies in CD-1 mice: a host-mediated assay, cytogenetic study, and dominant lethal assay.

Timolol maleate was devoid of mutagenic potential when tested in vivo (mouse) in the micronucleus test and cytogenetic assay (doses up to 800 mg/kg) and in vitro in a neoplastic cell transformation assay (up to 100 mcg/mL). In Ames tests the highest concentrations of timolol employed, 5,000 or 10,000 mcg/plate, were associated with statistically significant elevations of revertants observed with tester strain TA100 (in seven replicate assays), but not in the remaining three strains. In the assays with tester strain TA100, no consistent dose response relationship was observed, and the ratio of test to control revertants did not reach 2. A ratio of 2 is usually considered the criterion for a positive Ames test.

Reproduction and fertility studies in rats with timolol maleate and in rats with brimonidine tartrate demonstrated no adverse effect on male or female fertility at doses up to approximately 100 times the systemic exposure following the maximum recommended human ophthalmic dose of **COMBIGAN®**.

14   CLINICAL STUDIES
Clinical studies were conducted to compare the IOP-lowering effect over the course of the day of **COMBIGAN®** administered twice a day (BID) to individually-administered brimonidine tartrate ophthalmic solution, 0.2% administered three times per day (TID) and timolol maleate ophthalmic solution, 0.5% BID in patients with glaucoma or ocular hypertension. **COMBIGAN®** BID provided an additional 1 to 3 mm Hg decrease in IOP over brimonidine treatment TID and an additional 1 to 2 mm Hg decrease over timolol treatment BID during the first 7 hours post dosing. However, the IOP-lowering of **COMBIGAN®** BID was less (approximately 1-2 mm Hg) than that seen with the concomitant administration of 0.5% timolol BID and 0.2% brimonidine tartrate TID. **COMBIGAN®** administered BID had a favorable safety profile versus concurrently administered brimonidine TID and timolol BID in the self-reported level of severity of sleepiness for patients over age 40.

16   HOW   SUPPLIED/STORAGE   AND HANDLING
COMBIGAN® is supplied sterile, in white opaque plastic LDPE bottles and tips, with blue high impact polystyrene (HIPS) caps as follows:
5 mL in 10 mL bottle NDC 0023-9211-05
10 mL in 10 mL bottle NDC 0023-9211-10
Storage: Store between 15°-25°C (59°-77°F). Protect from light.

17   PATIENT   COUNSELING INFORMATION
Patients with bronchial asthma, a history of bronchial asthma, severe chronic obstructive

pulmonary disease, sinus bradycardia, second or third degree atrioventricular block, or cardiac failure should be advised not to take this product (see **CONTRAINDICATIONS**, 4).

Patients should be instructed that ocular solutions, if handled improperly or if the tip of the dispensing container contacts the eye or surrounding structures, can become contaminated by common bacteria known to cause ocular infections. Serious damage to the eye and subsequent loss of vision may result from using contaminated solutions (see **WARNINGS AND PRECAUTIONS**, 5.9).

Patients also should be advised that if they have ocular surgery or develop an intercurrent ocular condition (e.g., trauma or infection), they should immediately seek their physician's advice concerning the continued use of the present multidose container.

If more than one topical ophthalmic drug is being used, the drugs should be administered at least five minutes apart.

Patients should be advised that **COMBIGAN®** contains benzalkonium chloride which may be absorbed by soft contact lenses. Contact lenses should be removed prior to administration of the solution. Lenses may be reinserted 15 minutes following administration of **COMBIGAN®**.

As with other similar medications, **COMBIGAN®** may cause fatigue and/or drowsiness in some patients. Patients who engage in hazardous activities should be cautioned of the potential for a decrease in mental alertness.

© 2011 Allergan, Inc., Irvine, CA 92612, U.S.A.
® marks owned by Allergan, Inc.
U.S. Patents 6,194,415; 6,465,464; 7,030,149; 7,320,976; 7,323,463; and 7,642,258
Made in the U.S.A. 72060US12C

Shown in Product Identification
Guide, page 103

LUMIGAN®   ℞
(bimatoprost ophthalmic solution) 0.03%

HIGHLIGHTS OF PRESCRIBING INFORMATION
These highlights do not include all the information needed to use LUMIGAN® 0.01% and 0.03% (bimatoprost ophthalmic solution) safely and effectively. See full prescribing information for LUMIGAN®.
LUMIGAN® 0.01% and 0.03% (bimatoprost ophthalmic solution)
Initial U.S. Approval: 2001

——————— INDICATIONS AND USAGE ———————

LUMIGAN® is a prostaglandin analog indicated for the reduction of elevated intraocular pressure in patients with open angle glaucoma or ocular hypertension. (1)

——— DOSAGE AND ADMINISTRATION ———

One drop in the affected eye(s) once daily in the evening. (2)

——— DOSAGE FORMS AND STRENGTHS ———

Solution containing 0.1 mg/mL bimatoprost (LUMIGAN® 0.01%) or containing 0.3 mg/mL bimatoprost (LUMIGAN® 0.03%). (3)

——— WARNINGS AND PRECAUTIONS ———

• Pigmentation.
  Pigmentation of the iris, periorbital tissue (eyelid) and eyelashes can occur. Iris pigmentation is likely to be permanent (5.1).
• Eyelash Changes.
  Gradual change to eyelashes including increased length, thickness and number of lashes. Usually reversible. (5.2)

——————— ADVERSE REACTIONS ———————

Most common adverse reaction (range 25% - 45%) is conjunctival hyperemia. (6.1)

Continued on next page

Lumigan—Cont.

—— USE IN SPECIFIC POPULATIONS ——

Use in pediatric patients below the age of 16 years is not recommended because of potential safety concerns related to increased pigmentation following long-term chronic use. (8.4)

See 17 for PATIENT COUNSELING INFORMATION

Revised: 08/2010

FULL PRESCRIBING INFORMATION: CONTENTS*

FULL PRESCRIBING INFORMATION

1   INDICATIONS AND USAGE

LUMIGAN® 0.01% and 0.03% (bimatoprost ophthalmic solution) is indicated for the reduction of elevated intraocular pressure in patients with open angle glaucoma or ocular hypertension.

2   DOSAGE AND ADMINISTRATION

The recommended dosage is one drop in the affected eye(s) once daily in the evening. LUMIGAN® 0.01% and 0.03% (bimatoprost ophthalmic solution) should not be administered more than once daily since it has been shown that more frequent administration of prostaglandin analogs may decrease the intraocular pressure lowering effect.

Reduction of the intraocular pressure starts approximately 4 hours after the first administration with maximum effect reached within approximately 8 to 12 hours.

LUMIGAN® may be used concomitantly with other topical ophthalmic drug products to lower intraocular pressure. If more than one topical ophthalmic drug is being used, the drugs should be administered at least five (5) minutes apart.

3   DOSAGE FORMS AND STRENGTHS

Ophthalmic solution containing bimatoprost 0.1 mg/mL (LUMIGAN® 0.01%) or containing bimatoprost 0.3 mg/mL (LUMIGAN® 0.03%).

4   CONTRAINDICATIONS

None

5   WARNINGS AND PRECAUTIONS

5.1   Pigmentation

Bimatoprost ophthalmic solution has been reported to cause changes to pigmented tissues. The most frequently reported changes have been increased pigmentation of the iris, periorbital tissue (eyelid) and eyelashes. Pigmentation is expected to increase as long as bimatoprost is administered. The pigmentation change is due to increased melanin content in the melanocytes rather than to an increase in the number of melanocytes. After discontinuation of bimatoprost, pigmentation of the iris is likely to be permanent, while pigmentation of the periorbital tissue and eyelash changes have been reported to be reversible in some patients. Patients who receive treatment should be informed of the possibility of increased pigmentation. The long term effects of increased pigmentation are not known.

Iris color change may not be noticeable for several months to years. Typically, the brown pigmentation around the pupil spreads concentrically towards the periphery of the iris and the entire iris or parts of the iris become more brownish. Neither nevi nor freckles of the iris appear to be affected by treatment. While treatment with LUMIGAN® 0.01% and 0.03% (bimatoprost ophthalmic solution) can be continued in patients who develop noticeably increased iris pigmentation, these patients should be examined regularly. (see PATIENT COUNSELING INFORMATION, 17.1).

5.2   Eyelash Changes

LUMIGAN® 0.01% and 0.03% may gradually change eyelashes and vellus hair in the treated eye. These changes include increased length, thickness, and number of lashes. Eyelash changes are usually reversible upon discontinuation of treatment.

5.3   Intraocular Inflammation

LUMIGAN® 0.01% and 0.03% should be used with caution in patients with active intraocular inflammation (e.g., uveitis) because the inflammation may be exacerbated.

5.4   Macular Edema

Macular edema, including cystoid macular edema, has been reported during treatment with bimatoprost ophthalmic solution. LUMIGAN® 0.01% and 0.03% should be used with caution in aphakic patients, in pseudophakic patients with a torn posterior lens capsule, or in patients with known risk factors for macular edema.

5.5   Angle-closure, Inflammatory, or Neovascular Glaucoma

LUMIGAN® 0.01% and 0.03% has not been evaluated for the treatment of angle-closure, inflammatory or neovascular glaucoma.

5.6   Bacterial Keratitis

There have been reports of bacterial keratitis associated with the use of multiple-dose containers of topical ophthalmic products. These containers had been inadvertently contaminated by patients who, in most cases, had a concurrent corneal disease or a disruption of the ocular epithelial surface (see PATIENT COUNSELING INFORMATION, 17.3).

5.7   Use with Contact Lenses

Contact lenses should be removed prior to instillation of LUMIGAN® 0.01% and 0.03% and may be reinserted 15 minutes following its administration.

6   ADVERSE REACTIONS

6.1   Clinical Studies Experience

Because clinical studies are conducted under widely varying conditions, adverse reaction rates observed in the clinical studies of a drug cannot be directly compared to rates in the clinical studies of another drug and may not reflect the rates observed in practice.

In clinical studies with bimatoprost ophthalmic solutions (0.01% or 0.03%) the most common adverse event was conjunctival hyperemia (range 25% – 45%). Approximately 0.5% to 3% of patients discontinued therapy due to conjunctival hypere-

mia with 0.01% or 0.03% bimatoprost ophthalmic solutions. Other common events (>10%) included growth of eyelashes, and ocular pruritus.

Additional ocular adverse events (reported in 1 to 10% of patients) with bimatoprost ophthalmic solutions included ocular dryness, visual disturbance, ocular burning, foreign body sensation, eye pain, pigmentation of the periocular skin, blepharitis, cataract, superficial punctate keratitis, eyelid erythema, ocular irritation, eyelash darkening, eye discharge, tearing, photophobia, allergic conjunctivitis, asthenopia, increases in iris pigmentation, conjunctival edema, conjunctival hemorrhage, and abnormal hair growth. Intraocular inflammation, reported as iritis was reported in less than 1% of patients.

Systemic adverse events reported in approximately 10% of patients with bimatoprost ophthalmic solutions were infections (primarily colds and upper respiratory tract infections). Other systemic adverse events (reported in 1 to 5% of patients) included headaches, abnormal liver function tests and asthenia.

8   USE IN SPECIFIC POPULATIONS

8.1   Pregnancy

Pregnancy Category C

Teratogenic effects: In embryo/fetal developmental studies in pregnant mice and rats, abortion was observed at oral doses of bimatoprost which achieved at least 33 or 97 times, respectively, the maximum intended human exposure based on blood AUC levels.

At doses at least 41 times the maximum intended human exposure based on blood AUC levels, the gestation length was reduced in the dams, the incidence of dead fetuses, late resorptions, peri- and postnatal pup mortality was increased, and pup body weights were reduced.

There are no adequate and well-controlled studies of LUMIGAN® 0.01% and 0.03% (bimatoprost ophthalmic solution) administration in pregnant women. Because animal reproductive studies are not always predictive of human response, LUMIGAN® should be administered during pregnancy only if the potential benefit justifies the potential risk to the fetus.

8.3   Nursing Mothers

It is not known whether LUMIGAN® 0.01% and 0.03% is excreted in human milk, although in animal studies, bimatoprost has been shown to be excreted in breast milk. Because many drugs are excreted in human milk, caution should be exercised when LUMIGAN® is administered to a nursing woman.

8.4   Pediatric Use

Use in pediatric patients below the age of 16 years is not recommended because of potential safety concerns related to increased pigmentation following long-term chronic use.

8.5   Geriatric Use

No overall clinical differences in safety or effectiveness have been observed between elderly and other adult patients.

8.6   Hepatic Impairment

In patients with a history of liver disease or abnormal ALT, AST and/or bilirubin at baseline, bimatoprost 0.03% had no adverse effect on liver function over 48 months.

10   OVERDOSAGE

No information is available on overdosage in humans. If overdose with LUMIGAN® 0.01% and 0.03% (bimatoprost ophthalmic solution) occurs, treatment should be symptomatic.

In oral (by gavage) mouse and rat studies, doses up to 100 mg/kg/day did not produce any toxicity. This dose expressed as mg/m^2 is at least 70 times higher than the accidental dose of one bottle of LUMIGAN® 0.03% for a 10 kg child.

11   DESCRIPTION

LUMIGAN® 0.01% and 0.03% (bimatoprost ophthalmic solution) is a synthetic prostamide analog with ocular hypotensive activity. Its chemical name is (Z)-7-[(1R,2R,3R,5S)-3,5-Dihydroxy-2-[(1E,3S)-3-hydroxy-5-phenyl-1-pentenyl]cyclopen-

...yl-5-*N*-ethylheptenamide, and its molecular weight is 415.58. Its molecular formula is $C_{25}H_{37}NO_4$. Its chemical structure is:

Bimatoprost is a powder, which is very soluble in ethyl alcohol and methyl alcohol and slightly soluble in water. **LUMIGAN®** 0.01% and 0.03% is a clear, isotonic, colorless, sterile ophthalmic solution with an osmolality of approximately 290 mOsmol/kg.

LUMIGAN® 0.01% contains **Active**: bimatoprost 0.1 mg/mL; **Preservative**: benzalkonium chloride 0.2 mg/mL; **Inactives**: sodium chloride; sodium phosphate, dibasic; citric acid; and purified water. Sodium hydroxide and/or hydrochloric acid may be added to adjust pH. The pH during its shelf life ranges from 6.8-7.8.

LUMIGAN® 0.03% contains **Active**: bimatoprost 0.3 mg/mL; **Preservative**: benzalkonium chloride 0.05 mg/mL; **Inactives**: sodium chloride; sodium phosphate, dibasic; citric acid; and purified water. Sodium hydroxide and/or hydrochloric acid may be added to adjust pH. The pH during its shelf life ranges from 6.8-7.8.

2 CLINICAL PHARMACOLOGY

2.1 Mechanism of Action

Bimatoprost, a prostaglandin analog, is a synthetic structural analog of prostaglandin with ocular hypotensive activity. It selectively mimics the effects of naturally occurring substances, prostamides. Bimatoprost is believed to lower intraocular pressure (IOP) in humans by increasing outflow of aqueous humor through both the trabecular meshwork and uveoscleral routes. Elevated IOP presents a major risk factor for glaucomatous field loss. The higher the level of IOP, the greater the likelihood of optic nerve damage and visual field loss.

2.3 Pharmacokinetics

Absorption: After one drop of bimatoprost ophthalmic solution 0.03% was administered once daily to both eyes of 15 healthy subjects for two weeks, blood concentrations peaked within 10 minutes after dosing and were below the lower limit of detection (0.025 ng/mL) in most subjects within 1.5 hours after dosing. Mean C_{max} and AUC_{0-24hr} values were similar on days 7 and 14 at approximately 0.08 ng/mL and 0.09 ng•hr/mL, respectively, indicating that steady state is reached during the first week of ocular dosing. There was no significant systemic drug accumulation over time.

Distribution: Bimatoprost is moderately distributed into body tissues with a steady-state volume of distribution of 0.67 L/kg. In human blood, bimatoprost resides mainly in the plasma. Approximately 12% of bimatoprost remains unbound in human plasma.

Metabolism: Bimatoprost is the major circulating species in the blood once it reaches the systemic circulation following ocular dosing. Bimatoprost then undergoes oxidation, N-deethylation and glucuronidation to form a diverse variety of metabolites.

Elimination: Following an intravenous dose of radiolabeled bimatoprost (3.12 μg/kg) to six healthy subjects, the maximum blood concentration of unchanged drug was 12.2 ng/mL and decreased rapidly with an elimination half-life of approximately 45 minutes. The total blood clearance of bimatoprost was 1.5 L/hr/kg. Up to 67% of the administered dose was excreted in the urine while 25% of the dose was recovered in the feces.

13 NONCLINICAL TOXICOLOGY

13.1 Carcinogenesis, Mutagenesis, Impairment of Fertility

Bimatoprost was not carcinogenic in either mice or rats when administered by oral gavage at doses of up to 2 mg/kg/day and 1 mg/kg/day respectively (at least 192 and 291 times the recommended human exposure based on blood AUC levels respectively) for 104 weeks.

Bimatoprost was not mutagenic or clastogenic in the Ames test, in the mouse lymphoma test, or in the *in vivo* mouse micronucleus tests.

Bimatoprost did not impair fertility in male or female rats up to doses of 0.6 mg/kg/day (at least 103 times the recommended human exposure based on blood AUC levels).

14 CLINICAL STUDIES

In clinical studies of patients with open angle glaucoma or ocular hypertension with a mean baseline IOP of 26 mmHg, the IOP-lowering effect of **LUMIGAN®** 0.03% (bimatoprost ophthalmic solution) once daily (in the evening) was 7-8 mmHg. In a 3 month clinical study of patients with open angle glaucoma or ocular hypertension with an average baseline IOP of 23.5 mmHg, the IOP-lowering effect of **LUMIGAN®** 0.01% once daily (in the evening) was up to 7.5 mmHg and was approximately 0.5 mmHg less effective than **LUMIGAN®** 0.03%. In this same study, **LUMIGAN®** 0.01% also had a similar overall safety profile compared with **LUMIGAN®** 0.03%. After 12 months of treatment, discontinuations were 8.1% for **LUMIGAN®** 0.01% and 13.4% for **LUMIGAN®** 0.03%.

16 HOW SUPPLIED/STORAGE AND HANDLING

LUMIGAN® (bimatoprost ophthalmic solution) 0.01% is supplied sterile in opaque white low density polyethylene ophthalmic dispenser bottles and tips with turquoise polystyrene caps in the following sizes:
2.5 mL fill in a 5 mL container - NDC 0023-3205-03
5 mL fill in a 10 mL container - NDC 0023-3205-05
7.5 mL fill in a 10 mL container - NDC 0023-3205-08

LUMIGAN® (bimatoprost ophthalmic solution) 0.03% is supplied sterile in opaque white low density polyethylene ophthalmic dispenser bottles and tips with turquoise polystyrene caps in the following sizes:
2.5 mL fill in 5 mL container - NDC 0023-9187-03
5 mL fill in 10 mL container - NDC 0023-9187-05
7.5 mL fill in 10 mL container - NDC 0023-9187-07

Storage: **LUMIGAN®** 0.01% and 0.03% should be stored at 2° to 25°C (36° to 77°F).

17 PATIENT COUNSELING INFORMATION

17.1 Potential for Pigmentation

Patients should be advised about the potential for increased brown pigmentation of the iris, which may be permanent. Patients should also be informed about the possibility of eyelid skin darkening, which may be reversible after discontinuation of **LUMIGAN®** 0.01% and 0.03% (bimatoprost ophthalmic solution).

17.2 Potential for Eyelash Changes

Patients should also be informed of the possibility of eyelash and vellus hair changes in the treated eye during treatment with **LUMIGAN®** 0.01% and 0.03%. These changes may result in a disparity between eyes in length, thickness, pigmentation, number of eyelashes or vellus hairs, and/or direction of eyelash growth. Eyelash changes are usually reversible upon discontinuation of treatment.

17.3 Handling the Container

Patients should be instructed to avoid allowing the tip of the dispensing container to contact the eye, surrounding structures, fingers, or any other surface in order to avoid contamination of the solution by common bacteria known to cause ocular infections. Serious damage to the eye and subsequent loss of vision may result from using contaminated solutions.

17.4 When to Seek Physician Advice

Patients should also be advised that if they develop an intercurrent ocular condition (e.g., trauma or infection), have ocular surgery, or develop any ocular reactions, particularly conjunctivitis and eyelid reactions, they should immediately seek their physician's advice concerning the continued use of **LUMIGAN®** 0.01% and 0.03%.

17.5 Use with Contact Lenses

Patients should be advised that **LUMIGAN®** 0.01% and 0.03% contains benzalkonium chloride, which may be absorbed by soft contact lenses. Contact lenses should be removed prior to instillation of **LUMIGAN®** and may be reinserted 15 minutes following its administration.

17.6 Use with Other Ophthalmic Drugs

If more than one topical ophthalmic drug is being used, the drugs should be administered at least five (5) minutes between applications.

© 2010 Allergan, Inc., Irvine, CA 92612
® marks owned by Allergan, Inc.
U.S. Patents 5,688,819 and 6,403,649
71807US12B

Shown in Product Identification Guide, page 103

OZURDEX® ℞
(dexamethasone intravitreal implant)

HIGHLIGHTS OF PRESCRIBING INFORMATION
These highlights do not include all the information needed to use OZURDEX® safely and effectively. See full prescribing information for OZURDEX®.
OZURDEX® (dexamethasone intravitreal implant)
Initial U.S. Approval: 1958

——— **INDICATIONS AND USAGE** ———
OZURDEX® is a corticosteroid indicated for the treatment of macular edema following branch retinal vein occlusion (BRVO) or central retinal vein occlusion (CRVO) (1.1) and for the treatment of non-infectious uveitis affecting the posterior segment of the eye. (1.2)

——— **DOSAGE AND ADMINISTRATION** ———
• For ophthalmic intravitreal injection only. (2.1)
• The intravitreal injection procedure should be carried out under controlled aseptic conditions. Following the intravitreal injection, patients should be monitored for elevation in intraocular pressure and for endophthalmitis. (2.2)

——— **DOSAGE FORMS AND STRENGTHS** ———
• Intravitreal implant containing dexamethasone 0.7 mg in the **NOVADUR®** solid polymer drug delivery system. (3)

——— **CONTRAINDICATIONS** ———
• Ocular or periocular infections. (4.1)
• Advanced glaucoma. (4.2)

——— **WARNINGS AND PRECAUTIONS** ———
• Intravitreal injections have been associated with endophthalmitis, eye inflammation, increased intraocular pressure, and retinal detachments. Patients should be monitored following the injection. (5.1)
• Use of corticosteroids may produce posterior subcapsular cataracts, increased intraocular pressure, glaucoma, and may enhance the establishment of secondary ocular infections due to bacteria, fungi, or viruses. (5.2)

——— **ADVERSE REACTIONS** ———
In controlled studies, the most common adverse reactions reported by ≥ 20% of patients were increased intraocular pressure and conjunctival hemorrhage. (6.1)
To report SUSPECTED ADVERSE REACTIONS, contact Allergan at 1-800-433-8871 or FDA at 1-800-FDA-1088 or www.fda.gov/medwatch.

Continued on next page

Ozurdex—Cont.

See 17 for PATIENT COUNSELING INFORMA-
TION

Revised: 10/2011

FULL PRESCRIBING INFORMATION: CONTENTS*

FULL PRESCRIBING INFORMATION

1 INDICATIONS AND USAGE

1.1 Retinal Vein Occlusion

OZURDEX® (dexamethasone intravitreal implant) is indicated for the treatment of macular edema following branch retinal vein occlusion (BRVO) or central retinal vein occlusion (CRVO).

1.2 Posterior Segment Uveitis

OZURDEX® is indicated for the treatment of non-infectious uveitis affecting the posterior segment of the eye.

2 DOSAGE AND ADMINISTRATION

2.1 General Dosing Information

For ophthalmic intravitreal injection only.

2.2 Administration

The intravitreal injection procedure should be carried out under controlled aseptic conditions which include the use of sterile gloves, a sterile drape, and a sterile eyelid speculum (or equivalent). Adequate anesthesia and a broad-spectrum microbicide are recommended to be given prior to the injection.

Remove the foil pouch from the carton and examine for damage. Then, open the foil pouch over a sterile field and gently drop the applicator on a sterile tray. Carefully remove the cap from the applicator. Hold the applicator in one hand and pull the safety tab straight off the applicator. **Do not twist or flex the tab**. The long axis of the applicator should be held parallel to the limbus, and the sclera should be engaged at an oblique angle with the bevel of the needle up (away from the sclera) to create a shelved scleral path. The tip of the needle is advanced within the sclera for about 1 mm (parallel to the limbus), then re-directed toward the center of the eye and advanced until penetration of the sclera is completed and the vitreous cavity is entered. The needle should not be advanced past the point where the sleeve touches the conjunctiva.

Slowly depress the actuator button until an audible click is noted. Before withdrawing the applicator from the eye, make sure that the actuator button is fully depressed and has locked flush with the applicator surface. Remove the needle in the same direction as used to enter the vitreous.

Following the intravitreal injection, patients should be monitored for elevation in intraocular pressure and for endophthalmitis. Monitoring may consist of a check for perfusion of the optic nerve head immediately after the injection, tonometry within 30 minutes following the injection, and biomicroscopy between two and seven days following the injection. Patients should be instructed to report any symptoms suggestive of endophthalmitis without delay.

Each applicator can only be used for the treatment of a single eye. If the contralateral eye requires treatment, a new applicator must be used, and the sterile field, syringe, gloves, drapes, and eyelid speculum should be changed before **OZURDEX®** is administered to the other eye.

3 DOSAGE FORMS AND STRENGTHS

Intravitreal implant containing dexamethasone 0.7 mg in the **NOVADUR®** solid polymer drug delivery system.

4 CONTRAINDICATIONS

4.1 Ocular or Periocular Infections

OZURDEX® (dexamethasone intravitreal implant) is contraindicated in patients with active or suspected ocular or periocular infections including most viral diseases of the cornea and conjunctiva, including active epithelial herpes simplex keratitis (dendritic keratitis), vaccinia, varicella, mycobacterial infections, and fungal diseases.

4.2 Advanced Glaucoma

OZURDEX® is contraindicated in patients with advanced glaucoma.

4.3 Hypersensitivity

OZURDEX® is contraindicated in patients with known hypersensitivity to any components of this product.

5 WARNINGS AND PRECAUTIONS

5.1 Intravitreal Injection-related Effects

Intravitreal injections have been associated with endophthalmitis, eye inflammation, increased intraocular pressure, and retinal detachments. Patients should be monitored following the injection (see **PATIENT COUNSELING INFORMATION**, 17).

5.2 Potential Steroid-related Effects

Use of corticosteroids may produce posterior subcapsular cataracts, increased intraocular pressure, glaucoma, and may enhance the establishment of secondary ocular infections due to bacteria, fungi, or viruses.

Corticosteroids should be used cautiously in patients with a history of ocular herpes simplex.

6 ADVERSE REACTIONS

6.1 Clinical Studies Experience

Because clinical studies are conducted under widely varying conditions, adverse reaction rates observed in the clinical studies of a drug cannot be directly compared to rates in the clinical studies of another drug and may not reflect the rates observed in practice.

Adverse reactions associated with ophthalmic steroids include elevated intraocular pressure, which may be associated with optic nerve damage, visual acuity and field defects, posterior subcapsular cataract formation, secondary ocular infection from pathogens including herpes simplex, and perforation of the globe where there is thinning of the cornea or sclera.

The following information is based on the combined clinical trial results from 3 initial, randomized, 6-month, sham-controlled studies (2 for retinal vein occlusion and 1 for posterior segment uveitis):

Adverse Reactions Reported by Greater than 2% of Patients in the First Six Months

MedDRA Term	OZURDEX® N=497 (%)	Sham N=498 (%)
Intraocular pressure increased	125 (25%)	10 (2%)
Conjunctival hemorrhage	108 (22%)	79 (16%)
Eye pain	40 (8%)	26 (5%)
Conjunctival hyperemia	33 (7%)	27 (5%)
Ocular hypertension	23 (5%)	3 (1%)
Cataract	24 (5%)	10 (2%)
Vitreous detachment	12 (2%)	8 (2%)
Headache	19 (4%)	12 (2%)

Increased IOP with **OZURDEX®** peaked at approximately week 8. During the initial treatment period, 1% (3/421) of the patients who received **OZURDEX®** required surgical procedures for management of elevated IOP.

Following a second injection of **OZURDEX®** in cases where a second injection was indicated, the overall incidence of cataracts was higher after 1 year.

8 USE IN SPECIFIC POPULATIONS

8.1 Pregnancy

Teratogenic Effects: Pregnancy Category C

Topical dexamethasone has been shown to be teratogenic in mice producing fetal resorptions and cleft palate. In the rabbit, dexamethasone produced fetal resorptions and multiple abnormalities involving the head, ears, limbs, palate, etc. Pregnant rhesus monkeys treated with dexamethasone sodium phosphate intramuscularly at 1 mg/kg/day every other day for 28 days or at 10 mg/kg/day once or every other day at 3 or 5 days between gestation days 23 and 49 had fetuses with minor cranial abnormalities. A 1 mg/kg/dose in pregnant rhesus monkeys would be approximately 85 times higher than an **OZURDEX®** injection in humans (assuming 60 kg body weight).

There are no adequate and well-controlled studies in pregnant women. OZURDEX® (dexamethasone intravitreal implant) should be used during pregnancy only if the potential benefit justifies the potential risk to the fetus.

8.3 Nursing Mothers

It is not known whether ocular administration of corticosteroids could result in sufficient systemic absorption to produce detectable quantities in human milk. Systemically administered corticosteroids appear in human milk and could suppress growth, interfere with endogenous corticosteroid production, or cause other untoward effects. Caution should be exercised when corticosteroids are administered to a nursing woman.

8.4 Pediatric Use

Safety and effectiveness of **OZURDEX®** in pediatric patients have not been established.

8.5 Geriatric Use

No overall differences in safety or effectiveness have been observed between elderly and younger patients.

11 DESCRIPTION

OZURDEX® is an intravitreal implant containing 0.7 mg (700 µg) dexamethasone in the **NOVADUR®** solid polymer drug delivery system. OZURDEX® is preloaded into a single-use, specially designed **DDS®** applicator to facilitate injection of the rod-shaped implant directly into the vitreous. The **NOVADUR®** system contains poly (D,L-lactide-co-glycolide) PLGA intravitreal polymer matrix without a preservative. The chemical name for

exemethasone is Pregna-1,4-diene-3,20-dione,
-fluoro-11,17,21-trihydroxy-16-methyl-, (11β,16α)-.
ts structural formula is:

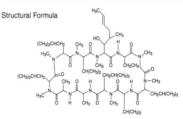

W 392.47; molecular formula: $C_{22}H_{29}FO_5$
Dexamethasone occurs as a white to cream-colored
crystalline powder having not more than a slight
odor, and is practically insoluble in water and very
soluble in alcohol.
The PLGA matrix slowly degrades to lactic acid and
glycolic acid.

12 CLINICAL PHARMACOLOGY

12.1 Mechanism of Action
Dexamethasone, a potent corticosteroid, has been
known to suppress inflammation by inhibiting
multiple inflammatory cytokines resulting in
decreased edema, fibrin deposition, capillary
leakage and migration of inflammatory cells.

12.3 Pharmacokinetics
Plasma concentrations were obtained from 21
patients in two 6 month studies prior to dosing and
on Days 7, 30, 60, and 90 following the intravitreal
implant containing 0.35 mg or 0.7 mg
dexamethasone. In both studies, the majority of
plasma dexamethasone concentrations were below
the lower limit of quantitation (LLOQ = 50 pg/mL).
Plasma dexamethasone concentrations from 10 of
73 samples in the 0.7 mg dose group and from 2 of
72 samples in the 0.35 mg dose group were above
the LLOQ, ranging from 52 pg/mL to 94 pg/mL. The
highest plasma concentration value of 94 pg/mL
was observed in one subject from the 0.7 mg group.
Plasma dexamethasone concentration did not
appear to be related to age, body weight, or sex of
patients.
In an in vitro metabolism study, following the
incubation of $[^{14}C]$-dexamethasone with human
cornea, iris-ciliary body, choroid, retina, vitreous
humor, and sclera tissues for 18 hours, no
metabolites were observed.

13 NONCLINICAL TOXICOLOGY

13.1 Carcinogenesis, Mutagenesis, Impairment of Fertility
No adequate studies in animals have been
conducted to determine whether **OZURDEX**®
(dexamethasone intravitreal implant) has the
potential for carcinogenesis.
Although no adequate studies have been conducted
to determine the mutagenic potential of
OZURDEX®, dexamethasone has been shown to
have no mutagenic effects in bacterial and
mammalian cells in vitro or in the in vivo mouse
micronucleus test.

14 CLINICAL STUDIES

Retinal Vein Occlusion
The efficacy of **OZURDEX**® for the treatment of
macular edema following branch retinal vein
occlusion (BRVO) or central retinal vein occlusion
(CRVO) was assessed in two, multicenter, double-
masked, randomized, parallel studies.
Following a single injection, **OZURDEX**®
demonstrated the following clinical results for the
percent of patients with ≥ 15 letters of improvement from baseline in best-corrected visual acuity
(BCVA):
[See table above]
In each individual study and in a pooled analysis,
time to achieve ≥ 15 letters (3-line) improvement in
BCVA cumulative response rate curves were
significantly faster with **OZURDEX**® compared to
sham
(p < 0.01), with **OZURDEX**® treated patients
achieving a 3-line improvement in BCVA earlier
than sham-treated patients.
The onset of a ≥ 15 letter (3-line) improvement in
BCVA with **OZURDEX**® occurs within the first two
months after implantation in approximately

	Number (Percent) of Patients with ≥ 15 Letters Improvement from Baseline in BCVA					
	Study 1			**Study 2**		
Study Day	**DEX 700** N=201	**Sham** N=202	**p-value***	**DEX 700** N=226	**Sham** N=224	**p-value***
Day 30	40 (20%)	15 (7%)	< 0.01	51 (23%)	17 (8%)	< 0.01
Day 60	58 (29%)	21 (10%)	< 0.01	67 (30%)	27 (12%)	< 0.01
Day 90	45 (22%)	25 (12%)	< 0.01	48 (21%)	31 (14%)	0.039
Day 180	39 (19%)	37 (18%)	0.780	53 (24%)	38 (17%)	0.087

*P-values were based on the Pearson's chi-square test.

20-30% of subjects. The duration of effect persists
approximately one to three months after onset of
this effect.

Posterior Segment Uveitis
The efficacy of **OZURDEX**® was assessed in a single,
multicenter, masked, randomized study of 153
patients with non-infectious uveitis affecting the
posterior segment of the eye.
After a single injection, the percent of patients
reaching a vitreous haze score of 0 (where a score of
0 represents no inflammation) was statistically
significantly greater for patients receiving
OZURDEX® versus sham at week 8 (primary time
point) (47% vs. 12%). The percent of patients
achieving a 3-line improvement from baseline
BCVA was 43% for patients receiving **OZURDEX**®
vs. 7% for sham at week 8.

16 HOW SUPPLIED/STORAGE AND HANDLING
OZURDEX® (dexamethasone intravitreal implant)
0.7 mg is supplied in a foil pouch with 1 single-use
plastic applicator, NDC 0023-3348-07.
Storage: Store at 15°-30°C (59°-86°F).

17 PATIENT COUNSELING INFORMATION
In the days following intravitreal injection of
OZURDEX®, patients are at risk for potential
complications including in particular, but not
limited to, the development of endophthalmitis or
elevated intraocular pressure. If the eye becomes
red, sensitive to light, painful, or develops a change
in vision, the patients should seek immediate care
from an ophthalmologist.
Patients may experience temporary visual blurring
after receiving an intravitreal injection. They
should not drive or use machines until this has
resolved.
© 2011 Allergan, Inc., Irvine, CA 92612, U.S.A.
® marks owned by Allergan, Inc.
U.S. Patents 6,726,918; 6,899,717; 7,033,605; and
7,767,223
Made in Ireland 72212US12C

RESTASIS®   ℞
(cyclosporine ophthalmic emulsion) 0.05%
Sterile, Preservative-Free

DESCRIPTION
RESTASIS® (cyclosporine ophthalmic emulsion)
0.05% contains a topical immunomodulator with
anti-inflammatory effects. Cyclosporine's chemical
name is Cyclo[[(E)-($2S,3R,4R$)-3-hydroxy-4-methyl-
2-(methylamino)-6-octenoyl]-L-2-aminobutyryl-N-
methylglycyl-N-methyl-L-leucyl-L-valyl-N-methyl-
L-leucyl-L-alanyl-D-alanyl-N-methyl-L-leucyl-N-
methyl-L-leucyl-N-methyl-L-valyl] and it has the
following structure:
[See chemical structure at top of next column]
Cyclosporine is a fine white powder. **RESTASIS**®
appears as a white opaque to slightly translucent
homogeneous emulsion. It has an osmolality of 230
to 320 mOsmol/kg and a pH of 6.5-8.0. Each mL of
RESTASIS® ophthalmic emulsion contains: **Active:**
cyclosporine 0.05%. **Inactives:** glycerin; castor oil;
polysorbate 80; carbomer copolymer type A; purified
water; and sodium hydroxide to adjust pH.

Structural Formula

Formula: $C_{62}H_{111}N_{11}O_{12}$ Mol. Wt.: 1202.6

CLINICAL PHARMACOLOGY
Mechanism of Action
Cyclosporine is an immunosuppressive agent when
administered systemically.
In patients whose tear production is presumed to be
suppressed due to ocular inflammation associated
with keratoconjunctivitis sicca, cyclosporine
emulsion is thought to act as a partial
immunomodulator. The exact mechanism of action
is not known.

Pharmacokinetics
Blood cyclosporin A concentrations were measured
using a specific high pressure liquid
chromatography-mass spectrometry assay. Blood
concentrations of cyclosporine, in all the samples
collected, after topical administration of
RESTASIS® 0.05%, BID, in humans for up to 12
months, were below the quantitation limit of 0.1 ng/
mL. There was no detectable drug accumulation in
blood during 12 months of treatment with
RESTASIS® ophthalmic emulsion.

Clinical Evaluations
Four multicenter, randomized, adequate and
well-controlled clinical studies were performed in
approximately 1200 patients with moderate to
severe keratoconjunctivitis sicca. **RESTASIS**®
demonstrated statistically significant increases in
Schirmer wetting of 10 mm versus vehicle at six
months in patients whose tear production was
presumed to be suppressed due to ocular
inflammation. This effect was seen in
approximately 15% of **RESTASIS**® ophthalmic
emulsion treated patients versus approximately 5%
of vehicle treated patients. Increased tear
production was not seen in patients currently
taking topical anti-inflammatory drugs or using
punctal plugs.
No increase in bacterial or fungal ocular infections
was reported following administration of
RESTASIS®.

INDICATIONS AND USAGE
RESTASIS® ophthalmic emulsion is indicated to
increase tear production in patients whose tear
production is presumed to be suppressed due to
ocular inflammation associated with
keratoconjunctivitis sicca. Increased tear
production was not seen in patients currently
taking topical anti-inflammatory drugs or using
punctal plugs.

CONTRAINDICATIONS
RESTASIS® is contraindicated in patients with
active ocular infections and in patients with known
or suspected hypersensitivity to any of the
ingredients in the formulation.

Continued on next page

Restasis—Cont.

WARNING

RESTASIS® ophthalmic emulsion has not been studied in patients with a history of herpes keratitis.

PRECAUTIONS

General: For ophthalmic use only.

Information for Patients

The emulsion from one individual single-use vial is to be used immediately after opening for administration to one or both eyes, and the remaining contents should be discarded immediately after administration.

Do not allow the tip of the vial to touch the eye or any surface, as this may contaminate the emulsion.

RESTASIS® should not be administered while wearing contact lenses. Patients with decreased tear production typically should not wear contact lenses. If contact lenses are worn, they should be removed prior to the administration of the emulsion. Lenses may be reinserted 15 minutes following administration of **RESTASIS®** ophthalmic emulsion.

Carcinogenesis, Mutagenesis, and Impairment of Fertility

Systemic carcinogenicity studies were carried out in male and female mice and rats. In the 78-week oral (diet) mouse study, at doses of 1, 4, and 16 mg/kg/day, evidence of a statistically significant trend was found for lymphocytic lymphomas in females, and the incidence of hepatocellular carcinomas in mid-dose males significantly exceeded the control value.

In the 24-month oral (diet) rat study, conducted at 0.5, 2, and 8 mg/kg/day, pancreatic islet cell adenomas significantly exceeded the control rate in the low dose level. The hepatocellular carcinomas and pancreatic islet cell adenomas were not dose related. The low doses in mice and rats are approximately 1000 and 500 times greater, respectively, than the daily human dose of one drop (28 μL) of 0.05% **RESTASIS®** BID into each eye of a 60 kg person (0.001 mg/kg/day), assuming that the entire dose is absorbed.

Cyclosporine has not been found mutagenic/genotoxic in the Ames Test, the V79-HGPRT Test, the micronucleus test in mice and Chinese hamsters, the chromosome-aberration tests in Chinese hamster bone-marrow, the mouse dominant lethal assay, and the DNA-repair test in sperm from treated mice. A study analyzing sister chromatid exchange (SCE) induction by cyclosporine using human lymphocytes *in vitro* gave indication of a positive effect (i.e., induction of SCE).

No impairment in fertility was demonstrated in studies in male and female rats receiving oral doses of cyclosporine up to 15 mg/kg/day (approximately 15,000 times the human daily dose of 0.001 mg/kg/day) for 9 weeks (male) and 2 weeks (female) prior to mating.

Pregnancy-Teratogenic Effects

Pregnancy category C.

Teratogenic Effects: No evidence of teratogenicity was observed in rats or rabbits receiving oral doses of cyclosporine up to 300 mg/kg/day during organogenesis. These doses in rats and rabbits are approximately 300,000 times greater than the daily human dose of one drop (28 μL) 0.05% **RESTASIS®** BID into each eye of a 60 kg person (0.001mg/kg/day), assuming that the entire dose is absorbed.

Non-Teratogenic Effects: Adverse effects were seen in reproduction studies in rats and rabbits only at dose levels toxic to dams. At toxic doses (rats at 30 mg/kg/day and rabbits at 100 mg/kg/day), cyclosporine oral solution, USP, was embryo- and fetotoxic as indicated by increased pre- and postnatal mortality and reduced fetal weight together with related skeletal retardations. These doses are 30,000 and 100,000 times greater, respectively than the daily human dose of one drop (28 μL) of 0.05% **RESTASIS®** BID into each eye of a 60 kg person (0.001 mg/kg/day), assuming that the entire dose is absorbed. No evidence of embryofetal toxicity was observed in rats or rabbits receiving cyclosporine at oral doses up to 17 mg/kg/day or 30 mg/kg/day, respectively, during organogenesis. These doses in rats and rabbits are approximately 17,000 and 30,000 times greater, respectively, than the daily human dose.

Offspring of rats receiving a 45 mg/kg/day oral dose of cyclosporine from Day 15 of pregnancy until Day 21 postpartum, a maternally toxic level, exhibited an increase in postnatal mortality; this dose is 45,000 times greater than the daily human topical dose, 0.001 mg/kg/day, assuming that the entire dose is absorbed. No adverse events were observed at oral doses up to 15 mg/kg/day (15,000 times greater than the daily human dose).

There are no adequate and well-controlled studies of **RESTASIS®** in pregnant women. **RESTASIS®** should be administered to a pregnant woman only if clearly needed.

Nursing Mothers

Cyclosporine is known to be excreted in human milk following systemic administration but excretion in human milk after topical treatment has not been investigated. Although blood concentrations are undetectable after topical administration of **RESTASIS®** ophthalmic emulsion, caution should be exercised when **RESTASIS®** is administered to a nursing woman.

Pediatric Use

The safety and efficacy of **RESTASIS®** ophthalmic emulsion have not been established in pediatric patients below the age of 16.

Geriatric Use

No overall difference in safety or effectiveness has been observed between elderly and younger patients.

ADVERSE REACTIONS

The most common adverse event following the use of **RESTASIS®** was ocular burning (17%).

Other events reported in 1% to 5% of patients included conjunctival hyperemia, discharge, epiphora, eye pain, foreign body sensation, pruritus, stinging, and visual disturbance (most often blurring).

DOSAGE AND ADMINISTRATION

Invert the unit dose vial a few times to obtain a uniform, white, opaque emulsion before using. Instill one drop of **RESTASIS®** ophthalmic emulsion twice a day in each eye approximately 12 hours apart. **RESTASIS®** can be used concomitantly with artificial tears, allowing a 15 minute interval between products. Discard vial immediately after use.

HOW SUPPLIED

RESTASIS® ophthalmic emulsion is packaged in single use vials. Each vial contains 0.4 mL fill in a 0.9 mL LDPE vial; 30 vials are packaged in a polypropylene tray with an aluminum peelable lid. The entire contents of each tray (30 vials) must be dispensed intact. **RESTASIS®** is also provided in a 60 count (2 × 30) package (one month supply) that must be dispensed intact.

30 Vials 0.4 mL each - NDC 0023-9163-30
60 (2 × 30) Vials 0.4 mL each - NDC 0023-9163-60

Storage: Store **RESTASIS®** ophthalmic emulsion at 15 - 25° C (59 - 77° F).

KEEP OUT OF THE REACH OF CHILDREN.

Rx Only

Revised: 02/2010

© 2010 Allergan, Inc. Irvine, CA 92612, U.S.A.
® marks owned by Allergan, Inc.
U.S. Patent 5,474,979
Made in the U.S.A. 71876US14B

Shown in Product Identification Guide, page 103

Bausch & Lomb Incorporated

ONE BAUSCH & LOMB PLACE
ROCHESTER NY 14604

7 GIRALDA FARMS
MADISON, NJ 07940

Direct Inquiries to:
(800) 323-0000
Consumer Affairs
1-800-553-5340

Product List-Bausch & Lomb Pharma

NDC 24208	PRODUCT	
-601-10	**ALAWAY®** Ketotifen Fumarate Ophthalmic Solution Antihistamine Eye Drops 10 mL	OTC
-353-	**ALREX®** loteprednol etabonate ophthalmic suspension, 0.2% 5 mL: -05 10 mL: -10	℞
-825-55	**ATROPINE SULFATE OPHTHALMIC OINTMENT USP, 1%** 3.5 gram tubes	℞
-750-	**ATROPINE SULFATE OPHTHALMIC SOLUTION USP, 1%** 5 mL: -60 15 mL: -06	℞
-446-05	**BESIVANCE™** Besifloxacin ophthalmic suspension, 0.6% 5 mL	℞
411-	**BRIMONIDINE TARTRATE OPHTHALMIC SOLUTION, 0.2%** 5 mL: -05 10 mL: -10 15 mL: -15	℞
555-55	**BACITRACIN ZINC & POLYMYXIN B SULFATE OPHTHALMIC OINTMENT USP** 3.5 g tube	℞
367-	**CARTEOLOL HYDROCHLORIDE OPHTHALMIC SOLUTION, USP, 1%** 5 mL: -05 10 mL: -10 15 mL: -15	℞
-735-	**CYCLOPENTOLATE HYDROCHLORIDE OPHTHALMIC SOLUTION USP, 1%** 2 mL: -01 15 mL: -06	℞
-720-02	**DEXAMETHASONE SODIUM PHOSPHATE** Ophthalmic Solution, USP, 0.1% 5 mL	℞
457-	**DICLOFENAC SODIUM OPHTHALMIC SOLUTION, 0.1%** 2.5 mL: -25 5 mL: -05	℞
485-10	**DORZOLAMIDE HCl OPHTHALMIC SOLUTION, 2%** 10 mL	℞
486-10	**DORZOLAMIDE HCl/ TIMOLOL MALEATE OPHTHALMIC SOLUTION** 10 mL	℞

Code	Product	Type
10-	**ERYTHROMYCIN OPHTHALMIC** Ointment USP, 0.5% 50 × 1 g tube -19 3.5 g tube -55	℞
32-05	**FLUORESCEIN SODIUM & BENOXINATE HCl OPHTHALMIC SOLUTION** USP, 0.25%/0.4% 5 ml	℞
14-25	**FLURBIPROFEN** Sodium Ophthalmic Solution USP, 0.03% 2.5 ml	℞
580-	**GENTAMICIN SULFATE Ophthalmic Solution** USP, 0.3% 5 mL: -60 15 mL: -64	℞
63-25	**LATANOPROST OPHTHALMIC SOLUTION, 0.005%** 2.5 mL - 25	℞
505-	**LEVOBUNOLOL HYDROCHLORIDE OPHTHALMIC SOLUTION USP, 0.5%** 5 mL: -05 10 mL: -10 15 mL: -15	℞
299-	**LOTEMAX®** loteprednol etabonate ophthalmic suspension, 0.5% 5 mL -05 10 mL -10 15 mL -15	℞
43-35	**LOTEMAX® OINTMENT** loteprednol etabonate opthalmic ointment 0.5% 3.5 g tube - 35	℞
539-20	**MIOCHOL®-E** acetylcholine chloride intraocular solution 1 Kit in 1 Blister Pack - 20	℞
385	**MURO 128® 5% OINTMENT** Sodium Chloride Hypertonicity Ophthalmic Ointment, 5% 3.5g: -55 TWIN PACK 2×3.5g: -56	OTC
276-15	**MURO 128® 2% SOLUTION** Sodium Chloride Hypertonicity Ophthalmic Solution, 2% 15 mL	OTC
277-	**MURO 128® 5% SOLUTION** Sodium Chloride Hypertonicity Ophthalmic Solution, 5% 15 mL: -15 30 mL: -30	OTC
785-55	**NEOMYCIN & POLYMYXIN B SULFATES, BACITRACIN ZINC AND HYDROCORTISONE OPHTHALMIC** Ointment USP 3.5 g tube	℞
780-55	**NEOMYCIN AND POLYMYXIN B SULFATES AND BACITRACIN ZINC OPHTHALMIC** Ointment USP 3.5 gram tubes	℞
795-35	**NEOMYCIN AND POLYMYXIN B SULFATES AND DEXAMETHASONE OPHTHALMIC OINTMENT USP** 3.5 gram tubes	℞

Code	Product	Type
830-60	**NEOMYCIN AND POLYMYXIN B SULFATES AND DEXAMETHASONE Ophthalmic Suspension USP** 5 mL	℞
790-62	**NEOMYCIN AND POLYMYXIN B SULFATES AND GRAMICIDIN Ophthalmic Solution USP** 10 mL	℞
465-30	**OCUVITE® ADULT 50+** Eye Vitamin and Mineral Supplement 50 soft gels	OTC
465-40	30 soft gels	
387-62	**OCUVITE® LUTEIN** Eye Vitamin & Mineral Supplement 120 tablets	OTC
387-60	60 tablets	
403-19	**OCUVITE® LUTEIN & ZEAXANTHIN** Eye Vitamin and Mineral Supplement Bottle of 36 capsules	OTC
403-73	Bottle of 72 capsules	
434-	**OFLOXACIN OPHTHALMIC SOLUTION** 5 mL -05 10 mL -10	℞
430-15	**OPCON-A®** pheniramine maleate 0.315% and naphazoline hydrochloride 0.02675% ophthalmic solution Itching and Redness reliever eye drops 15 mL TWIN PACK 2 × 15 mL	OTC
-275-	**OPTIPRANOLOL®** (metipranolol ophthalmic solution) 0.3% 5 mL -07 10 mL -09	℞
-740-	**PHENYLEPHRINE HYDROCHLORIDE OPHTHALMIC SOLUTION USP, 2.5%** 2 mL: -59 5 mL: -02 15 mL: -06	℞
315-10	**POLYMYXIN B SULFATE AND TRIMETHOPRIM OPHTHALMIC SOLUTION USP** 10 mL	℞
-715-10	**PREDNISOLONE SODIUM PHOSPHATE OPHTHALMIC SOLUTION USP, 1%** 10 mL:	℞
432-62	**PRESERVISION® AREDS** Eye Vitamin and Mineral Supplement 120s tablets	OTC
432-72	**PRESERVISION® AREDS** Eye Vitamin and Mineral Supplement 240s tablets	OTC
625-04	**PRESERVISION® EYE VITAMIN AREDS 2 FORMULA** Eye Vitamin and Mineral Supplement 120 soft gels	OTC
632-10	**PRESERVISION® LUTEIN** Eye Vitamin and Mineral Supplement 50 soft gels	OTC
632-11	120 soft gels	
632-61	180 soft gels	

Code	Product	Type
532	**PRESERVISION® AREDS** Eye Vitamin and Mineral Supplement 60 soft gels - 20 120 soft gels - 30 150 soft gels - 40	OTC
730-06	**PROPARACAINE HYDROCHLORIDE OPHTHALMIC SOLUTION USP, 0.5%** 15 mL	℞
495-28	**SOOTHE® PRESERVATIVE FREE LUBRICANT EYE DROPS** 28 ct	OTC
	SOOTHE® HYDRATION Lubricant Eye Drops 15 mL	OTC
-313-34	**SOOTHE® NIGHT TIME LUBRICANT EYE OINTMENT** 1/8 oz (3.5g)	OTC
317-	**SULFACETAMIDE SODIUM AND PREDNISOLONE SODIUM PHOSPHATE Ophthalmic Solution 10%/0.23%** (prednisolone phosphate) 5 mL: -05 10 mL: -10	℞
-670-04	**SULFACETAMIDE SODIUM OPHTHALMIC SOLUTION USP, 10%** 15mL	℞
-920-64	**TETRACAINE HYDROCHLORIDE OPHTHALMIC SOLUTION USP, 0.5%** 15mL	℞
-290-05	**TOBRAMYCIN OPHTHALMIC SOLUTION USP, 0.3%** 5mL	℞
-295-	**TOBRAMYCIN AND DEXAMETHASONE OPHTHALMIC SUSPENSION USP 0.3%/0.1%** -25 2.5 mL -05 5 mL -10 10 mL	℞
-590-64	**TROPICAMIDE OPHTHALMIC SOLUTION, USP 0.5%** 15 mL	℞
-585-	**TROPICAMIDE OPHTHALMIC SOLUTION, USP 1%** 2 mL: -59 15 mL: -64	℞
535-35	**ZIRGAN®** (ganciclovir ophthalmic gel) 0.15% 5 g Tube	℞
-358-	**ZYLET®** loteprednol etabonate 0.5% and tobramycin 0.3% ophthalmic suspension 5 mL: -05 10 mL: -10	℞

ALAWAY®   OTC
Ketotifen Fumarate Ophthalmic Solution
Antihistamine Eye Drops

Description: Alaway® (ketotifen fumarate ophthalmic solution 0.025%) Antihistamine Eye Drops are indicated for temporary relief for itchy eyes due to ragweed, pollen, grass, animal hair and dander. The original prescription strength, now available over-the-counter, stops the itch within minutes and provides up to 12 hours of symptom relief.

Drug Facts:

Active Ingredient: Ketotifen 0.025% (equivalent to ketotifen fumarate 0.035%)

Continued on next page

Alaway—Cont.

Purpose: Antihistamine

Inactive ingredients: Benzalkonium chloride, 0.01%, glycerin, sodium hydroxide and/or hydrochloric acid and water for injection.

Uses: For the temporary relief of itchy eyes due to ragweed, pollen, grass, animal hair and dander.

Warnings:

Do not use:
- if you are sensitive to any ingredient in this product
- if the solution changes color or becomes cloudy
- to treat contact lens related irritation

When using this product
- remove contact lenses before use
- wait at least 10 minutes before re-inserting contact lenses after use
- do not touch the tip of the container to any surface to avoid contamination
- replace cap after each use

Stop use and ask a doctor if you experience any of the following:
- eye pain
- changes in vision
- redness of the eyes
- itching that worsens or lasts for more than 72 hours

Keep out of reach of children. If swallowed, get medical help or contact a Poison Control Center right away.

Directions: Adults and children 3 years and older: put 1 drop in the affected eye(s) twice daily, every 8-12 hours, no more than twice per day.

Children under 3 years of age: consult a doctor

Other information

STORE AT 4–25°C (39–77°F)

How Supplied: NDC 24208-601-10 Sterile 0.34 FL OZ (10mL) plastic dispenser bottle

Questions or Comments?

Toll Free Product Information

Call: 1-800-553-5340

Distributed by: Bausch & Lomb Incorporated.

Rochester, NY 14609

Alaway is a registered trademark of Bausch & Lomb Incorporated.

© Bausch & Lomb Incorporated

Rochester, NY 14609

Shown in Product Identification Guide, page 103

ALREX® ℞

[ăl rĕx]

loteprednol etabonate

ophthalmic suspension 0.2%

STERILE OPHTHALMIC SUSPENSION

Rx only

Description: ALREX® (loteprednol etabonate ophthalmic suspension) contains a sterile, topical anti-inflammatory corticosteroid for ophthalmic use. Loteprednol etabonate is a white to off-white powder.

Loteprednol etabonate is represented by the following structural formula:

$C_{24}H_{31}ClO_7$ Mol. Wt. 466.96

Chemical Name:

chloromethyl 17α-[(ethoxycarbonyl)oxy]-11β-hydroxy-3-oxoandrosta-1,4-diene-17β-carboxylate.

Each mL contains:

ACTIVE: Loteprednol Etabonate 2 mg (0.2%);

INACTIVES: Edetate Disodium, Glycerin, Povidone, Purified Water and Tyloxapol. Hydrochloric Acid and/or Sodium Hydroxide may be added to adjust the pH to 5.4-5.5. The suspension is essentially isotonic with a tonicity of 250 to 310 mOsmol/kg.

PRESERVATIVE ADDED: Benzalkonium Chloride 0.01%.

Clinical Pharmacology: Corticosteroids inhibit the inflammatory response to a variety of inciting agents and probably delay or slow healing. They inhibit the edema, fibrin deposition, capillary dilation, leukocyte migration, capillary proliferation, fibroblast proliferation, deposition of collagen, and scar formation associated with inflammation. There is no generally accepted explanation for the mechanism of action of ocular corticosteroids. However, corticosteroids are thought to act by the induction of phospholipase A_2 inhibitory proteins, collectively called lipocortins. It is postulated that these proteins control the biosynthesis of potent mediators of inflammation such as prostaglandins and leukotrienes by inhibiting the release of their common precursor arachidonic acid. Arachidonic acid is released from membrane phospholipids by phospholipase A_2. Corticosteroids are capable of producing a rise in intraocular pressure.

Loteprednol etabonate is structurally similar to other corticosteroids. However, the number 20 position ketone group is absent. It is highly lipid soluble which enhances its penetration into cells. Loteprednol etabonate is synthesized through structural modifications of prednisolone-related compounds so that it will undergo a predictable transformation to an inactive metabolite. Based upon *in vivo* and *in vitro* preclinical metabolism studies, loteprednol etabonate undergoes extensive metabolism to inactive carboxylic acid metabolites. Results from a bioavailability study in normal volunteers established that plasma levels of loteprednol etabonate and Δ^1 cortienic acid etabonate (PJ 91), its primary, inactive metabolite, were below the limit of quantitation (1 ng/mL) at all sampling times. The results were obtained following the ocular administration of one drop in each eye of 0.5% loteprednol etabonate 8 times daily for 2 days or 4 times daily for 42 days. This study suggests that limited (<1 ng/mL) systemic absorption occurs with ALREX.

Clinical Studies:

In two double-masked, placebo-controlled six-week environmental studies of 268 patients with seasonal allergic conjunctivitis, ALREX, when dosed four times per day was superior to placebo in the treatment of the signs and symptoms of seasonal allergic conjunctivitis. ALREX provided reduction in bulbar conjunctival injection and itching, beginning approximately 2 hours after instillation of the first dose and throughout the first 14 days of treatment.

Indications and Usage: ALREX Ophthalmic Suspension is indicated for the temporary relief of the signs and symptoms of seasonal allergic conjunctivitis.

Contraindications: ALREX, as with other ophthalmic corticosteroids, is contraindicated in most viral diseases of the cornea and conjunctiva including epithelial herpes simplex keratitis (dendritic keratitis), vaccinia, and varicella, and also in mycobacterial infection of the eye and fungal diseases of ocular structures. ALREX is also contraindicated in individuals with known or suspected hypersensitivity to any of the ingredients of this preparation and to other corticosteroids.

Warnings: Prolonged use of corticosteroids may result in glaucoma with damage to the optic nerve, defects in visual acuity and fields of vision, and in posterior subcapsular cataract formation. Steroids should be used with caution in the presence of glaucoma.

Prolonged use of corticosteroids may suppress the host response and thus increase the hazard of secondary ocular infections. In those diseases causing thinning of the cornea or sclera, perforations have been known to occur with the use of topical steroids. In acute purulent conditions of the eye, steroids may mask infection or enhance existing infection.

Use of ocular steroids may prolong the course and may exacerbate the severity of many viral infections of the eye (including herpes simplex). Employment of a corticosteroid medication in the treatment of patients with a history of herpes simplex requires great caution.

Precautions:

General: For ophthalmic use only. The initial prescription and renewal of the medication order beyond 14 days should be made by a physician only after examination of the patient with the aid of magnification, such as slit lamp biomicroscopy and where appropriate, fluorescein staining.

If signs and symptoms fail to improve after two days, the patient should be re-evaluated.

If this product is used for 10 days or longer, intraocular pressure should be monitored.

Fungal infections of the cornea are particularly prone to develop coincidentally with long-term local steroid application. Fungus invasion must be considered in any persistent corneal ulceration where a steroid has been used or is in use. Fungal cultures should be taken when appropriate.

Information for Patients: This product is sterile when packaged. Patients should be advised not to allow the dropper tip to touch any surface, as this may contaminate the suspension. If redness or itching becomes aggravated, the patient should be advised to consult a physician.

Patients should be advised not to wear a contact lens if their eye is red. ALREX should not be used to treat contact lens related irritation. The preservative in ALREX, benzalkonium chloride, may be absorbed by soft contact lenses. Patients who wear soft contact lenses and whose eyes are not red should be instructed to wait at least ten minutes after instilling ALREX before they insert their contact lenses.

Carcinogenesis, mutagenesis, impairment of fertility: Long-term animal studies have not been conducted to evaluate the carcinogenic potential of loteprednol etabonate. Loteprednol etabonate was not genotoxic *in vitro* in the Ames test, the mouse lymphoma tk assay, or in a chromosome aberration test in human lymphocytes, or *in vivo* in the single dose mouse micronucleus assay. Treatment of male and female rats with up to 50 mg/kg/day and 25 mg/kg/day of loteprednol etabonate, respectively, (1500 and 750 times the maximum clinical dose, respectively) prior to and during mating did not impair fertility in either gender.

Pregnancy: Teratogenic effects: Pregnancy Category C. Loteprednol etabonate has been shown to be embryotoxic (delayed ossification) and teratogenic (increased incidence of meningocele, abnormal left common carotid artery, and limb flexures) when administered orally to rabbits during organogenesis at a dose of 3 mg/kg/day (85 times the maximum daily clinical dose), a dose which caused no maternal toxicity. The no-observed-effect-level (NOEL) for these effects was 0.5 mg/kg/day (15 times the maximum daily clinical dose). Oral treatment of rats during organogenesis resulted in teratogenicity (absent innominate artery at ≥5 mg/kg/day doses, and cleft palate and umbilical hernia at ≥50 mg/kg/day) and embryotoxicity (increased post-implantation losses at 100 mg/kg/day and decreased fetal body weight and skeletal ossification with ≥50 mg/kg/day). Treatment of rats with 0.5 mg/kg/day (15 times the maximum clinical dose) during organogenesis did not result in any reproductive toxicity. Loteprednol etabonate was maternally toxic (significantly reduced body weight gain during treatment) when administered to pregnant rats during organogenesis at doses of ≥5 mg/kg/day.

Oral exposure of female rats to 50 mg/kg/day of loteprednol etabonate from the start of the fetal period through the end of lactation, a maternally toxic treatment regimen (significantly decreased body weight gain), gave rise to decreased growth and survival, and retarded development in the offspring during lactation; the NOEL for these effects was 5 mg/kg/day. Loteprednol etabonate had no effect on the duration of gestation or parturition when administered orally to pregnant rats at doses up to 50 mg/kg/day during the fetal period.

There are no adequate and well controlled studies in pregnant women. ALREX Ophthalmic Suspension should be used during pregnancy only if the potential benefit justifies the potential risk to the fetus.

Nursing Mothers: It is not known whether topical ophthalmic administration of corticosteroids could result in sufficient systemic absorption to produce detectable quantities in human milk. Systemic steroids appear in human milk and could suppress growth, interfere with endogenous corticosteroid production, or cause other untoward effects. Caution should be exercised when ALREX is administered to a nursing woman.

Pediatric Use: Safety and effectiveness in pediatric patients have not been established.

Adverse Reactions: Reactions associated with ophthalmic steroids include elevated intraocular pressure, which may be associated with optic nerve damage, visual acuity and field defects, posterior subcapsular cataract formation, secondary ocular infection from pathogens including herpes simplex, and perforation of the globe where there is thinning of the cornea or sclera.

Ocular adverse reactions occurring in 5–15% of patients treated with loteprednol etabonate ophthalmic suspension (0.2%–0.5%) in clinical studies included abnormal vision/blurring, burning on instillation, chemosis, discharge, dry eyes, epiphora, foreign body sensation, itching, injection, and photophobia. Other ocular adverse reactions occurring in less than 5% of patients include conjunctivitis, corneal abnormalities, eyelid erythema, keratoconjunctivitis, ocular irritation/pain/discomfort, papillae, and uveitis. Some of these events were similar to the underlying ocular disease being studied.

Non-ocular adverse reactions occurred in less than 15% of patients. These include headache, rhinitis and pharyngitis.

In a summation of controlled, randomized studies of individuals treated for 28 days or longer with loteprednol etabonate, the incidence of significant elevation of intraocular pressure (≥10 mm Hg) was 2% (15/901) among patients receiving loteprednol etabonate, 7% (11/164) among patients receiving 1% prednisolone acetate and 0.5% (3/583) among patients receiving placebo. Among the smaller group of patients who were studied with ALREX, the incidence of clinically significant increases in IOP (≥10 mm Hg) was 1% (1/133) with ALREX and 1% (1/135) with placebo.

Dosage and Administration: SHAKE VIGOROUSLY BEFORE USING.

One drop instilled into the affected eye(s) four times daily.

How Supplied: ALREX® (loteprednol etabonate ophthalmic suspension, 0.2%) is supplied in a plastic bottle with a controlled drop tip in the following sizes:

5 mL (NDC 24208-353-05) - AB35307
10 mL (NDC 24208-353-10) - AB35309

DO NOT USE IF NECKBAND IMPRINTED WITH

"Protective Seal" AND YELLOW ⚕ IS NOT INTACT

Storage: Store upright between 15°–25°C (59°–77°F). DO NOT FREEZE.

KEEP OUT OF REACH OF CHILDREN.

Revised August 2008.

Bausch & Lomb Incorporated, Tampa, Florida 33637

U.S. Patent No. 4,996,335
U.S. Patent No. 5,540,930
U.S. Patent No. 5,747,061
©Bausch & Lomb Incorporated
Alrex® is a registered trademark of Bausch & Lomb Incorporated
9007902 (Folded)
9005502 (Flat)

Shown in Product Identification Guide, page 103

BESIVANCE™   ℞
(besifloxacin ophthalmic suspension, 0.6%)

HIGHLIGHTS OF PRESCRIBING INFORMATION
These highlights do not include all the information needed to use Besivance safely and effectively. See full prescribing information for Besivance.
Besivance™ (besifloxacin ophthalmic suspension) 0.6%
Sterile topical ophthalmic drops
Initial U.S. Approval: 2009

---------- INDICATIONS AND USAGE ----------

Besivance™ (besifloxacin ophthalmic suspension) 0.6%, is a quinolone antimicrobial indicated for the treatment of bacterial conjunctivitis caused by susceptible isolates of the following bacteria:
CDC coryneform group G
Corynebacterium pseudodiphtheriticum*, Corynebacterium striatum*, Haemophilus influenzae, Moraxella lacunata*, Staphylococcus aureus, Staphylococcus epidermidis, Staphylococcus hominis*, Staphylococcus lugdunensis*, Streptococcus mitis group, Streptococcus oralis, Streptococcus pneumoniae, Streptococcus salivarius*
*Efficacy for this organism was studied in fewer than 10 infections. (1)

------- DOSAGE AND ADMINISTRATION -------

Instill one drop in the affected eye(s) 3 times a day, four to twelve hours apart for 7 days. (2)

------ DOSAGE FORMS AND STRENGTHS ------

7.5 mL size bottle filled with 5 mL of besifloxacin ophthalmic suspension, 0.6% (3)

------------ CONTRAINDICATIONS ------------

None

-------- WARNINGS AND PRECAUTIONS --------

Topical Ophthalmic Use Only. (5.1)
Growth of Resistant Organisms with Prolonged Use. (5.2)
Avoidance of Contact Lenses. Patients should not wear contact lenses if they have signs or symptoms of bacterial conjunctivitis or during the course of therapy with Besivance™ (5.3)

------------ ADVERSE REACTIONS ------------

The most common adverse event reported in 2% of patients treated with Besivance™ was conjunctival redness. (6)
To report SUSPECTED ADVERSE REACTIONS, contact Bausch & Lomb Incorporated at 1-800-323-0000 or FDA at 1-800-FDA-1088 or www.fda.gov/medwatch
See 17 for PATIENT COUNSELING INFORMATION

                       Revised: 04/2009

FULL PRESCRIBING INFORMATION

1.   INDICATIONS AND USAGE
Besivance™ (besifloxacin ophthalmic suspension) 0.6%, is indicated for the treatment of bacterial conjunctivitis caused by susceptible isolates of the following bacteria:
CDC coryneform group G
Corynebacterium pseudodiphtheriticum[1]
Corynebacterium striatum[1]
Haemophilus influenzae
Moraxella lacunata[1]
Staphylococcus aureus
Staphylococcus epidermidis
Staphylococcus hominis[1]
Staphylococcus lugdunensis[1]
Streptococcus mitis group
Streptococcus oralis
Streptococcus pneumoniae
Streptococcus salivarius[1]

[1]Efficacy for this organism was studied in fewer than 10 infections.

2.   DOSAGE AND ADMINISTRATION
Invert closed bottle and shake once before use.
Instill one drop in the affected eye(s) 3 times a day, four to twelve hours apart for 7 days.

3.   DOSAGE FORMS AND STRENGTHS
7.5 mL bottle filled with 5 mL of besifloxacin ophthalmic suspension, 0.6%.

4.   CONTRAINDICATIONS
None

5.   WARNINGS AND PRECAUTIONS
5.1   Topical Ophthalmic Use Only
NOT FOR INJECTION INTO THE EYE.
Besivance™ is for topical ophthalmic use only, and should not be injected subconjunctivally, nor should it be introduced directly into the anterior chamber of the eye.
5.2   Growth of Resistant Organisms with Prolonged Use
As with other anti-infectives, prolonged use of Besivance™ (besifloxacin ophthalmic suspension) 0.6% may result in overgrowth of non-susceptible organisms, including fungi. If super-infection occurs, discontinue use and institute alternative therapy. Whenever clinical judgment dictates, the patient should be examined with the aid of magnification, such as slit-lamp biomicroscopy, and, where appropriate, fluorescein staining.
5.3   Avoidance of Contact Lenses
Patients should not wear contact lenses if they have signs or symptoms of bacterial conjunctivitis or during the course of therapy with Besivance™.

6.   ADVERSE REACTIONS
Because clinical trials are conducted under widely varying conditions, adverse reaction rates observed in one clinical trial of a drug cannot be directly compared with the rates in the clinical trials of the same or another drug and may not reflect the rates observed in practice. The data described below reflect exposure to Besivance™ in approximately 1,000 patients between 1 and 98 years old with clinical signs and symptoms of bacterial conjunctivitis. The most frequently reported ocular adverse event was conjunctival redness, reported in approximately 2% of patients.
Other adverse events reported in patients receiving Besivance™ occurring in approximately 1–2% of patients included: blurred vision, eye pain, eye irritation, eye pruritus and headache.

Continued on next page

Besivance—Cont.

8. USE IN SPECIFIC POPULATIONS

8.1 Pregnancy

Pregnancy Category C. Oral doses of besifloxacin up to 1000 mg/kg/day were not associated with visceral or skeletal malformations in rat pups in a study of embryo-fetal development, although this dose was associated with maternal toxicity (reduced body weight gain and food consumption) and maternal mortality. Increased post-implantation loss, decreased fetal body weights, and decreased fetal ossification were also observed. At this dose, the mean C_{max} in the rat dams was approximately 20 mcg/mL, >45,000 times the mean plasma concentrations measured in humans. The No Observed Adverse Effect Level (NOAEL) for this embryo-fetal development study was 100 mg/kg/day (C_{max}, 5 mcg/mL, >11,000 times the mean plasma concentrations measured in humans).

In a prenatal and postnatal development study in rats, the NOAELs for both fetal and maternal toxicity were also 100 mg/kg/day. At 1000 mg/kg/day, the pups weighed significantly less than controls and had a reduced neonatal survival rate. Attainment of developmental landmarks and sexual maturation were delayed, although surviving pups from this dose group that were reared to maturity did not demonstrate deficits in behavior, including activity, learning and memory, and their reproductive capacity appeared normal.

Since there are no adequate and well-controlled studies in pregnant women, Besivance™ should be used during pregnancy only if the potential benefit justifies the potential risk to the fetus.

8.3 Nursing Mothers

Besifloxacin has not been measured in human milk, although it can be presumed to be excreted in human milk. Caution should be exercised when Besivance™ is administered to a nursing mother.

8.4 Pediatric Use

The safety and effectiveness of Besivance™ in infants below one year of age have not been established. The efficacy of Besivance™ in treating bacterial conjunctivitis in pediatric patients one year or older has been demonstrated in controlled clinical trials [see 14 CLINICAL STUDIES]. There is no evidence that the ophthalmic administration of quinolones has any effect on weight bearing joints, even though systemic administration of some quinolones has been shown to cause arthropathy in immature animals.

8.5 Geriatric Use

No overall differences in safety and effectiveness have been observed between elderly and younger patients.

11. DESCRIPTION

Besivance™ (besifloxacin ophthalmic suspension) 0.6%, is a sterile ophthalmic suspension of besifloxacin formulated with DuraSite®[2] (polycarbophil, edetate disodium dihydrate and sodium chloride). Each mL of Besivance™ contains 6.63 mg besifloxacin hydrochloride equivalent to 6 mg besifloxacin base. It is an 8-chloro fluoroquinolone anti-infective for topical ophthalmic use.

$C_{19}H_{21}ClFN_3O_3 \cdot HCl$
Mol Wt 430.30

Chemical Name: (+)-7-[(3R)-3-aminohexahydro-1H-azepin-1-yl]-8-chloro-1-cyclopropyl-6-fluoro-4-oxo-1,4-dihydroquinoline-3-carboxylic acid hydrochloride.

Besifloxacin hydrochloride is a white to pale yellowish-white powder.

Each mL Contains:
Active: besifloxacin 0.6% (6 mg/mL);
Preservative: benzalkonium chloride 0.01%
Inactives: polycarbophil, mannitol, poloxamer 407, sodium chloride, edetate disodium dihydrate, sodium hydroxide and water for injection.
Besivance™ is an isotonic suspension with an osmolality of approximately 290 mOsm/kg.

---

[2]DuraSite is a trademark of InSite Vision Incorporated

12. CLINICAL PHARMACOLOGY

12.1 Mechanism Of Action

Besifloxacin is a fluoroquinolone antibacterial [see 12.4 Clinical Pharmacology, Microbiology].

12.3 Pharmacokinetics

Plasma concentrations of besifloxacin were measured in adult patients with suspected bacterial conjunctivitis who received Besivance™ bilaterally three times a day (16 doses total). Following the first and last dose, the maximum plasma besifloxacin concentration in each patient was less than 1.3 ng/mL. The mean besifloxacin C_{max} was 0.37 ng/mL on day 1 and 0.43 ng/mL on day 6. The average elimination half-life of besifloxacin in plasma following multiple dosing was estimated to be 7 hours.

12.4 Microbiology

Besifloxacin is an 8-chloro fluoroquinolone with a N-1 cyclopropyl group. The compound has activity against Gram-positive and Gram-negative bacteria due to the inhibition of both bacterial DNA gyrase and topoisomerase IV. DNA gyrase is an essential enzyme required for replication, transcription and repair of bacterial DNA. Topoisomerase IV is an essential enzyme required for partitioning of the chromosomal DNA during bacterial cell division. Besifloxacin is bactericidal with minimum bactericidal concentrations (MBCs) generally within one dilution of the minimum inhibitory concentrations (MICs).

The mechanism of action of fluoroquinolones, including besifloxacin, is different from that of aminoglycoside, macrolide, and β-lactam antibiotics. Therefore, besifloxacin may be active against pathogens that are resistant to these antibiotics and these antibiotics may be active against pathogens that are resistant to besifloxacin. In vitro studies demonstrated cross-resistance between besifloxacin and some fluoroquinolones.

In vitro resistance to besifloxacin develops via multiple-step mutations and occurs at a general frequency of $< 3.3 \times 10^{-10}$ for Staphylococcus aureus and $< 7 \times 10^{-10}$ for Streptococcus pneumoniae.

Besifloxacin has been shown to be active against most isolates of the following bacteria both in vitro and in conjunctival infections treated in clinical trials as described in the INDICATIONS AND USAGE section:

CDC coryneform group G
Corynebacterium pseudodiphtheriticum[3]
Corynebacterium striatum[3]
Haemophilus influenzae
Moraxella lacunata[3]
Staphylococcus aureus
Staphylococcus epidermidis
Staphylococcus hominis[3]
Staphylococcus lugdunensis[3]
Streptococcus mitis group
Streptococcus oralis
Streptococcus pneumoniae
Streptococcus salivarius[3]

---

[3]Efficacy for this organism was studied in fewer than 10 infections.

13. NONCLINICAL TOXICOLOGY

13.1 Carcinogenesis, Mutagenesis, Impairment Of Fertility

Long-term studies in animals to determine the carcinogenic potential of besifloxacin have not been performed.

No in vitro mutagenic activity of besifloxacin was observed in an Ames test (up to 3.33 mcg/plate) on bacterial tester strains Salmonella typhimurium TA98, TA100, TA1535, TA1537 and Escherichia coli WP2uvrA. However, it was mutagenic in S. typhimurium strain TA102 and E. coli strain WP2(pKM101). Positive responses in these strains have been observed with other quinolones and are likely related to topoisomerase inhibition. Besifloxacin induced chromosomal aberrations in CHO cells in vitro and it was positive in an in vivo mouse micronucleus assay at oral doses ≥ 1500 mg/kg. Besifloxacin did not induce unscheduled DNA synthesis in hepatocytes cultured from rats given the test compound up to 2,000 mg/kg by the oral route. In a fertility and early embryonic development study in rats, besifloxacin did not impair the fertility of male or female rats at oral doses of up to 500 mg/kg/day. This is over 10,000 times higher than the recommended total daily human ophthalmic dose.

14. CLINICAL STUDIES

In a randomized, double-masked, vehicle controlled, multicenter clinical trial, in which patients 1–98 years of age were dosed 3 times a day for 5 days, Besivance™ was superior to its vehicle in patients with bacterial conjunctivitis. Clinical resolution was achieved in 45% (90/198) for the Besivance™ treated group versus 33% (63/191) for the vehicle treated group (difference 12%, 95% CI 3%-22%). Microbiological outcomes demonstrated a statistically significant eradication rate for causative pathogens of 91% (181/198) for the Besivance™ treated group versus 60% (114/191) for the vehicle treated group (difference 31%, 95% CI 23%-40%). Microbiologic eradication does not always correlate with clinical outcome in anti-infective trials.

16. HOW SUPPLIED/STORAGE AND HANDLING

Besivance™ (besifloxacin ophthalmic suspension, 0.6%, is supplied as a sterile ophthalmic suspension in a white low density polyethylene (LDPE) bottle with a controlled dropper tip and tan polypropylene cap. Tamper evidence is provided with a shrink band around the cap and neck area of the package
5 mL in 7.5 mL bottle
NDC 24208-446-05
Storage: Store at 15°–25°C (59°–77°F). Protect from Light.
Invert closed bottle and shake once before use.
Rx Only

17. PATIENT COUNSELING INFORMATION

Patients should be advised to avoid contaminating the applicator tip with material from the eye, fingers or other source.

Although Besivance™ is not intended to be administered systemically, quinolones administered systemically have been associated with hypersensitivity reactions, even following a single dose. Patients should be advised to discontinue use immediately and contact their physician at the first sign of a rash or allergic reaction.

Patients should be told that although it is common to feel better early in the course of the therapy, the medication should be taken exactly as directed. Skipping doses or not completing the full course of therapy may (1) decrease the effectiveness of the immediate treatment and (2) increase the likelihood that bacteria will develop resistance and will not be treatable by Besivance™ or other antibacterial drugs in the future.

Patients should be advised not to wear contact lenses if they have signs or symptoms of bacterial conjunctivitis or during the course of therapy with Besivance™.

Patients should be advised to thoroughly wash hands prior to using Besivance™.

Patients should be instructed to invert closed bottle (upside down) and shake once before each use. Remove cap with bottle still in the inverted position. Tilt head back, and with bottle inverted, gently squeeze bottle to instill one drop into the affected eye(s).

MANUFACTURER INFORMATION

Manufactured by: Bausch & Lomb Incorporated
Tampa, Florida 33637
©Bausch & Lomb Incorporated
U.S. Patent No. 6,685,958

.S. Patent No. 6,699,492
.S. Patent No. 5,447,926
esivance is a registered trademark of Bausch &
omb Incorporated.
pril 2009
142602 (flat)
142702 (folded)

*Shown in Product Identification
Guide, page 103*

OTEMAX®   ℞
[Lō tē max]
oteprednol etabonate
ophthalmic ointment 0.5%

IGHLIGHTS OF PRESCRIBING INFORMATION

hese highlights do not include all the information
eeded to use Lotemax® ointment safely and effec-
vely. See full prescribing information for Lotemax
oteprednol etabonate ophthalmic ointment)
5%.

itial U.S. Approval: 1998

———— INDICATIONS AND USAGE ————

OTEMAX ointment is a corticosteroid indicated
or the treatment of post-operative inflammation
nd pain following ocular surgery.

—— DOSAGE AND ADMINISTRATION ——

.pply a small amount (approximately ½ inch rib-
on) into the conjunctival sac(s) four times daily be-
nning 24 hours after surgery and continuing
hroughout the first 2 weeks of the post-operative
eriod.

– DOSAGE FORMS AND STRENGTHS —

.5 gram tube filled with loteprednol etabonate
phthalmic ointment, 0.5%.

———— CONTRAINDICATIONS ————

OTEMAX ointment, as with other ophthalmic cor-
costeroids, is contraindicated in most viral dis-
ases of the cornea and conjunctiva including epi-
helial herpes simplex keratitis (dendritic
eratitis), vaccinia, and varicella, and also in myco-
acterial infection of the eye and fungal diseases of
cular structures. (4)

—— WARNINGS AND PRECAUTIONS ——

Intraocular pressure (IOP) increase–Prolonged
use of corticosteroids may result in glaucoma with
damage to the optic nerve, defects in visual acuity
and fields of vision. If this product is used for 10
days or longer, IOP should be monitored even
though it may be difficult in children and uncooperative patients. (5.1)
Cataracts–Use of corticosteroids may result in
posterior subcapsular cataract formation. (5.2)
Delayed healing–The use of steroids after cataract
surgery may delay healing and increase the incidence of bleb formation. In those diseases causing
thinning of the cornea or sclera, perforations have
been known to occur with the use of topical steroids. (5.3)
Bacterial infections–Prolonged use of corticosteroids may suppress the host response and thus increase the hazard of secondary ocular infections.
In acute purulent conditions, steroids may mask
infection or enhance existing infection. (5.4)
Viral infections–Employment of a corticosteroid
medication in the treatment of patients with a
history of herpes simplex requires great caution.
Use of ocular steroids may prolong the course and
may exacerbate the severity of many viral infections of the eye (including herpes simplex). (5.5)
Fungal infections–Fungal infections of the cornea
are particularly prone to develop coincidentally
with long-term local steroid application. Fungus
invasion must be considered in any persistent corneal ulceration where a steroid has been used or
is in use. (5.6)

———— ADVERSE REACTIONS ————

he most common ocular adverse event, reported in
pproximately 25% of subjects in clinical studies, is

---

anterior chamber inflammation. Other common adverse events, with an incidence of 4-5%, are conjunctival hyperemia, corneal edema, and eye pain.
(6)
**To report SUSPECTED ADVERSE REACTIONS, con-
tact Bausch & Lomb at 1-800-323-0000 or FDA at
1-800-FDA-1088 or www.fda.gov/medwatch.**
**See 17 for PATIENT COUNSELING INFORMA-
TION**

Revised: 04/2011

FULL PRESCRIBING INFORMATION: CONTENTS*

FULL PRESCRIBING INFORMATION

1   INDICATIONS AND USAGE

LOTEMAX® ointment is a corticosteroid indicated
for the treatment of post-operative inflammation
and pain following ocular surgery.

2   DOSAGE AND ADMINISTRATION

Apply a small amount (approximately ½ inch rib-
bon) into the conjunctival sac(s) four times daily beginning 24 hours after surgery and continuing
throughout the first 2 weeks of the post-operative
period.

3   DOSAGE FORMS AND STRENGTHS

LOTEMAX is supplied sterile in a 3.5 gram tube
filled with loteprednol etabonate ophthalmic
ointment, 0.5%.

4   CONTRAINDICATIONS

LOTEMAX ointment, as with other ophthalmic corticosteroids, is contraindicated in most viral diseases of the cornea and conjunctiva including epithelial herpes simplex keratitis (dendritic
keratitis), vaccinia, and varicella, and also in mycobacterial infection of the eye and fungal diseases of
ocular structures.

5   WARNINGS AND PRECAUTIONS

5.1   Intraocular pressure (IOP) increase
Prolonged use of corticosteroids may result in glaucoma with damage to the optic nerve, defects in visual acuity and fields of vision. If this product is
used for 10 days or longer, IOP should be monitored
even though it may be difficult in children and uncooperative patients.

5.2   Cataracts
Use of corticosteroids may result in posterior subcapsular cataract formation.

5.3   Delayed healing
The use of steroids after cataract surgery may delay
healing and increase the incidence of bleb formation. In those diseases causing thinning of the cornea or sclera, perforations have been known to occur with the use of topical steroids.
The initial prescription and renewal of the medication order beyond 14 days should be made by a physician only after examination of the patient with
the aid of magnification such as slit lamp biomicroscopy and, where appropriate, fluorescein staining.
5.4   Bacterial infections
Prolonged use of corticosteroids may suppress the
host response and thus increase the hazard of
secondary ocular infections. In acute purulent conditions, steroids may mask infection or enhance existing infection. If signs and symptoms fail to improve after 2 days, the patient should be re-
evaluated.
5.5   Viral infections
Employment of a corticosteroid medication in the
treatment of patients with a history of herpes simplex requires great caution. Use of ocular steroids
may prolong the course and may exacerbate the severity of many viral infections of the eye (including
herpes simplex).
5.6   Fungal infections
Fungal infections of the cornea are particularly
prone to develop coincidentally with long-term local
steroid application. Fungus invasion must be considered in any persistent corneal ulceration where a
steroid has been used or is in use. Fungal culture
should be taken when appropriate.
5.7   Contact Lens Wear
Patients should not wear contact lenses during
their course of therapy with LOTEMAX ointment.
5.8   Amblyopia
LOTEMAX (loteprednol etabonate ophthalmic
ointment), 0.5% should not be used in children following ocular surgery. Its use may interfere with
amblyopia treatment by hindering the child's ability to see out of the operated eye (see Pediatric Use,
8.4).
5.9   Topical ophthalmic use only
Lotemax is not indicated for intraocular administration.

6   ADVERSE REACTIONS

Adverse reactions associated with ophthalmic steroids include elevated intraocular pressure, which
may be associated with optic nerve damage, visual
acuity and field defects, posterior subcapsular cataract formation, secondary ocular infection from
pathogens including herpes simplex, and perforation of the globe where there is thinning of the cornea or sclera.
The most common ocular adverse event reported at
approximately 25% in subjects in clinical studies
with Lotemax ointment was anterior chamber inflammation. Other common adverse events, with an
incidence of 4-5%, were conjunctival hyperemia,
corneal edema, and eye pain. Many of these events
may have been the consequence of the surgical procedure. The only non-ocular adverse event occurring at ≥ 1% was headache (1.5%).

8   USE IN SPECIFIC POPULATIONS

8.1   Pregnancy
Teratogenic effects: Pregnancy Category C.
Loteprednol etabonate has been shown to be embryotoxic (delayed ossification) and teratogenic (increased incidence of meningocele, abnormal left
common carotid artery, and limb flexures) when administered orally to rabbits during organogenesis
at a dose of 3 mg/kg/day (150 times the maximum
daily clinical dose), a dose which caused no maternal toxicity. The no-observed-effect-level (NOEL) for
these effects was 0.5 mg/kg/day (25 times the maximum daily clinical dose). Oral treatment of rats
during organogenesis resulted in teratogenicity (absent innominate artery at ≥ 5 mg/kg/day doses, and
cleft palate and umbilical hernia at ≥ 50 mg/kg/
day) and embryotoxicity (increased post-
implantation losses at 100 mg/kg/day and decreased fetal body weight and skeletal ossification

Continued on next page

Lotemax Ointment—Cont.

with $\geq$ 50 mg/kg/day). Treatment of rats with 0.5 mg/kg/day (25 times the maximum daily clinical dose) during organogenesis did not result in any reproductive toxicity. Loteprednol etabonate was maternally toxic (significantly reduced body weight gain during treatment) when administered to pregnant rats during organogenesis at doses of $\geq$ 5 mg/kg/day.

Oral exposure of female rats to 50 mg/kg/day of loteprednol etabonate from the start of the fetal period through the end of lactation, a maternally toxic treatment regimen (significantly decreased body weight gain), gave rise to decreased growth and survival, and retarded development in the offspring during lactation; the NOEL for these effects was 5 mg/kg/day. Loteprednol etabonate had no effect on the duration of gestation or parturition when administered orally to pregnant rats at doses up to 50 mg/kg/day during the fetal period.

LOTEMAX should be used during pregnancy only if the potential benefit justifies the potential risk to the embryo or fetus.

8.3   Nursing Mothers

It is not known whether topical ophthalmic administration of corticosteroids could result in sufficient systemic absorption to produce detectable quantities in human milk. Systemically administered steroids appear in human milk and could suppress growth, interfere with endogenous corticosteroid production, or cause other untoward effects. Caution should be exercised when LOTEMAX ointment is administered to a nursing woman.

8.4   Pediatric Use

Safety and effectiveness in pediatric patients have not been established.

LOTEMAX (loteprednol etabonate ophthalmic ointment) 0.5% should not be used in children following ocular surgery. Its use may interfere with amblyopia treatment by hindering the child's ability to see out of the operated eye.

8.5   Geriatric Use

No overall differences in safety and effectiveness have been observed between elderly and younger patients.

11   DESCRIPTION

LOTEMAX (loteprednol etabonate ophthalmic ointment) 0.5% is a sterile, topical corticosteroid for ophthalmic use. Loteprednol etabonate is a white to off-white powder.

Loteprednol etabonate is represented by the following structural formula:

Chemical Name:
chloromethyl   17α-[(ethoxycarbonyl)oxy]-11β-hydroxy-3-oxoandrosta-1,4-diene-17β-carboxylate

Each gram contains:
ACTIVE: Loteprednol Etabonate 5 mg (0.5%);
INACTIVES: Mineral Oil and White Petrolatum.

12   CLINICAL PHARMACOLOGY

12.1   Mechanism of Action

Corticosteroids inhibit the inflammatory response to a variety of inciting agents and probably delay or slow healing. They inhibit the edema, fibrin deposition, capillary dilation, leukocyte migration, capillary proliferation, fibroblast proliferation, deposition of collagen, and scar formation associated with inflammation. While glucocorticoids are known to bind to and activate the glucocorticoid receptor, the molecular mechanisms involved in glucocorticoid/glucocorticoid receptor-dependent modulation of inflammation are not clearly established. However, corticosteroids are thought to inhibit prostaglandin production through several independent mechanisms.

12.3   Pharmacokinetics

The systemic exposure to loteprednol etabonate following ocular administration of LOTEMAX ointment has not been studied in humans. However, results from a bioavailability study with LOTEMAX suspension in normal volunteers established that plasma concentrations of loteprednol etabonate and Δ^1 cortienic acid etabonate (PJ 91), its primary, inactive metabolite, were below the limit of quantitation (1 ng/mL) at all sampling times. The results were obtained following the ocular administration of one drop in each eye of 0.5% loteprednol etabonate suspension, 8 times daily for 2 days or 4 times daily for 42 days. The maximum systemic exposure to loteprednol following administration of the ointment product dosed four times daily is not expected to exceed exposures attained with LOTEMAX suspension dosed up to two drops four times daily.

13   NONCLINICAL TOXICOLOGY

13.1   Carcinogenesis, Mutagenesis, and Impairment of Fertilty

Long-term animal studies have not been conducted to evaluate the carcinogenic potential of loteprednol etabonate. Loteprednol etabonate was not genotoxic *in vitro* in the Ames test, the mouse lymphoma tk assay, or in a chromosome aberration test in human lymphocytes, or *in vivo* in the single dose mouse micronucleus assay. Treatment of male and female rats with up to 50 mg/kg/day and 25 mg/kg/day of loteprednol etabonate, respectively, (2500 and 1250 times the maximum daily clinical dose, respectively) prior to and during mating did not impair fertility in either gender.

14   CLINICAL STUDIES

In two independent, randomized, multicenter, double-masked, parallel-group, vehicle-controlled studies in 805 subjects meeting a protocol-specified threshold amount of anterior chamber inflammation, LOTEMAX ointment was more effective compared to its vehicle for complete resolution of postoperative anterior chamber cell, flare, and pain following cataract surgery. Primary endpoint was complete resolution of anterior chamber cells and flare (cell count of 0 and no flare) and no pain at post-operative day 8. The individual clinical trial results are provided below.

In the 2 studies, Lotemax had statistically significant higher incidence of complete clearing of anterior chamber cells and flare at post-operative day 8 (24-32% vs. 11-14%) and also had a statistically significant higher incidence of subjects that were pain free at post-operative day 8 (73-78% vs. 41-45%).

16   HOW SUPPLIED/STORAGE AND HANDLING

LOTEMAX (loteprednol etabonate ophthalmic ointment), 0.5% is a sterile ointment supplied in a tin tube with a pink polypropylene cap in the following size:
3.5 gram (NDC 24208-443-35)

Do not use if tamper evident skirt is visible on bottom of cap.

Storage: Store between 15°–25°C (59°–77°F).
Rx only.

17   PATIENT COUNSELING INFORMATION

17.1   Risk of Contamination

Patients should be advised not to touch the eyelid or surrounding areas with the tip of the tube. The cap should remain on the tube when not in use. Patients should be advised to wash hands prior to using LOTEMAX ointment.

Do not use if tamper evident skirt is visible on bottom of cap.

17.2   Contact Lens Wear

Patients should also be advised not to wear contact lenses during their course of therapy.

17.3   Risk of Secondary Infection

If pain, redness, itching or inflammation becomes aggravated, the patient should be advised to consult a physician.

MANUFACTURER INFORMATION

Bausch & Lomb Incorporated
Tampa, Florida 33637 USA
©Bausch & Lomb Incorporated

U.S. Patent No. 4,996,335
Lotemax is a registered trademark of Bausch & Lomb Incorporated
Shown in Product Identification Guide, page 103

LOTEMAX®

[Lō tĕ max]
loteprednol etabonate
ophthalmic suspension 0.5%
STERILE OPHTHALMIC SUSPENSION
Rx only

Description: LOTEMAX® (loteprednol etabonate ophthalmic suspension) contains a sterile, topical anti-inflammatory corticosteroid for ophthalmic use. Loteprednol etabonate is a white to off-white powder.

Loteprednol etabonate is represented by the following structural formula:

Chemical Name:
chloromethyl   17α-[(ethoxycarbonyl)oxy]-11β-hydroxy-3-oxoandrosta-1,4-diene-17β-carboxylate

Each mL contains:
ACTIVE: Loteprednol Etabonate 5 mg (0.5%);
INACTIVES: Edetate   Disodium,   Glycerin, Povidone,   Purified   Water   and   Tyloxapo. Hydrochloric Acid and/or Sodium Hydroxide may be added to adjust the pH to 5.5-5.6. The suspension is essentially isotonic with a tonicity of 250 to 31 mOsmol/kg.
PRESERVATIVE   ADDED: Benzalkonium Chloride 0.01%.

Clinical Pharmacology: Corticosteroids inhibit the inflammatory response to a variety of inciting agents and probably delay or slow healing. They inhibit the edema, fibrin deposition, capillary dilation, leukocyte migration, capillary proliferation, fibroblast proliferation, deposition of collagen, and scar formation associated with inflammation. There is no generally accepted explanation for the mechanism of action of ocular corticosteroids. However, corticosteroids are thought to act by the induction of phospholipase A_2 inhibitory proteins, collectively called lipocortins. It is postulated that these proteins control the biosynthesis of potent mediators of inflammation such as prostaglandins and leukotrienes by inhibiting the release of their common precursor arachidonic acid. Arachidonic acid is released from membrane phospholipids by phospholipase A_2. Corticosteroids are capable of producing a rise in intraocular pressure.

Loteprednol etabonate is structurally similar to other corticosteroids. However, the number 20 position ketone group is absent. It is highly lipid soluble which enhances its penetration into cells. Loteprednol etabonate is synthesized through structural modifications of prednisolone-related compounds so that it will undergo a predictable transformation to an inactive metabolite. Based upon *in vivo* and *in vitro* preclinical metabolism studies, loteprednol etabonate undergoes extensive metabolism to inactive carboxylic acid metabolites. Results from a bioavailability study in normal volunteers established that plasma levels of loteprednol etabonate and Δ^1 cortienic acid etabonate (PJ 91), its primary, inactive metabolite, were below the limit of quantitation (1 ng/mL) at all sampling times. The results were obtained following the ocular administration of one drop in each eye of 0.5% loteprednol etabonate 8 times daily for days or 4 times daily for 42 days. This study suggests that limited (<1 ng/ml) systemic absorption occurs with LOTEMAX.

Clinical Studies:
Post-Operative Inflammation: Placebo-controlled clinical studies demonstrated that LOTEMAX is effective for the treatment of anterior chamber inflammation as measured by cell and flare.

Giant Papillary Conjunctivitis: Placebo-controlled clinical studies demonstrated that LOTEMAX was effective in reducing the signs and symptoms of giant papillary conjunctivitis after 1 week of treatment and continuing for up to 6 weeks while on treatment.

Seasonal Allergic Conjunctivitis: A placebo-controlled clinical study demonstrated that LOTEMAX was effective in reducing the signs and symptoms of allergic conjunctivitis during peak periods of pollen exposure.

Uveitis: Controlled clinical studies of patients with uveitis demonstrated that LOTEMAX was less effective than prednisolone acetate 1%. Overall, 72% of patients treated with LOTEMAX experienced resolution of anterior chamber cell by day 28, compared to 87% of patients treated with 1% prednisolone acetate. The incidence of patients with clinically significant increases in IOP ($\geq$10 mmHg) was 1% with LOTEMAX and 6% with prednisolone acetate 1%.

Indications and Usage: LOTEMAX is indicated for the treatment of steroid responsive inflammatory conditions of the palpebral and bulbar conjunctiva, cornea and anterior segment of the globe such as allergic conjunctivitis, acne rosacea, superficial punctate keratitis, herpes zoster keratitis, iritis, cyclitis, selected infective conjunctivitides, when the inherent hazard of steroid use is accepted to obtain an advisable diminution in edema and inflammation.

LOTEMAX is less effective than prednisolone acetate 1% in two 28-day controlled clinical studies in acute anterior uveitis, where 72% of patients treated with LOTEMAX experienced resolution of anterior chamber cells, compared to 87% of patients treated with prednisolone acetate 1%. The incidence of patients with clinically significant increases in IOP ($\geq$10 mmHg) was 1% with LOTEMAX and 6% with prednisolone acetate 1%. LOTEMAX should not be used in patients who require a more potent corticosteroid for this indication.

LOTEMAX is also indicated for the treatment of post-operative inflammation following ocular surgery.

Contraindications: LOTEMAX, as with other ophthalmic corticosteroids, is contraindicated in most viral diseases of the cornea and conjunctiva including epithelial herpes simplex keratitis (dendritic keratitis), vaccinia, and varicella, and also in mycobacterial infection of the eye and fungal diseases of ocular structures. LOTEMAX is also contraindicated in individuals with known or suspected hypersensitivity to any of the ingredients of this preparation and to other corticosteroids.

Warnings: Prolonged use of corticosteroids may result in glaucoma with damage to the optic nerve, defects in visual acuity and fields of vision, and in posterior subcapsular cataract formation. Steroids should be used with caution in the presence of glaucoma.

Prolonged use of corticosteroids may suppress the host response and thus increase the hazard of secondary ocular infections. In those diseases causing thinning of the cornea or sclera, perforations have been known to occur with the use of topical steroids. In acute purulent conditions of the eye, steroids may mask infection or enhance existing infection.

Use of ocular steroids may prolong the course and may exacerbate the severity of many viral infections of the eye (including herpes simplex). Employment of a corticosteroid medication in the treatment of patients with a history of herpes simplex requires great caution.

The use of steroids after cataract surgery may delay healing and increase the incidence of bleb formation.

Precautions: General: For ophthalmic use only. The initial prescription and renewal of the medication order beyond 14 days should be made by a physician only after examination of the patient with the aid of magnification, such as slit lamp biomicroscopy and, where appropriate, fluorescein staining.

If signs and symptoms fail to improve after two days, the patient should be re-evaluated.

If this product is used for 10 days or longer, intraocular pressure should be monitored even though it may be difficult in children and uncooperative patients *(see WARNINGS)*.

Fungal infections of the cornea are particularly prone to develop coincidentally with long-term local steroid application. Fungus invasion must be considered in any persistent corneal ulceration where a steroid has been used or is in use. Fungal cultures should be taken when appropriate.

Information for Patients: This product is sterile when packaged. Patients should be advised not to allow the dropper tip to touch any surface, as this may contaminate the suspension. If pain develops, redness, itching or inflammation becomes aggravated, the patient should be advised to consult a physician. As with all ophthalmic preparations containing benzalkonium chloride, patients should be advised not to wear soft contact lenses when using LOTEMAX®.

Carcinogenesis, mutagenesis, impairment of fertility: Long-term animal studies have not been conducted to evaluate the carcinogenic potential of loteprednol etabonate. Loteprednol etabonate was not genotoxic *in vitro* in the Ames test, the mouse lymphoma tk assay, or in a chromosome aberration test in human lymphocytes, or *in vivo* in the single dose mouse micronucleus assay. Treatment of male and female rats with up to 50 mg/kg/day and 25 mg/kg/day of loteprednol etabonate, respectively, (600 and 300 times the maximum clinical dose, respectively) prior to and during mating did not impair fertility in either gender.

Pregnancy: Teratogenic effects: Pregnancy Category C. Loteprednol etabonate has been shown to be embryotoxic (delayed ossification) and teratogenic (increased incidence of meningocele, abnormal left common carotid artery, and limb flexures) when administered orally to rabbits during organogenesis at a dose of 3 mg/kg/day (35 times the maximum daily clinical dose), a dose which caused no maternal toxicity. The no-observed-effect-level (NOEL) for these effects was 0.5 mg/kg/day (6 times the maximum daily clinical dose). Oral treatment of rats during organogenesis resulted in teratogenicity (absent innominate artery at $\geq$5 mg/kg/day doses, and cleft palate and umbilical hernia at $\geq$50 mg/kg/day) and embryotoxicity (increased post-implantation losses at 100 mg/kg/day and decreased fetal body weight and skeletal ossification with $\geq$50 mg/kg/day). Treatment of rats with 0.5 mg/kg/day (6 times the maximum clinical dose) during organogenesis did not result in any reproductive toxicity. Loteprednol etabonate was maternally toxic (significantly reduced body weight gain during treatment) when administered to pregnant rats during organogenesis at doses of $\geq$5 mg/kg/day.

Oral exposure of female rats to 50 mg/kg/day of loteprednol etabonate from the start of the fetal period through the end of lactation, a maternally toxic treatment regimen (significantly decreased body weight gain), gave rise to decreased growth and survival, and retarded development in the offspring during lactation; the NOEL for these effects was 5 mg/kg/day. Loteprednol etabonate had no effect on the duration of gestation or parturition when administered orally to pregnant rats at doses up to 50 mg/kg/day during the fetal period.

Nursing Mothers: It is not known whether topical ophthalmic administration of corticosteroids could result in sufficient systemic absorption to produce detectable quantities in human milk. Systemic steroids appear in human milk and could suppress growth, interfere with endogenous corticosteroid production, or cause other untoward effects. Caution should be exercised when LOTEMAX is administered to a nursing woman.

Pediatric Use: Safety and effectiveness in pediatric patients have not been established.

Adverse Reactions: Reactions associated with ophthalmic steroids include elevated intraocular pressure, which may be associated with optic nerve damage, visual acuity and field defects, posterior subcapsular cataract formation, secondary ocular infection from pathogens including herpes simplex, and perforation of the globe where there is thinning of the cornea or sclera.

Ocular adverse reactions occurring in 5-15% of patients treated with loteprednol etabonate ophthalmic suspension (0.2%-0.5%) in clinical studies included abnormal vision/blurring, burning on instillation, chemosis, discharge, dry eyes, epiphora, foreign body sensation, itching, injection, and photophobia. Other ocular adverse reactions occurring in less than 5% of patients include conjunctivitis, corneal abnormalities, eyelid erythema, keratoconjunctivitis, ocular irritation/pain/discomfort, papillae, and uveitis. Some of these events were similar to the underlying ocular disease being studied.

Non-ocular adverse reactions occurred in less than 15% of patients. These include headache, rhinitis and pharyngitis.

In a summation of controlled, randomized studies of individuals treated for 28 days or longer with loteprednol etabonate, the incidence of significant elevation of intraocular pressure ($\geq$10 mmHg) was 2% (15/901) among patients receiving loteprednol etabonate, 7% (11/164) among patients receiving 1% prednisolone acetate and 0.5% (3/583) among patients receiving placebo.

Dosage and Administration: SHAKE VIGOROUSLY BEFORE USING.

Steroid Responsive Disease Treatment: Apply one to two drops of LOTEMAX into the conjunctival sac of the affected eye(s) four times daily. During the initial treatment within the first week, the dosing may be increased, up to 1 drop every hour, if necessary. Care should be taken not to discontinue therapy prematurely. If signs and symptoms fail to improve after two days, the patient should be re-evaluated (See PRECAUTIONS).

Post-Operative Inflammation: Apply one to two drops of LOTEMAX into the conjunctival sac of the operated eye(s) four times daily beginning 24 hours after surgery and continuing throughout the first 2 weeks of the post-operative period.

How Supplied: LOTEMAX® (loteprednol etabonate ophthalmic suspension) is supplied in a plastic bottle with a controlled drop tip in the following sizes:

2.5 mL (NDC 24208-299-25) - AB29904
5 mL (NDC 24208-299-05) - AB29907
10 mL (NDC 24208-299-10) - AB29909
15 mL (NDC 24208-299-15) - AB29911

DO NOT USE IF NECKBAND IMPRINTED WITH

"Protective Seal" AND YELLOW ⚕ IS NOT INTACT

Storage: Store upright between 15°–25°C (59°–77°F). DO NOT FREEZE.

KEEP OUT OF REACH OF CHILDREN.

Revised April 2006
Bausch & Lomb Incorporated, Tampa, Florida 33637
U.S. Patent No. 4,996,335
U.S. Patent No. 5,540,930
U.S. Patent No. 5,747,061
©Bausch & Lomb Incorporated
Lotemax is a registered trademark of Bausch & Lomb Incorporated.
9007802 (Folded)
9005902 (Flat)

Shown in Product Identification Guide, page 103

MIOCHOL®-E   ℞
acetylcholine chloride intraocular solution
1:100 with Electrolyte Diluent
Rx only

Prescribing Information

DESCRIPTION
Miochol®-E (acetylcholine chloride intraocular solution) is a parasympathomimetic preparation for

Continued on next page

Miochol-E—Cont.

intraocular use. It is packaged in a blister pack containing one vial and one ampoule. The vial contains 20 mg acetylcholine chloride and 56 mg mannitol. The accompanying ampoule contains 2 mL of a modified diluent of sodium acetate trihydrate, potassium chloride, magnesium chloride hexahydrate, calcium chloride dihydrate and sterile water for injection.

The reconstituted liquid will be a sterile isotonic solution (275–330 milliosmoles/Kg) containing 20 mg acetylcholine chloride (1:100 solution) and 2.8% mannitol. The pH range is 5.0–8.2. Mannitol is used in the process of lyophilizing acetylcholine chloride, and is not considered an active ingredient. The chemical name for acetylcholine chloride, $C_7H_{16}ClNO_2$, is Ethanaminium, 2-(acetyloxy)-*N,N,N*-trimethyl-, chloride and is represented by the following chemical structure:

$$CH_3CO(CH_2)_2N^+(CH_3)_3 \ Cl^-$$

CLINICAL PHARMACOLOGY

Acetylcholine is a naturally occurring neurohormone which mediates nerve impulse transmission at all cholinergic sites involving somatic and autonomic nerves. After release from the nerve ending, acetylcholine is rapidly inactivated by the enzyme acetylcholinesterase by hydrolysis to acetic acid and choline.

Direct application of acetylcholine to the iris will cause rapid miosis of short duration. Topical ocular instillation of acetylcholine to the intact eye causes no discernible response as cholinesterase destroys the molecule more rapidly than it can penetrate the cornea.

INDICATIONS AND USAGE

To obtain miosis of the iris in seconds after delivery of the lens in cataract surgery, in penetrating keratoplasty, iridectomy and other anterior segment surgery where rapid miosis may be required

CONTRAINDICATIONS

Miochol®-E (acetylcholine chloride intraocular solution) is contraindicated in persons with a known hypersensitivity to any component of this product.

WARNINGS

DO NOT GAS STERILIZE. If blister or peelable backing is damaged or broken, sterility of the enclosed vial and ampoule cannot be assured. Open under aseptic conditions only.

PRECAUTIONS

General

If miosis is to be obtained quickly with Miochol®-E (acetylcholine chloride intraocular solution), anatomical hindrances to miosis, such as anterior or posterior synechiae, must be released, prior to administration of Miochol-E. During cataract surgery, use Miochol-E only after delivery of the lens.

Aqueous solutions of acetylcholine chloride are unstable. Prepare solution immediately before use. Do not use solution which is not clear and colorless. Discard any solution that has not been used.

Drug Interactions

Although clinical studies with acetylcholine chloride and animal studies with acetylcholine or carbachol revealed no interference, and there is no known pharmacological basis for an interaction, there have been reports that acetylcholine chloride and carbachol have been ineffective when used in patients treated with topical nonsteroidal anti-inflammatory agents.

Pediatric Use

Safety and effectiveness in pediatric patients have not been established.

ADVERSE REACTIONS

Infrequent cases of corneal edema, corneal clouding, and corneal decompensation have been reported with the use of intraocular acetylcholine.

Adverse reactions have been reported rarely which are indicative of systemic absorption. These include bradycardia, hypotension, flushing, breathing difficulties and sweating.

OVERDOSAGE

Atropine sulfate (0.5 to 1 mg) should be given intramuscularly or intravenously and should be readily available to counteract possible overdosage. Epinephrine (0.1 to 1 mg subcutaneously) is also of value in overcoming severe cardiovascular or bronchoconstrictor responses.

DOSAGE AND ADMINISTRATION

Miochol®-E (acetylcholine chloride intraocular solution) is instilled into the anterior chamber before or after securing one or more sutures.

Instillation should be gentle and parallel to the iris face and tangential to pupil border.

If there are no mechanical hindrances, the pupil starts to constrict in seconds and the peripheral iris is drawn away from the angle of the anterior chamber. Any anatomical hindrance to miosis must be released to permit the desired effect of the drug. In most cases, 0.5 to 2 mL produces satisfactory miosis. Note that the syringe filter supplied with Miochol-E has a priming volume of 0.6 mL (approximately).

In cataract surgery, use Miochol-E only after delivery of the lens.

Aqueous solutions of acetylcholine chloride are unstable. Prepare solution immediately before use. Do not use solution which is not clear and colorless. Discard any solution that has not been used.

DIRECTIONS FOR PREPARING MIOCHOL®-E:

STERILE UNLESS PACKAGE OPEN OR BROKEN

1. Inspect the unopened blister, vial and ampoule to ensure that they are all intact. Peel open the blister under a sterile field. Maintain sterility of the outer containers of the vial and ampoule during preparation of solution.
2. Aseptically attach a sterile 18–20 gauge, beveled needle to the luer tip of a sterile disposable syringe with a twisting motion to assure a secure fit.
3. Break open the ampoule containing the diluent. The One Point Cut (OPC) ampoule must be opened as follows: Hold the bottom part of the ampoule with the thumb pointing to the colored dot. Grasp the top of the ampoule with the other hand, positioning the thumb at the colored dot, and press back to break at the existing cut under the dot.
4. Remove the needle protector and withdraw the diluent from the ampoule into the syringe. Discard the ampoule.
5. Remove and discard the cap from the top of the vial.
6. Insert the needle through the center of the vial stopper, and transfer the diluent from the syringe to the vial. Shake gently to dissolve the powder.
7. Slowly withdraw the solution from the vial through the needle into the syringe. Discard the needle.
8. Aseptically open the syringe filter pouch, and attach the filter onto the luer tip of the syringe with a twisting motion to assure a secure fit.
9. Aseptically attach a sterile blunt tip irrigation cannula to the male luer of the filter prior to intraocular irrigation

Discard the filter appropriately after use.

Do not reuse the syringe filter.

Do not aspirate and inject through the same filter.

HOW SUPPLIED

Miochol®-E
(acetylcholine chloride
intraocular solution)   NDC 24208-539-20

One blister pack containing the following components:

• Vial of 20 mg acetylcholine chloride powder for intraocular solution
• Ampoule of 2 mL diluent

One 0.2 micron sterile filter
• Priming volume 0.6 mL (approximately)
Store at 4°–25°C (39°–77°F).
KEEP FROM FREEZING.
REV: MARCH 2007   T2007-10
MIOCHOL is a registered trademark of Bausch Lomb Incorporated.
Distributed by:
Bausch & Lomb Incorporated
Rochester, NY 14609
© Bausch & Lomb Incorporated
9214900   AB53920
2074024 **US**

MURO 128®
sodium chloride hypertonicity ophthalmic ointment, 5%

Drug Facts

Active ingredient	*Purpo*
Sodium chloride, 50 mg (5%)	Hypertonici age

Uses

temporary relief of corneal edema

Warnings

Do not use except under the advice and supervisic of a doctor

When using this product

■ it may cause temporary burning and irritation
■ replace cap after use
■ to avoid contamination do not touch tip of co tainer to any surface

Stop use and ask a doctor if

■ condition worsens or persists for more than ? hours
■ you experience eye pain, changes in vision, co tinued redness or irritation of the eye

Keep out of reach of children. If swallowed, ge medical help or contact a Poison Control Cente right away.

Directions

■ pull down the lower lid of the affected eye
■ apply a small amount (1/4 inch) of ointment to th inside of eyelid
■ apply every 3 or 4 hours or as directed by a docto

Other information

■ store at 15°-30°C (59°-86°F)
■ keep tightly closed
■ do not freeze
■ see crimp of tube or carton for Lot Number an Expiration Date
■ serious side effects associated with use of th product may be reported to the phone number be low

Inactive ingredients

lanolin, mineral oil, purified water, white petrola tum

Questions?

Call: 1-800-323-0000

Bausch & Lomb Incorporated

Tampa, FL 33637

Muro 128 is a registered trademark of Bausch Lomb Incorporated

---

MURO 128® 2% & 5% SOLUTION

Description: Muro 128® 2% Solution is a steril ophthalmic solution hypertonicity agent.

Each mL Contains: ACTIVE: Sodium Chloride 2% INACTIVES: Boric Acid, Hypromellose, Propylen Glycol, Purified Water, Sodium Borate. Sodium Hy droxide and/or Hydrochloric Acid may be added t adjust pH.

PRESERVATIVES: Methylparaben   0.028% Propylparaben 0.012%

Description: Muro 128® 5% Solution is a steril ophthalmic solution hypertonicity agent.

Drug Facts

Active ingredient — **Purpose**
Sodium chloride 2% — Hypertonicity agent
Sodium Chloride 5%

Inactive ingredients
boric acid, hypromellose, propylene glycol, purified water, sodium borate. Sodium hydroxide and/or hydrochloric acid may be added to adjust pH.
PRESERVATIVES ADDED:
methylparaben 0.028%, propylparaben 0.012%.
PRESERVATIVES ADDED FOR 5%:
methylparaben 0.023% propylparaben 0.01%

Uses
temporary relief of corneal edema

Warnings
Do not use
- except under the advice and supervision of a doctor
- if solution changes color or becomes cloudy

When using this product
- it may cause temporary burning and irritation
- to avoid contamination do not touch tip of container to any surface
- replace cap after use

Stop use and ask a doctor if
- condition worsens or persists for more than 72 hours
- you experience eye pain, changes in vision, continued redness or irritation of the eye

Keep out of reach of children.
If swallowed, get medical help or contact a Poison Control Center right away.

Directions
instill 1 or 2 drops in the affected eye(s) every 3 or 4 hours, or as directed by a physician.

How Supplied:
NDC 24208-276-15
NDC 24208-277-15
NDC 24208-277-30
½ FL. OZ. (15 mL)
1 FL. OZ. (30mL)

Other Information
- store upright at 15°-30°C (59°-86°F)
- keep tightly closed
- serious side effects associated with use of the product may be reported to the phone number provided below

Questions?
Call 1-800-323-0000
Muro 128 is a registered trademark of Bausch & Lomb Incorporated
9082302
9081702
9082102

OCUVITE® ADULT 50+   DS
Eye Vitamin and Mineral Supplement

Directions for Use: Take 1 soft gel daily, in the morning with a full glass of water during a meal. [See table above]
Other Ingredients: Gelatin, Fish Oil (anchovy, sardine), Glycerin, Yellow Beeswax, Silicon Dioxide, Soy Lecithin, FD&C Red # 40, FD&C Blue # 1, Titanium Dioxide, Natural Flavoring
How Supplied: NDC 24208-465-40 (30 ct) and NDC 24208-465-30 (50 ct) Oblong, burgundy, soft gels. Available in bottles of 30 and 50 count soft gels.
Marketed by Bausch & Lomb Incorporated, Rochester, NY 14609 Made in USA
Ocuvite® Eye Vitamin Adult 50+ Formula helps replenish essential eye protecting nutrients that you can lose as you age.[1]
Bausch + Lomb has developed this unique formulation of essential eye nutrients not found in leading multivitamins and often not obtained in sufficient quantities through diet alone.

Supplement Facts
Serving Size: 1 Soft Gel
Amount per Soft Gel

		%DV
Calories	5	
Calories from Fat	5	
Total Fat	0.5 g	1%*
Cholesterol	<5 mg	2%
Vitamin C (ascorbic acid)	150 mg	250%
Vitamin E (d-alpha tocopherol)	30 IU	100%
Zinc (as zinc oxide)	9 mg	60%
Copper (as copper gluconate)	1 mg	50%
Omega-3 fatty acids (160 mg EPA, 90 mg DHA)	250 mg	†
Lutein	5 mg	†
Zeaxanthin	1 mg	†

*Percent Daily Values (DV) are based on a 2,000 calorie diet.
†Daily Value not established.

The role of nutrients in the eye:
Lutein & Zeaxanthin – Help to filter harmful blue light and support macular health.[1]
Omega -3 – Essential nutrients that are important for proper retinal function.[1]
For more information, go to: Ocuvite.com

[1]These statements have not been evaluated by the food and Drug Administration. This product is not intended to diagnose, treat, cure or prevent any disease.
KEEP OUT OF REACH OF CHILDREN
STORE AT ROOM TEMPERATURE
For product information or to report a serious side effect call 1-800-553-5340
Ocuvite, Eye Vitamin Adult 50+ Formula contains antioxidants and nutrients, including Vitamin C, E and Zinc, to help protect eye health.[2]
Bausch+Lomb
Committed to research and leadership in ocular nutritionals
Ocuvite is a registered trademark of Bausch & Lomb Incorporated.
©Bausch & Lomb Incorporated.
DO NOT USE IF SEAL UNDER CLOSURE IS BROKEN OR MISSING

[2]This statement has not been evaluated by the food and Drug Administration. This product is not intended to diagnose, treat, cure or prevent any disease.

Shown in Product Identification Guide, page 103

OCUVITE® LUTEIN   DS
Eye Vitamin and Mineral Supplement

Supplement Facts
Serving Size: 1 tablet

Amount per Serving		%DV
Vitamin A (beta carotene)	1000 IU	20%
Vitamin C (ascorbic acid)	200 mg	333%
Vitamin E (dl-alpha tocopherol acetate)	60 IU	200%
Zinc (from zinc oxide)	40 mg	267%
Selenium (from sodium selenate)	55 mcg	79%
Copper (from cupric oxide)	2 mg	100%
Lutein	2 mg	†

†Daily Value not established.

RECOMMENDED INTAKE: Adults: One tablet per day, or as directed by your doctor.
Other Ingredients: Dibasic calcium phosphate, microcrystalline cellulose, Hypromellose, crospovidone, titanium dioxide, magnesium sterate, silicon dioxide, stearic acid, triethyl citrate, polysorbate 80, FD&C Yellow # 6 Dye, FD&C Yellow #6 Lake
How Supplied: NDC 24208-387-60 (60 ct) and NDC 24208-387-62 (120 ct) Orange, film-coated, modified-oval shaped tablet. One side is engraved with "OCUVITE" and the other side is engraved with a 02 divided by a 90° bisect. Available in bottles of 60 count and 120 count Tablets.
Marketed by: Bausch & Lomb Incorporated, Rochester, NY 14609 Made in USA
OCUVITE HELPS REPLENISH ESSENTIAL NUTRIENTS TO HELP PROTECT THE HEALTH OF YOUR EYES*
- Lutein supports macular health by helping filter harmful blue light*
- Formulation with 2 mg Lutein and other key eye nutrients helps protect eye health*
- Uses FloraGLO®, the Lutein brand most trusted by doctors[1]
OCUVITE® - IS A DOCTOR RECOMMENDED VITAMIN-MINERAL SUPPLEMENT. [2]
For more information, go to: Ocuvite.com
Reference: 1. Based on the results of the National Disease and Therapeutic Index syndicated report among physicians who recommend a dietary supplement with lutein for eye health-Sept. 2009-Sept. 2010 (USA data)
2. Data on file, Bausch & Lomb Inc.
Keep this product out of the reach of children.
STORE AT ROOM TEMPERATURE
*These statements have not been evaluated by the food and Drug Administration. This product is not intended to diagnose, treat, cure or prevent any disease.
For more information or to report a serious side effect call 1-800-553-5340
®FloraGLO is a registered trademark of Kemin Industries, Inc.
Ocuvite is a registered trademark of Bausch & Lomb incorporated.
©Bausch & Lomb Incorporated
Shown in Product Identification Guide, page 103

Continued on next page

OCUVITE® LUTEIN & ZEAXANTHIN
DS
[lu'teen]
Eye Vitamin and Mineral Supplement

Directions for Use: One capsule per day, or as directed by your doctor.
[See table above]
Other Ingredients: Lactose monohydrate, Gelatin, Crospovidone, Magnesium Stearate, Titanium dioxide, Silicon dioxide, Yellow # 6, Blue # 2.
How Supplied: NDC 24208-403-19 (36 ct) and NDC 24208-403-73 (72 ct) Yellow, two-piece hardshell capsule, printed "OCUVITE" on cap and "Lutein" on body in black ink. Available in bottles of 36 count and 72 count Capsules.
Marketed by Bausch & Lomb Incorporated, Rochester, NY 14609 Made in USA
OCUVITE HELPS REPLENISH ESSENTIAL NUTRIENTS TO HELP PROTECT THE HEALTH OF YOUR EYES[1]
- Lutein supports macular health by helping filter harmful blue light[1]
- Formulation with 6 mg Lutein/Zeaxanthin and other key eye nutrients helps protect eye health[1]
- Uses FloraGLO®, the Lutein brand most trusted by doctors[1]
OCUVITE® - IS A DOCTOR RECOMMENED VITAMIN-MINERAL SUPPLEMENT.[2]
For more information, go to: Ocuvite.com
Reference: 1. Based on the results of the National Disease and Therapeutic Index syndicated report among physicians who recommend a dietary supplement with lutein for eye health-Sept. 2009-Sept. 2010 (USA data)
2. Data on file, Bausch & Lomb Inc.
Keep this product out of the reach of children.
STORE AT ROOM TEMPERATURE

[1]These statements have not been evaluated by the food and Drug Administration. This product is not intended to diagnose, treat, cure or prevent any disease.
For more information or to report a serious side effect call 1-800-553-5340
®FloraGLO is a registered trademark of Kemin Industries, Inc.
Ocuvite is a registered trademark of Bausch & Lomb incorporated.
©Bausch & Lomb Incorporated
Shown in Product Identification Guide, page 103

Supplement Facts
Serving Size: 1 Capsule
Amount per Serving

		%DV
Vitamin C (ascorbic acid)	60 mg	100%
Vitamin E (d-alpha tocopherol acetate)	30 IU	100%
Zinc (from zinc oxide)	15 mg	100%
Copper (from cupric oxide)	2 mg	100%
Crystalline Lutein Lutein, Zeaxanthin	6 mg	†

†Daily Value not established

Table A

Supplement Facts
Serving Size: 1 soft gel

Amount per serving	1 soft gel	% DV
Vitamin A (beta-carotene)	14,320 IU	286%
Vitamin C (ascorbic acid)	226 mg	377%
Vitamin E (dl-alpha tocopheryl acetate)	200 IU	667%
Zinc (zinc oxide)	34.8 mg	232%
Copper (cupric oxide)	0.8 mg	40%

OPCON-A®
OTC

Drug Facts

Active ingredients	Purpose
Naphazoline HCl (0.02675%)	Redness Reliever
Pheniramine maleate (0.315%)	Antihistamine

Uses
- temporarily relieves itching and redness caused by pollen, ragweed, grass, animal hair and dander.

Warnings
Do not use
- if you are sensitive to any ingredient in this product
- if solution changes color or becomes cloudy
Ask a doctor before use if you have
- heart disease
- high blood pressure
- trouble urinating due to an enlarged prostate gland
- narrow angle glaucoma
When using this product
- overuse may cause more eye redness
- pupils may become enlarged temporarily
- do not touch tip of container to any surface to avoid contamination
- you may feel a brief tingling after putting drops in eye
- replace cap after use
- remove contact lenses before using

Stop use and ask a doctor if you experience
- eye pain
- changes in vision
- redness or irritation of the eye that worsens or lasts more than 72 hours.
Keep out of reach of children.
If swallowed, get medical help or contact a Poison Control Center right away. Accidental oral ingestion in infants and children may lead to coma and marked reduction in body temperature.
Directions
- **Adults and children 6 years of age and older:** Instill 1 or 2 drops in the affected eye(s) up to 4 times daily.
- **Children under 6 years:** ask a doctor
Other information
- store at 20°-25°C (68°-77°F)
- protect from light
- use before expiration date marked on the carton or bottle
Inactive ingredients
benzalkonium chloride, boric acid, edetate disodium, hypromellose, purified water, sodium borate, sodium chloride
Questions or Comments?
Call: 1-800-553-5340
Shown in Product Identification Guide, page 103

PRESERVISION® EYE VITAMIN
DS
AREDS FORMULA
AREDS: Soft Gels Formula.
2 per day Soft Gels Formula (AREDS daily dose)

Description: *see Supplement Facts (table A)*
[See table above]
Other Ingredients: Gelatin, Glycerin, Soybean Oil, Soy Lecithin, Yellow Beeswax, Silicon Dioxide, Titanium Dioxide, FD&C Yellow #6, FD&C Red #40, FD&C Blue #1. Contains Soy.
- Age-related macular degeneration (AMD) is the leading cause of vision loss and blindness in people over 65. The landmark National Institutes of Health AREDS trial proved that a high potency antioxidant vitamin and mineral supplement was effective in reducing risk of AMD-associated vision loss.[1]
- The patented Bausch & Lomb PreserVision® Eye Vitamin AREDS Formula Soft Gels are based on the original PreserVision® Eye Vitamin AREDS Formula that is the ONLY eye vitamin and mineral supplement clinically proven effective in the

10 year National Institutes of Health (NIH) Age Related Eye Disease Study (AREDS). US Paten 6,660,297.
- Bausch & Lomb PreserVision® Eye Vitamir AREDS Formula Soft Gels are a high potency antioxidant and mineral supplement with the anti oxidant vitamins A, C, E, and selected minerals in amounts above those in ordinary multivitamins and generally cannot be obtained through die alone.
- **Directions for Use:** Take 2 soft gels daily; 1 in the morning, 1 in the evening with a full glass o water and during meals.
Bausch & Lomb PreserVision® Eye Vitamin is the #1 recommended eye vitamin and mineral supplement among vitreoretinal eye doctors for AMD.[2]
CURRENT AND FORMER SMOKERS:
Consult your eye doctor or eye care professiona about the risks associated with smoking and Beta Carotene.

[1]This statement has not been evaluated by the Food and Drug Administration. This product is not intended to diagnose, treat, cure or prevent any disease.
[2]Data on file, Bausch & Lomb Incorporated.
How Supplied: NDC 24208-532-20 60 ct. NDC 24208-532-30 120 ct. NDC 24208-532-40 150 ct. Available in bottles of 60 count, 120 and 150 count soft gels.
Oval shaped soft gelatin capsule.
DO NOT USE IF SEAL UNDER CLOSURE IS BROKEN
Keep this product out of the reach of children.
STORE AT ROOM TEMPERATURE
For more information or to report a serious side effect, call 1-800-553-5340
Made in the USA
Marketed by:
Bausch & Lomb Incorporated, Rochester NY 14609
Preservision is a registered trademark of Bausch & Lomb Incorporated.
© Bausch & Lomb Incorporated. All rights reserved.
Shown in Product Identification Guide, page 103

PRESERVISION®
DS
EYE VITAMIN AREDS FORMULA TABLETS
High Potency Eye Vitamin and Mineral Supplement Original, 4 per day tablets

Description: *see Supplement Facts (table A)*
[See table at top of next page]

Other Ingredients: Lactose Monohydrate, Micro-crystalline Cellulose, Crospovidone, Stearic Acid, Magnesium Stearate, Silicon Dioxide, Polysorbate 80, Triethyl Citrate, Titanium Dioxide Yellow #6, Yellow 6 Lake, Red #40, Red 40 Lake. Contains Soy.

- Age-related macular degeneration is the leading cause of vision loss and blindness in people over 65. The National Institutes of Health (NIH) Age Related Eye Disease Study (AREDS) proved that a unique high-potency vitamin and mineral supplement was effective in reducing risk of AMD - associated vision loss.[1]
- Bausch & Lomb **PreserVision®** Eye Vitamin AREDS Formula was the only eye vitamin and mineral supplement clinically proven effective in the NIH AREDS Study.
- Bausch & Lomb **PreserVision®** Eye Vitamin AREDS Formula is a high-potency antioxidant supplement with the antioxidant vitamins A, C, E and select minerals at levels that are well above those in ordinary multivitamins and generally cannot be attained through diet alone.

For a FREE 16-page brochure on Age-Related Macular Degeneration call toll-free **1-866-467-3263 (1-866-HOPE-AMD)**

[1] This statement has not been evaluated by the Food and Drug Administration. This product is not intended to diagnose, treat, cure or prevent any disease.

Recommended Intake: To get the same levels proven in the NIH AREDS Study it is important to take 4 tablets per day – 2 in the morning, 2 in the evening with a full glass of water and during meals.

Smokers: Consult your eye care professional about the risks associated with smoking and using Beta-Carotene.

Bausch & Lomb PreserVision® is the #1 recommended eye vitamin and mineral supplement brand among Retinal Specialists.[1]

How Supplied: NDC 24208-432-62 (120 ct) NDC 24208-432-72 (240 ct) Eye shaped film coated tablet, engraved BL 01 on one side, scored on the other side. Available in bottles of 120 or 240 count tablets **DO NOT USE IF SEAL UNDER CLOSURE IS BROKEN.**

Keep this product out of the reach of children. **STORE AT ROOM TEMPERATURE.**

For more information or to report a serious side effect, call 1-800-553-5340
Made in USA
Marketed by
Bausch & Lomb Incorporated
Rochester, NY 14609
References: 1. Data on file, Bausch & Lomb, Incorporated
© Bausch & Lomb Incorporated. All Rights Reserved.
Preservision is a registered trademark of Bausch & Lomb Incorporated. Other brand names are trademarks of their respective owners.

Shown in Product Identification Guide, page 103

PRESERVISION® EYE VITAMIN AREDS 2 FORMULA — DS
Eye Vitamin and Mineral Supplement

Directions for Use: Take 4 Soft Gels per day, 2 in the morning, 2 in the evening with a full glass of water and during meals.
[See table above]
Other Ingredients: Gelatin, Fish Oil (anchovy, sardine), Glycerin, Yellow Beeswax, Silicon Dioxide, Soy Lecithin, FD&C Red # 40, FD&C Blue # 1, Titanium Dioxide, Natural Flavoring
How Supplied: NDC 24208-625-04 (120 ct) Oblong, dark red, soft gel. Available in bottles of 120 count soft gels.
Marketed by Bausch & Lomb Rochester, NY 14609
Made in USA
KEEP OUT OF REACH OF CHILDREN
STORE AT ROOM TEMPERATURE

Table A

Supplement Facts
Serving Size: 2 tablets

Contents	Two tablets Amount	% of Daily Value	Daily Dosage (4 tablets) Amount	% of Daily Value
Vitamin A (100% as beta-carotene)	14,320 IU	286%	28,640 IU	573%
Vitamin C (ascorbic acid)	226 mg	377%	452 mg	753%
Vitamin E (dl-alpha tocopheryl acetate)	200 IU	667%	400 IU	1333%
Zinc (zinc oxide)	34.8 mg	232%	69.6 mg	464%
Copper (cupric oxide)	0.8 mg	40%	1.6 mg	80%

Supplement Facts
Serving Size: 2 Soft Gels

	Per Serving Amount	%DV	Per Day Amount	%DV
Calories	10		20	
Calories from Fat	10		20	
Total Fat	1 g	1%‡	2 g	2%‡
Polyunsaturated Fat	0.5 g	**	1 g	**
Cholesterol	10 mg	3%	20 mg	6%
Vitamin C (ascorbic acid)	226 mg	377%	452 mg	753%
Vitamin E (d-alpha tocopherol)	200 IU	667%	400 IU	1333%
Zinc (as zinc oxide)	34.8 mg	232%	69.6 mg	464%
Copper (as copper gluconate)	0.8 mg	40%	1.6 mg	80%
Omega-3 fatty acids (325 mg EPA, 175 mg DHA)	500 mg	**	1000 mg	**
Lutein	5 mg	**	10 mg	**
Zeaxanthin	1 mg	**	2 mg	**

‡ Percent Daily Values (DV) are based on a 2,000 calorie diet.
** Daily Value (DV) not established

DO NOT USE IF SEAL UNDER CLOSURE IS BROKEN OR MISSING
†Bausch & Lomb PreserVision® Eye Vitamin AREDS 2 formula builds on the original PreserVision® Eye Vitamin AREDS formula, replacing beta-carotene with lutein (10 mg) and zeaxanthin (2 mg), and adding Omega-3 (1000 mg) per daily dosage.
Bausch & Lomb original PreserVision® Eye Vitamin AREDS formula is the one and only antioxidant vitamin and mineral supplement formula proven clinically effective in the Age-Related Eye Disease Study (AREDS).
One serving contains 325 mg EPA and 175 mg DHA, two important Omega-3 fatty acids. Compare levels to those of other fish oil supplements.
Bausch & Lomb was a proud sponsor of the original landmark AREDS study conducted by the National Institutes of Health.
Studies indicate that proper nutrition is important to help maintain eye health. As we age, our eyes may not get enough nutrition through diet alone. PreserVision® Eye Vitamin AREDS 2 formula contains 10 mg lutein, 2 mg zeaxanthin, 1000 mg of Omega-3 per daily dosage, and antioxidants vitamins C and E that are essential to the health of your eyes.[1] The leading multi-vitamins contain only a fraction of the amounts found to be beneficial.

[1] This statement has not been evaluated by the food and Drug Administration. This product is not intended to diagnose, treat, cure or prevent any disease.
To obtain product information or to report a serious side effect call 1-800-553-5340
AREDS 2 is a registered trademark of the United States Department of Health and Human Services.

AREDS2® is an ongoing study that is expected to end in 2013.
®Bausch & Lomb Incorporated.
Preservision is a registered trademark of Bausch & Lomb Incorporated.

Shown in Product Identification Guide, page 104

PRESERVISION® EYE VITAMIN LUTEIN FORMULA — DS
Eye Vitamin and Mineral Supplement
Beta-carotene free formulation.
Convenient to take 2 per day Soft Gels

Description: *see Supplement Facts (table A)*
[See table at top of next page]
Other Ingredients: Gelatin, Glycerin, Soybean Oil, Soy Lecithin, Yellow Beeswax, Silicon Dioxide, Titanium Dioxide, FD&C Red #40, FD&C Blue #1. Contains Soy.
This product is Vitamin A (beta-carotene) Free.
- The Bausch & Lomb PreserVision® Eye Vitamin Lutein Formula is based on the Bausch & Lomb PreserVision® Eye Vitamin AREDS Formula[1], with the beta-carotene substituted with 5 mg of FloraGlo® Lutein.
- Lutein is a carotenoid found in dark leafy green vegetables such as spinach. Carotenoids can be concentrated in the macula, the part of the eye responsible for central vision. Studies suggest that lutein may play an essential role in maintaining healthy central vision by protecting against free radical damage and filtering blue light.[2]
- Lutein levels in your eye are related to the amount in your diet. Bausch & Lomb PreserVision® Eye Vitamin Lutein Formula con-

Continued on next page

Supplement Facts
Serving Size: 1 soft gel

Amount per serving	1 Soft Gel	% Daily Value
Vitamin C (ascorbic acid)	226 mg	377%
Vitamin E (dl-alpha tocopheryl acetate)	200 IU	667%
Zinc (zinc oxide)	34.8 mg	232%
Copper (cupric oxide)	0.8 mg	40%
Lutein	5 mg	†

† Daily value not established

Preservision Lutein—Cont.

tains 5 mg of lutein per soft gel, which gives you 10 mg of lutein per day. The leading multivitamin contains only a fraction of the amount of lutein used in clinical studies.

[1]The original Bausch & Lomb PreserVision® Eye Vitamin AREDS Formula was the only antioxidant vitamin and mineral supplement proven effective in the 10-year National Institutes of Health (NIH) Age-Related Eye Disease Study (AREDS). AREDS was a 10-year, independent study conducted by the National Eye Institute (NEI) of the National Institutes of Health (NIH).
[2]**These statements have not been evaluated by the Food and Drug Administration. This product is not intended to diagnose, treat, cure or prevent any disease.**
Directions for Use: Take 2 soft gels daily; 1 in the morning, 1 in the evening with a full glass of water and during meals.
How Supplied: NDC 24208-632-10 (50 ct) NDC 24208-632-11 (120 ct) NDC 24208-632-61 (180 ct). Available in bottles of 50, 120 and 180 count soft gels. Oval shaped soft gelatin capsule.
DO NOT USE IF SEAL UNDER CLOSURE IS BROKEN.
Keep this product out of the reach of children.
STORE AT ROOM TEMPERATURE
For more information or to report a serious side effect, call 1-800-553-5340
®FloraGLO is a registered trademark of Kemin Industries, Inc.
Made in the USA
Marketed by:
Bausch & Lomb Incorporated, Rochester NY 14609
© Bausch & Lomb Incorporated. All rights reserved.
PreserVision is a registered trademark of Bausch & Lomb Incorporated.
Shown in Product Identification Guide, page 104

SOOTHE® HYDRATION LUBRICANT EYE DROPS   OTC

Drug Facts

Active ingredient	Purpose
Povidone (1.25%)	Lubricant

Uses
• relieves dryness of the eye
• prevents further irritation
Warnings
For external use only.
Do not use
• if solution changes color or becomes cloudy
When using this product
• do not touch tip of container to any surface to avoid contamination
• replace cap after using
Stop use and ask a doctor if you experience
• eye pain
• change in vision
• continued redness or irritation of the eye
• or if condition worsens or lasts more than 72 hours
If pregnant or breast feeding, ask a health professional before use.

Keep out of reach of children.
If swallowed, get medical help or contact a Poison Control Center right away.
Directions
• Put 1 to 2 drop(s) in the affected eye(s) as needed or directed by your doctor.
Other information
• Storage: 15° − 25°C (59° − 77°F)
• Use before expiration date marked on the carton or bottle
Inactive ingredients
boric acid, potassium chloride, sodium borate and sodium chloride; preserved with edetate disodium 0.1% and sorbic acid 0.1%
Questions or Comments?
Toll Free Product Information or to Report a Serious Side Effect Associated with use of the product Call: 1-800-533-5340
Soothe is a registered trademark of Bausch & Lomb Incorporated.
© Bausch & Lomb Incorporated.
Shown in Product Identification Guide, page 104

SOOTHE® NIGHT TIME   OTC

Drug Facts

Active ingredient	Purpose
Mineral oil (20%), White petrolatum (80%)	Lubricant

Uses
• relieves dryness of the eye
• prevents further irritation
Warnings
When using this product
• do not touch tip of container to any surface to avoid contamination
• do not use with contact lenses
• replace cap after use
Stop use and ask a doctor if
• you experience eye pain, change in vision, continued redness or irritation of the eye
• condition worsens or persists for more than 72 hours
Keep out of reach of children.
If swallowed, get medical help or contact a Poison Control Center right away.
Directions
• pull down the lower lid of the affected eye(s)
• apply a small amount (1/4 inch) of ointment to the inside of eyelid
• apply one or more times daily
Other information
• Storage: 15° − 25°C (59° − 77°F)
• keep tightly closed
• see crimp of tube or carton for Lot Number and Expiration Date
• use before expiration date marked on the carton and tube
• serious side effects associated with use of the product may be reported to the phone number below
Questions or Comments?
Call: 1-800-553-5340
Shown in Product Identification Guide, page 104

SOOTHE® PRESERVATIVE FREE LUBRICANT EYE DROPS   OTC
Lubricant Eye Drops

PERSISTENT DRY EYE
Ideal for sensitive eyes and LASIK dryness.
Description: *Preservative-Free,* Long Lasting Relief. This revolutionary advance in dry eye therapy provides soothing comfort and long lasting lubrication, keeping eyes feeling fresh throughout the day. This unique new formula restores the natural moisture in your eyes, providing effective, long lasting dry eye relief. Preservative-Free so it's gentle enough to use as often as needed

Drug Facts

Active Ingredients	Purpose
Glycerin (0.6%)	Lubricant
Propylene Glycol (0.6%)	Lubricant

Purpose: Lubricant Eye Drops

Inactive Ingredients
Boric acid, hydroxyalkylphosphonate, purified water, sodium alginate, sodium borate
Uses:
■ relieves dryness of the eye
■ prevents further irritation
Warnings:
Do not use
■ if solution changes color or becomes cloudy
■ if single-unit dispenser is not intact
When using this product
■ do not touch the tip of container to any surface to avoid contamination
■ once opened, discard
■ do not reuse
Stop and ask a doctor if
■ you experience eye pain, changes in vision, continued redness or irritation of the eye
■ condition worsens or persists for more than 72 hours
Keep out of reach of children. If swallowed, get medical help or contact a Poison Control Center right away.
Directions:
Easy to use sterile dispenser
■ To open, completely twist off tab
■ Instill 1 to 2 drops in the affected eye(s) as needed
Other Information
STORE AT 15°−25°C (59°−77°F)
DO NOT USE IF TAPE SEALS IMPRINTED WITH B&L TAPE SEAL ARE NOT INTACT
How Supplied:
NDC # 24208-495-28
4 ct. sample: 24208-495-95
28 sterile single-use dispensers 0.02 FL OZ EA (0.6mL EA)

Questions or Comments?
Toll Free product information or to report a serious side effect associated with use of this product call: 1-800-553-5340.
Soothe is a registered trademark of Bausch & Lomb Incorporated.
© Bausch & Lomb Incorporated
Patents pending.
Manufactured for:
Bausch & Lomb Incorporated
Rochester, NY 14609
Made in USA
www.bausch.com
Shown in Product Identification Guide, page 104

TOBRAMYCIN AND DEXAMETHASONE OPHTHALMIC SUSPENSION USP,   ℞
0.3%/0.1% (Sterile)
FOR OPHTHALMIC USE ONLY

DESCRIPTION:

Tobramycin and Dexamethasone Ophthalmic Suspension USP, 0.3%/0.1% is a sterile, multiple dose antibiotic and steroid combination for topical ophthalmic use. Tobramycin is represented by the following structural formula:

$C_{18}H_{37}N_5O_9$ Mol. Wt. 467.52

Chemical Name: O-3-Amino-3-deoxy-α-D-glucopyranosyl-(1→4)-O-[(2,6-diamino-2,3,6-tridexoxy-α-D-$ribo$-hexopyranosyl-(1→6)]-2-deoxy-L-streptamine

Dexamethasone is represented by the following structural formula:

$C_{22}H_{29}FO_5$ Mol. Wt. 392.47

Chemical Name: 9-Fluoro-11β,17,21-trihydroxy-16α-methylpregna-1,4-diene-3,20-dione

Each mL Contains: ACTIVES: Tobramycin 3 mg (0.3%) and Dexamethasone 1 mg (0.1%); INACTIVES: Sodium Sulfate, Sodium Chloride, Hydroxyethyl Cellulose, Tyloxapol, Edetate Disodium and Purified Water. Sulfuric Acid and/or Sodium Hydroxide may be added to adjust pH (5.0 - 6.0). PRESERVATIVE ADDED: Benzalkonium Chloride 0.01%.

CLINICAL PHARMACOLOGY: Corticoids suppress the inflammatory response to a variety of agents and they probably delay or slow healing. Since corticoids may inhibit the body's defense mechanism against infection, a concomitant antimicrobial drug may be used when this inhibition is considered to be clinically significant. Dexamethasone is a potent corticoid.

The antibiotic component in the combination (tobramycin) is included to provide action against susceptible organisms. *In vitro* studies have demonstrated that tobramycin is active against susceptible strains of the following microorganisms: Staphylococci, including *S. aureus* and *S. epidermidis* (coagulase-positive and coagulase-negative), including penicillin-resistant strains.

Streptococci, including some of the Group A-beta-hemolytic species, some nonhemolytic species, and some *Streptococcus pneumoniae*.

Pseudomonas aeruginosa, Escherichia coli, Klebsiella pneumoniae, Enterobacter aerogenes, Proteus mirabilis, Morganella morganii, most *Proteus vulgaris* strains, *Haemophilus influenzae* and *H. aegyptius, Moraxella lacunata, Acinetobacter calcoaceticus* and some *Neisseria* species.

Bacterial susceptibility studies demonstrate that in some cases microorganisms resistant to gentamicin remain susceptible to tobramycin.

No data are available on the extent of systemic absorption from tobramycin and dexamethasone ophthalmic suspension; however, it is known that some systemic absorption can occur with ocularly applied drugs. If the maximum dose of tobramycin and dexamethasone ophthalmic suspension is given for the first 48 hours (two drops in each eye every 2 hours) and complete systemic absorption occurs, which is highly unlikely, the daily dose of dexamethasone would be 2.4 mg. The usual physiologic replacement dose is 0.75 mg daily. If tobramycin and dexamethasone ophthalmic suspension is given after the first 48 hours as two drops in each eye every 4 hours, the administered dose of dexamethasone would be 1.2 mg daily.

INDICATIONS AND USAGE: Tobramycin and dexamethasone ophthalmic suspension is indicated for steroid responsive inflammatory ocular conditions for which a corticosteroid is indicated and where superficial bacterial ocular infection or a risk of bacterial ocular infection exists.

Ocular steroids are indicated in inflammatory conditions of the palpebral and bulbar conjunctiva, cornea and anterior segment of the globe where the inherent risk of steroid use in certain infective conjunctivitides is accepted to obtain a diminution in edema and inflammation. They are also indicated in chronic anterior uveitis and corneal injury from chemical, radiation or thermal burns, or penetration of foreign bodies.

The use of a combination drug with an anti-infective component is indicated where the risk of superficial ocular infection is high or where there is an expectation that potentially dangerous numbers of bacteria will be present in the eye.

The particular anti-infective drug in this product is active against the following common bacterial eye pathogens:

Staphylococci, including *S. aureus* and *S. epidermidis* (coagulase-positive and coagulase-negative), including penicillin-resistant strains.

Streptococci, including some of the Group A-beta-hemolytic species, some nonhemolytic species, and some *Streptococcus pneumoniae*.

Pseudomonas aeruginosa, Escherichia coli, Klebsiella pneumoniae, Enterobacter aerogenes, Proteus mirabilis, Morganella morganii, most *Proteus vulgaris* strains, *Haemophilus influenzae* and *H. aegyptius, Moraxella lacunata, Acinetobacter calcoaceticus* and some *Neisseria* species.

CONTRAINDICATIONS: Epithelial herpes simplex keratitis (dendritic keratitis), vaccinia, varicella, and many other viral diseases of the cornea and conjunctiva. Mycobacterial infection of the eye. Fungal diseases of ocular structures. Hypersensitivity to a component of the medication.

WARNINGS: FOR TOPICAL OPHTHALMIC USE ONLY. NOT FOR INJECTION INTO THE EYE.

Sensitivity to topically applied aminoglycosides may occur in some patients. If a sensitivity reaction does occur, discontinue use.

Prolonged use of steroids may result in glaucoma, with damage to the optic nerve, defects in visual acuity and fields of vision, and posterior subcapsular cataract formation. Intraocular pressure should be routinely monitored even though it may be difficult in pediatric patients and uncooperative patients. Prolonged use may suppress the host response and thus increase the hazard of secondary ocular infections. In those diseases causing thinning of the cornea or sclera, perforations have been known to occur with the use of topical steroids. In acute purulent conditions of the eye, steroids may mask infection or enhance existing infection.

PRECAUTIONS:

General The possibility of fungal infections of the cornea should be considered after long-term steroid dosing. As with other antibiotic preparations, prolonged use may result in overgrowth of nonsusceptible organisms, including fungi. If superinfection occurs, appropriate therapy should be initiated. When multiple prescriptions are required, or whenever clinical judgement dictates, the patient should be examined with the aid of magnification, such as slit lamp biomicroscopy and, where appropriate, fluorescein staining.

Cross-sensitivity to other aminoglycoside antibiotics may occur; if hypersensitivity develops with this product, discontinue use and institute appropriate therapy.

Information for Patients: Do not touch dropper tip to any surface, as this may contaminate the contents. Contact lenses should not be worn during the use of this product.

Carcinogenesis, Mutagenesis, Impairment of Fertility: No studies have been conducted to evaluate the carcinogenic or mutagenic potential. No impairment of fertility was noted in studies of subcutaneous tobramycin in rats at doses of 50 and 100 mg/kg/day.

Pregnancy Category C: Corticosteroids have been found to be teratogenic in animal studies. Ocular administration of 0.1% dexamethasone resulted in 15.6% and 32.3% incidence of fetal anomalies in two groups of pregnant rabbits. Fetal growth retardation and increased mortality rates have been observed in rats with chronic dexamethasone therapy. Reproduction studies have been performed in rats and rabbits with tobramycin at doses up to 100 mg/kg/day parenterally and have revealed no evidence of impaired fertility or harm to the fetus. There are no adequate and well controlled studies in pregnant women. Tobramycin and dexamethasone ophthalmic suspension should be used during pregnancy only if the potential benefit justifies the potential risk to the fetus.

Nursing Mothers: Systemically administered corticosteroids appear in human milk and could suppress growth, interfere with endogenous corticosteroid production, or cause other untoward effects. It is not known whether topical administration of corticosteroids could result in sufficient systemic absorption to produce detectable quantities in human milk. Because many drugs are excreted in human milk, caution should be exercised when tobramycin and dexamethasone ophthalmic suspension is administered to a nursing woman.

Pediatric Use: Safety and effectiveness in pediatric patients below the age of 2 years have not been established.

Geriatric Use: No overall differences in safety or effectiveness have been observed between elderly and younger patients.

ADVERSE REACTIONS: Adverse reactions have occurred with steroid/anti-infective combination drugs which can be attributed to the steroid component, the anti-infective component, or the combination. Exact incidence figures are not available. The most frequent adverse reactions to topical ocular tobramycin are hypersensitivity and localized ocular toxicity, including lid itching and swelling, and conjunctival erythema. These reactions occur in less than 4% of patients. Similar reactions may occur with the topical use of other aminoglycoside antibiotics. Other adverse reactions have not been reported; however, if topical ocular tobramycin is administered concomitantly with systemic aminoglycoside antibiotics, care should be taken to monitor the total serum concentration. The reactions due to the steroid component are: elevation of intraocular pressure (IOP) with possible development of glaucoma, and infrequent optic nerve damage; posterior subcapsular cataract formation; and delayed wound healing.

Secondary Infection: The development of secondary infection has occurred after use of combinations containing steroids and antimicrobials. Fungal infections of the cornea are particularly prone to develop coincidentally with long-term applications of steroids. The possibility of fungal invasion must be considered in any persistent corneal ulceration where steroid treatment has been used. Secondary bacterial ocular infection following suppression of host responses also occurs.

OVERDOSAGE: Clinically apparent signs and symptoms of an overdosage of tobramycin and dexamethasone ophthalmic suspension (punctate keratitis, erythema, increased lacrimation, edema and lid itching) may be similar to adverse reaction effects seen in some patients.

DOSAGE AND ADMINISTRATION: One or two drops instilled into the conjunctival sac(s) every four to six hours. During the initial 24 to 48 hours, the dosage may be increased to one or two drops every two (2) hours. Frequency should be decreased gradually as warranted by improvement in clinical signs. Care should be taken not to discontinue therapy prematurely.

Not more than 20 mL should be prescribed initially and the prescription should not be refilled without further evaluation as outlined in PRECAUTIONS above.

HOW SUPPLIED:

Tobramycin and Dexamethasone Ophthalmic Suspension USP, 0.3%/0.1% is supplied in a plastic bottle with a controlled drop tip in the following sizes:

Continued on next page

Tobramycin—Cont.

2.5 mL NDC 24208-295-25
5 mL NDC 24208-295-05
10 mL NDC 24208-295-10

DO NOT USE IF IMPRINTED NECKBAND IS NOT INTACT.

Storage: Store upright at 20° - 25°C (68° - 77°F) [See USP Controlled Room Temperature]. Shake well before using.
Rx only
Revised July 2008
Bausch & Lomb Incorporated
Tampa, Florida 33637
©Bausch & Lomb Incorporated
9090701 (folded)
9090601 (flat)

ZIRGAN®   ℞

[zir-gan]
(ganciclovir ophthalmic gel) 0.15%

HIGHLIGHTS OF PRESCRIBING INFORMATION
These highlights do not include all of the information needed to use ZIRGAN® safely and effectively. See full prescribing information for ZIRGAN.
ZIRGAN (ganciclovir ophthalmic gel) 0.15%
Initial U.S. approval: 1989

——————— INDICATIONS AND USAGE ———————

ZIRGAN is a topical ophthalmic antiviral that is indicated for the treatment of acute herpetic keratitis (dendritic ulcers). *(1)*

——— DOSAGE AND ADMINISTRATION ———

The recommended dosing regimen for ZIRGAN is 1 drop in the affected eye 5 times per day (approximately every 3 hours while awake) until the corneal ulcer heals, and then 1 drop 3 times per day for 7 days. *(2)*

——— DOSAGE FORMS AND STRENGTHS ———

ZIRGAN contains 0.15% of ganciclovir in a sterile preserved topical ophthalmic gel. *(3)*

——————— CONTRAINDICATIONS ———————

None.

——— WARNINGS AND PRECAUTIONS ———

• ZIRGAN is indicated for topical ophthalmic use only. *(5.1)*
• Patients should not wear contact lenses if they have signs or symptoms of herpetic keratitis or during the course of therapy with ZIRGAN. *(5.2)*

——————— ADVERSE REACTIONS ———————

Most common adverse reactions reported in patients were blurred vision (60%), eye irritation (20%), punctate keratitis (5%), and conjunctival hyperemia (5%). *(6)*
To report SUSPECTED ADVERSE REACTIONS, contact Bausch & Lomb at 1-800-323-0000 or FDA at 1-800-FDA-1088 or www.fda.gov/medwatch.
See 17 for PATIENT COUNSELING INFORMATION

Revised: 06/2010

FULL PRESCRIBING INFORMATION: CONTENTS*

FULL PRESCRIBING INFORMATION

1   INDICATIONS AND USAGE
ZIRGAN (ganciclovir ophthalmic gel) 0.15% is indicated for the treatment of acute herpetic keratitis (dendritic ulcers).

2   DOSAGE AND ADMINISTRATION
The recommended dosing regimen for ZIRGAN is 1 drop in the affected eye 5 times per day (approximately every 3 hours while awake) until the corneal ulcer heals, and then 1 drop 3 times per day for 7 days.

3   DOSAGE FORMS AND STRENGTHS
ZIRGAN contains 0.15% of ganciclovir in a sterile preserved topical ophthalmic gel.

4   CONTRAINDICATIONS
None.

5   WARNINGS AND PRECAUTIONS
5.1   Topical Ophthalmic Use Only
ZIRGAN is indicated for topical ophthalmic use only.

5.2   Avoidance of Contact Lenses
Patients should not wear contact lenses if they have signs or symptoms of herpetic keratitis or during the course of therapy with ZIRGAN.

6   ADVERSE REACTIONS
Most common adverse reactions reported in patients were blurred vision (60%), eye irritation (20%), punctate keratitis (5%), and conjunctival hyperemia (5%).

8   USE IN SPECIFIC POPULATIONS
8.1   Pregnancy: Teratogenic Effects
Pregnancy Category C: Ganciclovir has been shown to be embryotoxic in rabbits and mice following intravenous administration and teratogenic in rabbits. Fetal resorptions were present in at least 85% of rabbits and mice administered 60 mg/kg/day and 108 mg/kg/day (approximately 10,000× and 17,000× the human ocular dose of 6.25 mcg/kg/day), respectively, assuming complete absorption. Effects observed in rabbits included: fetal growth retardation, embryolethality, teratogenicity, and/or maternal toxicity. Teratogenic changes included cleft palate, anophthalmia/microphthalmia, aplastic organs (kidney and pancreas), hydrocephaly, and brachygnathia. In mice, effects observed were maternal/fetal toxicity and embryolethality. Daily intravenous doses of 90 mg/kg/day (14,000× the human ocular dose) administered to female mice prior to mating, during gestation, and during lactation caused hypoplasia of the testes and seminal vesicles in the month-old male offspring, as well as pathologic changes in the nonglandular region of the stomach *(see Carcinogenesis, Mutagenesis, and Impairment of Fertility)*.
There are no adequate and well-controlled studies in pregnant women. ZIRGAN should be used during pregnancy only if the potential benefit justifies the potential risk to the fetus.

8.3   Nursing Mothers
It is not known whether topical ophthalmic ganciclovir administration could result in sufficient systemic absorption to produce detectable quantities in breast milk. Caution should be exercised when ZIRGAN is administered to nursing mothers.

8.4   Pediatric Use
Safety and efficacy in pediatric patients below the age of 2 years have not been established.

8.5   Geriatric Use
No overall differences in safety or effectiveness have been observed between elderly and younger patients.

11   DESCRIPTION
ZIRGAN (ganciclovir ophthalmic gel) 0.15% contains a sterile, topical antiviral for ophthalmic use. The chemical name is 9-[[2-hydroxy-1-(hydroxymethyl)ethoxy]methyl]guanine (CAS number 82410-32-0). Ganciclovir is represented by the following structural formula:

Ganciclovir has a molecular weight of 255.23, and the empirical formula is $C_9H_{13}N_5O_4$.
Each gram of gel contains: ACTIVE: ganciclovir 1.5 mg (0.15%). INACTIVES: carbopol, water for injection, sodium hydroxide (to adjust the pH to 7.4), mannitol. PRESERVATIVE: benzalkonium chloride 0.075 mg.

12   CLINICAL PHARMACOLOGY
12.1   Mechanism of Action
ZIRGAN (ganciclovir ophthalmic gel) 0.15% contains the active ingredient, ganciclovir, which is a guanosine derivative that, upon phosphorylation, inhibits DNA replication by herpes simplex viruses (HSV). Ganciclovir is transformed by viral and cellular thymidine kinases (TK) to ganciclovir triphosphate, which works as an antiviral agent by inhibiting the synthesis of viral DNA in 2 ways: competitive inhibition of viral DNA-polymerase and direct incorporation into viral primer strand DNA, resulting in DNA chain termination and prevention of replication.

12.3   Pharmacokinetics
The estimated maximum daily dose of ganciclovir administered as 1 drop, 5 times per day is 0.375 mg. Compared to maintenance doses of systemically administered ganciclovir of 900 mg (oral valganciclovir) and 5 mg/kg (IV ganciclovir), the ophthalmically administered daily dose is approximately 0.04% and 0.1% of the oral dose and IV doses, respectively, thus minimal systemic exposure is expected.

13   NONCLINICAL TOXICOLOGY
13.1   Carcinogenesis, Mutagenesis, and Impairment of Fertility
Ganciclovir was carcinogenic in the mouse at oral doses of 20 and 1,000 mg/kg/day (approximately 3,000× and 160,000× the human ocular dose of 6.25 mcg/kg/day, assuming complete absorption). At the dose of 1,000 mg/kg/day there was a significant increase in the incidence of tumors of the preputial gland in males, forestomach (nonglandular mucosa) in males and females, and reproductive tissues (ovaries, uterus, mammary gland, clitoral gland, and vagina) and liver in females. At the dose of 20 mg/kg/day, a slightly increased incidence of tumors was noted in the preputial and harderian glands in males, forestomach in males and females, and liver in females. No carcinogenic effect was observed in mice administered ganciclovir at 1 mg/kg/day (160× the human ocular dose). Except for histocytic sarcoma of the liver, ganciclovir-induced tumors were generally of epithelial or vascular origin. Although the preputial and clitoral glands, forestomach and harderian glands of mice do not have human counterparts, ganciclovir should be considered a potential carcinogen in humans. Ganciclovir increased mutations in mouse lymphoma cells and DNA damage in human lymphocytes in vitro at concentrations between 50 to 500 and 250 to 2,000 mcg/mL, respectively.
In the mouse micronucleus assay, ganciclovir was clastogenic at doses of 150 and 500 mg/kg (IV)

24,000× to 80,000× human ocular dose) but not 50 mg/kg (8,000× human ocular dose). Ganciclovir was not mutagenic in the Ames Salmonella assay at concentrations of 500 to 5,000 mcg/mL. Ganciclovir caused decreased mating behavior, decreased fertility, and an increased incidence of embryolethality in female mice following intravenous doses of 90 mg/kg/day (approximately 14,000× the human ocular dose of 6.25 mcg/kg/day). Ganciclovir caused decreased fertility in male mice and hypospermatogenesis in mice and dogs following daily oral or intravenous administration of doses ranging from 0.2 to 10 mg/kg (30× to 1,600× the human ocular dose).

14   CLINICAL STUDIES

In one open-label, randomized, controlled, multicenter clinical trial which enrolled 164 patients with herpetic keratitis, ZIRGAN was non-inferior to acyclovir ophthalmic ointment, 3% in patients with dendritic ulcers. Clinical resolution (healed ulcers) at Day 7 was achieved in 77% (55/71) for ZIRGAN versus 72% (48/67) for acyclovir 3% (difference 5.8%, 95% CI - 9.6%-18.3%). In three randomized, single-masked, controlled, multicenter clinical trials which enrolled 213 total patients, ZIRGAN was non-inferior to acyclovir ophthalmic ointment 3% in patients with dendritic ulcers. Clinical resolution at Day 7 was achieved in 72% (41/57) for ZIRGAN versus 69% (34/49) for acyclovir (difference 2.5%, 95% CI - 15.6%-20.9%).

16   HOW SUPPLIED/STORAGE AND HANDLING

ZIRGAN is supplied as 5 grams of a sterile, preserved, clear, colorless, topical ophthalmic gel containing O.15% of ganciclovir in a polycoated aluminum tube with a white polyethylene tip and cap and protective band (NDC 24208-535-35).

Storage

Store at 15°C-25°C (59°F-77°F). Do not freeze.

17   PATIENT COUNSELING INFORMATION

This product is sterile when packaged. Patients should be advised not to allow the dropper tip to touch any surface, as this may contaminate the gel. If pain develops, or if redness, itching, or inflammation becomes aggravated, the patient should be advised to consult a physician. Patients should be advised not to wear contact lenses when using ZIRGAN.

Revised: June 2010
ZIRGAN is a trademark of Laboratoires Théa Corporation licensed by Bausch & Lomb Incorporated.
Bausch & Lomb Incorporated
Tampa, FL 33637
© Bausch & Lomb Incorporated
9187201

Shown in Product Identification Guide, page 104

ZYLET®   ℞
loteprednol etabonate 0.5%
and tobramycin 0.3%
ophthalmic suspension
STERILE

DESCRIPTION:

Zylet (loteprednol etabonate and tobramycin ophthalmic suspension), is a sterile, multiple dose topical anti-inflammatory corticosteroid and antibiotic combination for ophthalmic use. Both loteprednol etabonate and tobramycin are white to off-white powders. The chemical structures of loteprednol etabonate and tobramycin are shown below.

Loteprednol etabonate:

$C_{24}H_{31}ClO_7$ Mol. Wt. 466.96

Chemical name: chloromethyl 17α-[(ethoxycarbonyl)oxy]-11β-hydroxy-3-oxoandrosta-1,4-diene-17β -carboxylate

Tobramycin:

$C_{18}H_{37}N_5O_9$ Mol. Wt. 467.52

Chemical Name:
O-3-Amino-3-deoxy-α-D-glucopyranosyl-(1→ 4)-O- [2,6-diamino-2,3,6-trideoxy-α-D-*ribo*-hexopyranosyl- (1→ 6)] -2-deoxystreptamine

Each mL contains:

Actives: Loteprednol Etabonate 5 mg (0.5%) and Tobramycin 3 mg (0.3%). Inactives: Edetate Disodium, Glycerin, Povidone, Purified Water, Tyloxapol, and Benzalkonium Chloride 0.01% (preservative). Sulfuric Acid and/or Sodium Hydroxide may be added to adjust the pH to 5.7-5.9. The suspension is essentially isotonic with a tonicity of 260 to 320 mOsmol/kg.

CLINICAL PHARMACOLOGY:

Corticosteroids inhibit the inflammatory response to a variety of inciting agents and probably delay or slow healing. They inhibit the edema, fibrin deposition, capillary dilation, leukocyte migration, capillary proliferation, fibroblast proliferation, deposition of collagen, and scar formation associated with inflammation. There is no generally accepted explanation for the mechanism of action of ocular corticosteroids. However, corticosteroids are thought to act by the induction of phospholipase A_2 inhibitory proteins, collectively called lipocortins. It is postulated that these proteins control the biosynthesis of potent mediators of inflammation such as prostaglandins and leukotrienes by inhibiting the release of their common precursor arachidonic acid. Arachidonic acid is released from membrane phospholipids by phospholipase A_2. Corticosteroids are capable of producing a rise in intraocular pressure.
Loteprednol etabonate is structurally similar to other corticosteroids. However, the number 20 position ketone group is absent. It is highly lipid soluble which enhances its penetration into cells. Loteprednol etabonate is synthesized through structural modifications of prednisolone-related compounds so that it will undergo a predictable transformation to an inactive metabolite. Based upon *in vivo* and *in vitro* preclinical metabolism studies, loteprednol etabonate undergoes extensive metabolism to inactive carboxylic acid metabolites. The antibiotic component in the combination (tobramycin) is included to provide action against susceptible organisms. *In vitro* studies have demonstrated that tobramycin is active against susceptible strains of the following microorganisms:
Staphylococci, including *S. aureus* and *S. epidermidis* (coagulase-positive and coagulase-negative), including penicillin-resistant strains. Streptococci, including some of the Group A-beta-hemolytic species, some nonhemolytic species, and some *Streptococcus pneumoniae*. *Pseudomonas aeruginosa, Escherichia coli, Klebsiella pneumoniae, Enterobacter aerogenes, Proteus mirabilis, Morganella morganii*, most *Proteus vulgaris* strains, *Haemophilus influenzae* and *H. aegyptius*, *Moraxella lacunata, Acinetobacter calcoaceticus* and some *Neisseria* species.

Pharmacokinetics:

In a controlled clinical study of ocular penetration, the levels of loteprednol etabonate in the aqueous humor were found to be comparable between Lotemax and Zylet treatment groups.
Results from a bioavailability study in normal volunteers established that plasma levels of loteprednol etabonate and Δ^1 cortienic acid etabonate (PJ 91), its primary, inactive metabolite, were below the limit of quantitation (1 ng/mL) at all

sampling times. The results were obtained following the ocular administration of one drop in each eye of 0.5% loteprednol etabonate ophthalmic suspension 8 times daily for 2 days or 4 times daily for 42 days. This study suggests that limited (<1 ng/mL) systemic absorption occurs with 0.5% loteprednol etabonate.

INDICATIONS AND USAGE:

Zylet is indicated for steroid-responsive inflammatory ocular conditions for which a corticosteroid is indicated and where superficial bacterial ocular infection or a risk of bacterial ocular infection exists. Ocular steroids are indicated in inflammatory conditions of the palpebral and bulbar conjunctiva, cornea and anterior segment of the globe such as allergic conjunctivitis, acne rosacea, superficial punctate keratitis, herpes zoster keratitis, iritis, cyclitis, and where the inherent risk of steroid use in certain infective conjunctivitides is accepted to obtain a diminution in edema and inflammation. They are also indicated in chronic anterior uveitis and corneal injury from chemical, radiation or thermal burns, or penetration of foreign bodies.
The use of a combination drug with an anti-infective component is indicated where the risk of superficial ocular infection is high or where there is an expectation that potentially dangerous numbers of bacteria will be present in the eye.
The particular anti-infective drug in this product (tobramycin) is active against the following common bacterial eye pathogens: Staphylococci, including *S. aureus* and *S. epidermidis* (coagulase-positive and coagulase-negative), including penicillin-resistant strains. Streptococci, including some of the Group A-beta-hemolytic species, some nonhemolytic species, and some *Streptococcus pneumoniae. Pseudomonas aeruginosa, Escherichia coli, Klebsiella pneumoniae, Enterobacter aerogenes, Proteus mirabilis, Morganella morganii*, most *Proteus vulgaris* strains, *Haemophilus influenzae*, and *H. aegyptius, Moraxella lacunata, Acinetobacter calcoaceticus* and some *Neisseria* species.

CONTRAINDICATIONS:

Zylet, as with other steroid anti-infective ophthalmic combination drugs, is contraindicated in most viral diseases of the cornea and conjunctiva including epithelial herpes simplex keratitis (dendritic keratitis), vaccinia, and varicella, and also in mycobacterial infection of the eye and fungal diseases of ocular structures. Zylet is also contraindicated in individuals with known or suspected hypersensitivity to any of the ingredients of this preparation and to other corticosteroids.

WARNINGS:

NOT FOR INJECTION INTO THE EYE.
Prolonged use of corticosteroids may result in glaucoma with damage to the optic nerve, defects in visual acuity and fields of vision, and in posterior subcapsular cataract formation. Steroids should be used with caution in the presence of glaucoma. Sensitivity to topically applied aminoglycosides may occur in some patients. If sensitivity reaction does occur, discontinue use.
Prolonged use of corticosteroids may suppress the host response and thus increase the hazard of secondary ocular infections. In those diseases causing thinning of the cornea or sclera, perforations have been known to occur with the use of topical steroids.
In acute purulent conditions of the eye, steroids may mask infection or enhance existing infection. Use of ocular steroids may prolong the course and may exacerbate the severity of many viral infections of the eye (including herpes simplex). Employment of a corticosteroid medication in the treatment of patients with a history of herpes simplex requires great caution.
The use of steroids after cataract surgery may delay healing and increase the incidence of bleb formation.

PRECAUTIONS:

General: For ophthalmic use only. The initial prescription and renewal of the medication order be-

Continued on next page

Zylet—Cont.

yond 14 days should be made by a physician only after examination of the patient with the aid of magnification, such as slit lamp biomicroscopy and, where appropriate, fluorescein staining.

If signs and symptoms fail to improve after 2 days, the patient should be re-evaluated.

If this product is used for 10 days or longer, intraocular pressure should be monitored even though it may be difficult in children and uncooperative patients (See WARNINGS).

Fungal infections of the cornea are particularly prone to develop coincidentally with long-term local steroid application. Fungus invasion must be considered in any persistent corneal ulceration where a steroid has been used or is in use. Fungal cultures should be taken when appropriate.

As with other antibiotic preparations, prolonged use may result in overgrowth of nonsusceptible organisms, including fungi. If superinfection occurs, appropriate therapy should be initiated.

Cross-sensitivity to other aminoglycoside antibiotics may occur; if hypersensitivity develops with this product, discontinue use and institute appropriate therapy.

Information for Patients: This product is sterile when packaged. Patients should be advised not to allow the dropper tip to touch any surface, as this may contaminate the suspension. If pain develops, redness, itching or inflammation becomes aggravated, the patient should be advised to consult a physician. As with all ophthalmic preparations containing benzalkonium chloride, patients should be advised not to wear soft contact lenses when using Zylet.

Carcinogenesis, mutagenesis, impairment of fertility: Long-term animal studies have not been conducted to evaluate the carcinogenic potential of loteprednol etabonate or tobramycin.

Loteprednol etabonate was not genotoxic in vitro in the Ames test, the mouse lymphoma TK assay, a chromosome aberration test in human lymphocytes, or in an in vivo mouse micronucleus assay.

Oral treatment of male and female rats at 50 mg/kg/day and 25mg/kg/day of loteprednol etabonate, respectively, (500 and 250 times the maximum clinical dose, respectively) prior to and during mating did not impair fertility in either gender. No impairment of fertility was noted in studies of subcutaneous tobramycin in rats at 100 mg/kg/day (1700 times the maximum daily clinical dose).

Pregnancy: Teratogenic effects: Pregnancy Category C.

Loteprednol etabonate was shown to be teratogenic when administered orally to rats and rabbits during organogenesis at 5 and 3 mg/kg/day, respectively (50 and 30 times the maximum daily clinical dose in rats and rabbits, respectively). An oral dose of loteprednol etabonate in rats at 50 mg/kg/day (500 times the maximum daily clinical dose) during late pregnancy through the weaning period showed a decrease in the growth and survival of pups without dystocia. However, no adverse effect in the pups was observed at 5 mg/kg/day (50 times the maximum daily clinical dose).

Parenteral doses of tobramycin did not show any harm to fetuses up to 100 mg/kg/day (1700 times the maximum daily clinical dose) in rats and rabbits.

There are no adequate and well controlled studies in pregnant women. Zylet should be used during pregnancy only if the potential benefit justifies the potential risk to the fetus.

Nursing Mothers: It is not known whether topical ophthalmic administration of corticosteroids could result in sufficient systemic absorption to produce detectable quantities in human milk. Systemic steroids appear in human milk and could suppress growth, interfere with endogenous corticosteroid production, or cause other untoward effects. Caution should be exercised when Zylet is administered to a nursing woman.

Pediatric Use: In a trial to evaluate the safety and efficacy of Zylet in pediatric subjects age zero to six years with lid inflammation, Zylet with warm compresses did not demonstrate efficacy compared to vehicle with warm compresses. Patients received warm compress lid treatment plus Zylet or vehicle for 14 days. The majority of patients in both treatment groups showed reduced lid inflammation. There were no differences in safety assessments between the treatment groups.

Geriatric Use: No overall differences in safety and effectiveness have been observed between elderly and younger patients.

ADVERSE REACTIONS: Adverse reactions have occurred with steroid/anti-infective combination drugs which can be attributed to the steroid component, the anti-infective component, or the combination.

Zylet:

In a 42 day safety study comparing Zylet to placebo, the incidence of ocular adverse events reported in greater than 10% of subjects included injection (approximately 20%) and superficial punctate keratitis (approximately 15%). Increased intraocular pressure was reported in 10% (Zylet) and 4% (placebo) of subjects. Nine percent (9%) of Zylet subjects reported burning and stinging upon instillation. Ocular reactions reported with an incidence less than 4% include vision disorders, discharge, itching, lacrimation disorder, photophobia, corneal deposits, ocular discomfort, eyelid disorder, and other unspecified eye disorders.

The incidence of non-ocular adverse events reported in approximately 14% of subjects was headache; all other non-ocular events had an incidence of less than 5%.

Loteprednol etabonate ophthalmic suspension 0.2% - 0.5%:

Reactions associated with ophthalmic steroids include elevated intraocular pressure, which may be associated with infrequent optic nerve damage, visual acuity and field defects, posterior subcapsular cataract formation, delayed wound healing and secondary ocular infection from pathogens including herpes simplex, and perforation of the globe where there is thinning of the cornea or sclera.

In a summation of controlled, randomized studies of individuals treated for 28 days or longer with loteprednol etabonate, the incidence of significant elevation of intraocular pressure (≥ 10 mm Hg) was 2% (15/901) among patients receiving loteprednol etabonate, 7% (11/164) among patients receiving 1% prednisolone acetate and 0.5% (3/583) among patients receiving placebo.

Tobramycin ophthalmic solution 0.3%:

The most frequent adverse reactions to topical tobramycin are hypersensitivity and localized ocular toxicity, including lid itching and swelling and conjunctival erythema. These reactions occur in less than 4% of patients. Similar reactions may occur with the topical use of other aminoglycoside antibiotics. Other adverse reactions have not been reported; however, if topical ocular tobramycin is administered concomitantly with systemic aminoglycoside antibiotics, care should be taken to monitor the total serum concentration.

Secondary Infection: The development of secondary infection has occurred after use of combinations containing steroids and antimicrobials. Fungal infections of the cornea are particularly prone to develop coincidentally with long-term applications of steroids. The possibility of fungal invasion must be considered in any persistent corneal ulceration where steroid treatment has been used. Secondary bacterial ocular infection following suppression of host responses also occurs.

DOSAGE AND ADMINISTRATION:

SHAKE VIGOROUSLY BEFORE USING.

Apply one or two drops of Zylet into the conjunctival sac of the affected eye(s) every four to six hours. During the initial 24 to 48 hours, the dosing may be increased, to every one to two hours. Frequency should be decreased gradually as warranted by improvement in clinical signs. Care should be taken not to discontinue therapy prematurely. Not more than 20 mL should be prescribed initially and the

prescription should not be refilled without further evaluation as outlined in PRECAUTIONS above.

HOW SUPPLIED:

Zylet (loteprednol etabonate and tobramycin ophthalmic suspension) is supplied in a white low density polyethylene plastic bottle with a white controlled drop tip and a white polypropylene cap in the following sizes:

    2.5 mL   (NDC 24208-358-25) in a 7.5 mL bottle
    5 mL   (NDC 24208-358-05) in a 7.5 mL bottle
    10 mL   (NDC 24208-358-10) in a 10 mL bottle

USE ONLY IF IMPRINTED NECKBAND IS INTACT.

Storage: Store upright at 15°-25°C (59°-77°F). PROTECT FROM FREEZING.
KEEP OUT OF REACH OF CHILDREN.
Rx only
Revised May 2010
Manufactured by:
Bausch & Lomb Incorporated
Tampa, Florida 33637
©Bausch & Lomb Incorporated
U.S. Patent Numbers: 4,996,335; 5,540,930; 5,747,061
Zylet is a registered trademark of Bausch & Lomb Incorporated
9007702 (FOLDED)
9004402 (FLAT)

Shown in Product Identification Guide, page 104

FOCUS Laboratories, Inc.
**7645 COUNTS MASSIE ROAD
NORTH LITTLE ROCK, AR 72113**

Office Phone: 501-753-6006
Office Fax: 501-753-6021
website: www.focuslaboratories.com

FRESHKOTE®
STERILE OPHTHALMIC SOLUTION

Description: Each mL of FreshKote® Ophthalmic Solution contains:
Polyvinyl pyrrolidone 2.0%, Polyvinyl alcohol (87% hydrolyzed) 0.9%, Polyvinyl alcohol (99% hydrolyzed) 1.8%. Also contains Amisol® CLEAR. Other ingredients: Sodium chloride, Potassium chloride, Boric acid, Purified water and as preservatives Disodium edetate dihydrate, Polixetonium.

Indications: FreshKote® sterile ophthalmic solution is a lubricant indicated for the treatment of moderate to severe dry eye.

Contraindications: FreshKote® is contraindicated in patients with known severe hypersensitivity to any of the ingredients in the formulation.

Warnings:
- To avoid contamination, do not touch tip of container to any surface. Replace cap after using.
- If you experience eye pain, changes in vision, continued redness or irritation of the eye, or if the condition worsens or persists for more than 72 hours, discontinue use and consult a doctor.
- Do not use if solution changes color or becomes cloudy.
- Keep this and all medications out of the reach of children. In case of accidental ingestion, seek professional assistance or call a Poison Control Center immediately.
- Tamper Evident: For your protection, this bottle has an imprinted seal around the neck. Do Not Use if seal is damaged or missing at time of purchase.

Pregnancy: There are no adequate and well controlled studies in pregnant women. FreshKote® should be used during pregnancy only if the potential benefit justifies the potential risk.

Dosage and Administration: Instill 1 or 2 drops in the affected eye 3 or 4 times daily.

How Supplied: FreshKote® is packaged in 15 mL (NDC# 15821-101-15) and 1 mL (NDC# 15821-101-01) bottles; with a control dropper.
Storage: Store at controlled room temperature 15°–30°C (59°–86°F).
See box or dropper bottle for Lot Number and Expiration Date.
Rx Only
Protected by U.S. Patent Numbers:
5,300,296
7,758,883
Manufactured for:
FOCUS Laboratories, Inc.
North Little Rock, AR 72113
Rev. 02/08
MG #22080
Shown in Product Identification Guide, page 104

TOZAL®   ℞

DESCRIPTION:
TOZAL® is an orally administered Medical Food specially formulated for the Dietary Management of Age Related Macular Degeneration, Dry Eye Syndrome and Meibomian Gland Dysfunction. TOZAL® is intended to be used under the supervision of a doctor.

Serving Size: 3 Softgels
CONTAINS: (Each serving contains)

Vitamin A	(Palmitate) 10,000 IU
Vitamin A	(Natural Beta Carotene) 18,640 IU
Vitamin C	452 mg
Vitamin E	200 IU
Zinc	69 mg
Copper	1.6 mg
Taurine	400 mg
Lutein	10 mg
Zeaxanthin	2 mg
Vitamin D3	800 IU
Omega-3 Combination of EPA/DHA	600 mg

INDICATIONS:
TOZAL® is indicated for the distinct nutritional requirements of individuals diagnosed with or at risk for Age Related Macular Degeneration, Dry Eye Syndrome and Meibomian Gland Dysfunction. The clinically supported ingredients in TOZAL® aid in the treatment of inflammatory conditions of the eye.

CONTRAINDICATIONS:
TOZAL® is contraindicated in patients with a known hypersensitivity to any of the ingredients in the formulation. Smokers should consult with their doctor before taking products containing beta carotene.

WARNINGS:
Tamper Evident: For your protection, this bottle has an imprinted seal around the neck. Do Not Use if seal is damaged or missing at time of purchase.

PRECAUTIONS:
Avoid taking at the same time with other medication and/or supplements.
Pregnancy: Category C
There are no adequate and well-controlled studies in pregnant women. TOZAL® should be used during pregnancy only if the potential benefit justifies the potential risk.
Pediatric Use:
There are no adequate and well-controlled studies for pediatric use.

ADVERSE REACTIONS:
No serious side effects have been experienced with the consumption of normal amounts of these ingredients.

DOSAGE AND ADMINISTRATION:
Take one softgel three times daily or as directed by a physician. TOZAL® should be taken with food.

HOW SUPPLIED:
TOZAL® softgels are packed in a 90 count bottle (NDC 15821-501-90)

Storage:
Store at controlled room temperature 15°–30°C (59°–86°F). Keep container tightly closed.
See bottle or foil sample pouch for Lot Number and Expiration Date.
U.S. Patent Pending
TOZAL® is a registered trademark of Atlantic Medical, Inc.
KEEP THIS AND ALL DRUGS OUT OF REACH OF CHILDREN
In case of accidental ingestion, seek professional assistance or call a Poison Control Center immediately.
Rx Only
To report SUSPECTED ADVERSE REACTIONS, contact FOCUS Laboratories, Inc. at (501) 753-6006, 8am-5pm Monday-Friday CST.
Manufactured for:
FOCUS Laboratories, Inc.
North Little Rock, AR 72113
Rev 08/10
Shown in Product Identification Guide, page 104

Merck
One Merck Drive
P.O. Box 100
Whitehouse Station, NJ 08889

For updates to the product information listed below, please check the Merck Web site, http://www.merck.com, or call 1-866-342-5683. For complete product listing, please see the Manufacturers' Index.

Direct inquiries, including 24-hour emergency information to healthcare professionals, to:
The Merck National Service Center at
(800) NSC-MERCK
(800) 672-6372
Merck U.S. operating companies include:
Merck, Sharp & Dohme Corp.
Schering Corporation

TRUSOPT®   ℞
(dorzolamide hydrochloride ophthalmic solution)
Sterile Ophthalmic Solution 2%

DESCRIPTION
TRUSOPT[1] (dorzolamide hydrochloride ophthalmic solution) is a carbonic anhydrase inhibitor formulated for topical ophthalmic use.
Dorzolamide hydrochloride is described chemically as: (4S-*trans*)-4-(ethylamino)-5,6-dihydro-6-methyl-4H-thieno[2,3-*b*]thiopyran-2-sulfonamide 7,7-dioxide monohydrochloride. Dorzolamide hydrochloride is optically active. The specific rotation is

$$\alpha \; \frac{25°}{405} \quad (C=1, \text{water}) = \sim{-17°}.$$

Its empirical formula is $C_{10}H_{16}N_2O_4S_3 \cdot HCl$ and its structural formula is:

Dorzolamide hydrochloride has a molecular weight of 360.9 and a melting point of about 264°C. It is a white to off-white, crystalline powder, which is soluble in water and slightly soluble in methanol and ethanol.
TRUSOPT Sterile Ophthalmic Solution is supplied as a sterile, isotonic, buffered, slightly viscous, aqueous solution of dorzolamide hydrochloride. The pH of the solution is approximately 5.6, and the osmolarity is 260-330 mOsM. Each mL of TRUSOPT 2% contains 20 mg dorzolamide (22.3 mg of

dorzolamide hydrochloride). Inactive ingredients are hydroxyethyl cellulose, mannitol, sodium citrate dihydrate, sodium hydroxide (to adjust pH) and water for injection. Benzalkonium chloride 0.0075% is added as a preservative.

CLINICAL PHARMACOLOGY
Mechanism of Action
Carbonic anhydrase (CA) is an enzyme found in many tissues of the body including the eye. It catalyzes the reversible reaction involving the hydration of carbon dioxide and the dehydration of carbonic acid. In humans, carbonic anhydrase exists as a number of isoenzymes, the most active being carbonic anhydrase II (CA-II), found primarily in red blood cells (RBCs), but also in other tissues. Inhibition of carbonic anhydrase in the ciliary processes of the eye decreases aqueous humor secretion, presumably by slowing the formation of bicarbonate ions with subsequent reduction in sodium and fluid transport. The result is a reduction in intraocular pressure (IOP).
TRUSOPT Ophthalmic Solution contains dorzolamide hydrochloride, an inhibitor of human carbonic anhydrase II. Following topical ocular administration, TRUSOPT reduces elevated intraocular pressure. Elevated intraocular pressure is a major risk factor in the pathogenesis of optic nerve damage and glaucomatous visual field loss.
Pharmacokinetics/Pharmacodynamics
When topically applied, dorzolamide reaches the systemic circulation. To assess the potential for systemic carbonic anhydrase inhibition following topical administration, drug and metabolite concentrations in RBCs and plasma and carbonic anhydrase inhibition in RBCs were measured. Dorzolamide accumulates in RBCs during chronic dosing as a result of binding to CA-II. The parent drug forms a single N-desethyl metabolite, which inhibits CA-II less potently than the parent drug but also inhibits CA-I. The metabolite also accumulates in RBCs where it binds primarily to CA-I. Plasma concentrations of dorzolamide and metabolite are generally below the assay limit of quantitation (15nM). Dorzolamide binds moderately to plasma proteins (approximately 33%). Dorzolamide is primarily excreted unchanged in the urine; the metabolite also is excreted in urine. After dosing is stopped, dorzolamide washes out of RBCs nonlinearly, resulting in a rapid decline of drug concentration initially, followed by a slower elimination phase with a half-life of about four months.
To simulate the systemic exposure after long-term topical ocular administration, dorzolamide was given orally to eight healthy subjects for up to 20 weeks. The oral dose of 2 mg b.i.d. closely approximates the amount of drug delivered by topical ocular administration of TRUSOPT 2% t.i.d. Steady state was reached within 8 weeks. The inhibition of CA-II and total carbonic anhydrase activities was below the degree of inhibition anticipated to be necessary for a pharmacological effect on renal function and respiration in healthy individuals.
Clinical Studies
The efficacy of TRUSOPT was demonstrated in clinical studies in the treatment of elevated intraocular pressure in patients with glaucoma or ocular hypertension (baseline IOP ≥ 23 mmHg). The IOP-lowering effect of TRUSOPT was approximately 3 to 5 mmHg throughout the day and this was consistent in clinical studies of up to one year duration. The efficacy of TRUSOPT when dosed less frequently than three times a day (alone or in combination with other products) has not been established.

Continued on next page

Information on the Merck products listed on these pages is from the prescribing information in use August 1, 2011. For information, please call 1-800-NSC-Merck [1-800-672-6372].

Trusopt—Cont.

In a one year clinical study, the effect of TRUSOPT 2% t.i.d. on the corneal endothelium was compared to that of betaxolol ophthalmic solution b.i.d. and timolol maleate ophthalmic solution 0.5% b.i.d. There were no statistically significant differences between groups in corneal endothelial cell counts or in corneal thickness measurements. There was a mean loss of approximately 4% in the endothelial cell counts for each group over the one year period.

INDICATIONS AND USAGE
TRUSOPT Ophthalmic Solution is indicated in the treatment of elevated intraocular pressure in patients with ocular hypertension or open-angle glaucoma.

CONTRAINDICATIONS
TRUSOPT is contraindicated in patients who are hypersensitive to any component of this product.

WARNINGS
TRUSOPT is a sulfonamide and, although administered topically, is absorbed systemically. Therefore, the same types of adverse reactions that are attributable to sulfonamides may occur with topical administration with TRUSOPT. Fatalities have occurred, although rarely, due to severe reactions to sulfonamides including Stevens-Johnson syndrome, toxic epidermal necrolysis, fulminant hepatic necrosis, agranulocytosis, aplastic anemia, and other blood dyscrasias. Sensitization may recur when a sulfonamide is readministered irrespective of the route of administration. If signs of serious reactions or hypersensitivity occur, discontinue the use of this preparation.

PRECAUTIONS
General
The management of patients with acute angle-closure glaucoma requires therapeutic interventions in addition to ocular hypotensive agents. TRUSOPT has not been studied in patients with acute angle-closure glaucoma.
TRUSOPT has not been studied in patients with severe renal impairment (CrCl < 30 mL/min). Because TRUSOPT and its metabolite are excreted predominantly by the kidney, TRUSOPT is not recommended in such patients.
TRUSOPT has not been studied in patients with hepatic impairment and should therefore be used with caution in such patients.
In clinical studies, local ocular adverse effects, primarily conjunctivitis and lid reactions, were reported with chronic administration of TRUSOPT. Many of these reactions had the clinical appearance and course of an allergic-type reaction that resolved upon discontinuation of drug therapy. If such reactions are observed, TRUSOPT should be discontinued and the patient evaluated before considering restarting the drug. (See ADVERSE REACTIONS.)
There is a potential for an additive effect on the known systemic effects of carbonic anhydrase inhibition in patients receiving an oral carbonic anhydrase inhibitor and TRUSOPT. The concomitant administration of TRUSOPT and oral carbonic anhydrase inhibitors is not recommended.
There have been reports of bacterial keratitis associated with the use of multiple-dose containers of topical ophthalmic products. These containers had been inadvertently contaminated by patients who, in most cases, had a concurrent corneal disease or a disruption of the ocular epithelial surface.
Choroidal detachment has been reported with administration of aqueous suppressant therapy (e.g., dorzolamide) after filtration procedures.
There is an increased potential for developing corneal edema in patients with low endothelial cell counts. Precautions should be used when prescribing TRUSOPT to this group of patients.
Information for Patients
TRUSOPT is a sulfonamide and although administered topically is absorbed systemically. Therefore the same types of adverse reactions that are attributable to sulfonamides may occur with topical administration. Patients should be advised that if serious or unusual reactions including severe skin

reactions or signs of hypersensitivity occur, they should discontinue the use of the product (see WARNINGS).
Patients should be advised that if they develop any ocular reactions, particularly conjunctivitis and lid reactions, they should discontinue use and seek their physician's advice.
Patients should be instructed to avoid allowing the tip of the dispensing container to contact the eye or surrounding structures.
Patients should also be instructed that ocular solutions, if handled improperly or if the tip of the dispensing container contacts the eye or surrounding structures, can become contaminated by common bacteria known to cause ocular infections. Serious damage to the eye and subsequent loss of vision may result from using contaminated solutions.
Patients also should be advised that if they have ocular surgery or develop an intercurrent ocular condition (e.g., trauma or infection), they should immediately seek their physician's advice concerning the continued use of the present multidose container.
If more than one topical ophthalmic drug is being used, the drugs should be administered at least ten minutes apart.
Patients should be advised that TRUSOPT contains benzalkonium chloride which may be absorbed by soft contact lenses. Contact lenses should be removed prior to administration of the solution. Lenses may be reinserted 15 minutes following TRUSOPT administration.
Drug Interactions
Although acid-base and electrolyte disturbances were not reported in the clinical trials with TRUSOPT, these disturbances have been reported with oral carbonic anhydrase inhibitors and have, in some instances, resulted in drug interactions (e.g., toxicity associated with high-dose salicylate therapy). Therefore, the potential for such drug interactions should be considered in patients receiving TRUSOPT.
Carcinogenesis, Mutagenesis, Impairment of Fertility
In a two-year study of dorzolamide hydrochloride administered orally to male and female Sprague-Dawley rats, urinary bladder papillomas were seen in male rats in the highest dosage group of 20 mg/kg/day (250 times the recommended human ophthalmic dose). Papillomas were not seen in rats given oral doses equivalent to approximately 12 times the recommended human ophthalmic dose. No treatment-related tumors were seen in a 21-month study in female and male mice given oral doses up to 75 mg/kg/day (~900 times the recommended human ophthalmic dose).
The increased incidence of urinary bladder papillomas seen in the high-dose male rats is a class-effect of carbonic anhydrase inhibitors in rats. Rats are particularly prone to developing papillomas in response to foreign bodies, compounds causing crystalluria, and diverse sodium salts.
No changes in bladder urothelium were seen in dogs given oral dorzolamide hydrochloride for one year at 2 mg/kg/day (25 times the recommended human ophthalmic dose) or monkeys dosed topically to the eye at 0.4 mg/kg/day (~5 times the recommended human ophthalmic dose) for one year.
The following tests for mutagenic potential were negative: (1) *in vivo* (mouse) cytogenetic assay; (2) *in vitro* chromosomal aberration assay; (3) alkaline elution assay; (4) V-79 assay; and (5) Ames test.
In reproduction studies of dorzolamide hydrochloride in rats, there were no adverse effects on the reproductive capacity of males or females at doses up to 188 or 94 times, respectively, the recommended human ophthalmic dose.
Pregnancy
Teratogenic Effects
Pregnancy Category C
Developmental toxicity studies with dorzolamide hydrochloride in rabbits at oral doses of ≥ 2.5 mg/kg/day (31 times the recommended human ophthalmic dose) revealed malformations of the vertebral bodies. These malformations occurred at doses that caused metabolic acidosis with decreased body weight gain in dams and decreased fetal

weights. No treatment-related malformations were seen at 1.0 mg/kg/day (13 times the recommended human ophthalmic dose). There are no adequate and well-controlled studies in pregnant women. TRUSOPT should be used during pregnancy only if the potential benefit justifies the potential risk to the fetus.
Nursing Mothers
In a study of dorzolamide hydrochloride in lactating rats, decreases in body weight gain of 5 to 7% in offspring at an oral dose of 7.5 mg/kg/day (94 times the recommended human ophthalmic dose) were seen during lactation. A slight delay in postnatal development (incisor eruption, vaginal canalization and eye openings), secondary to lower fetal body weight, was noted.
It is not known whether this drug is excreted in human milk. Because many drugs are excreted in human milk and because of the potential for serious adverse reactions in nursing infants from TRUSOPT, a decision should be made whether to discontinue nursing or to discontinue the drug, taking into account the importance of the drug to the mother.
Pediatric Use
Safety and IOP-lowering effects of TRUSOPT have been demonstrated in pediatric patients in a 3-month, multicenter, double-masked, active-treatment-controlled trial.
Geriatric Use
No overall differences in safety or effectiveness have been observed between elderly and younger patients.

ADVERSE REACTIONS
Controlled clinical trials
The most frequent adverse events associated with TRUSOPT were ocular burning, stinging, or discomfort immediately following ocular administration (approximately one-third of patients). Approximately one-quarter of patients noted a bitter taste following administration. Superficial punctate keratitis occurred in 10-15% of patients and signs and symptoms of ocular allergic reaction in approximately 10%. Events occurring in approximately 1-5% of patients were conjunctivitis and lid reactions (see PRECAUTIONS, General), blurred vision, eye redness, tearing, dryness, and photophobia. Other ocular events and systemic events were reported infrequently, including headache, nausea, asthenia/fatigue; and, rarely, skin rashes, urolithiasis, and iridocyclitis.
In a 3-month, double-masked, active-treatment-controlled, multicenter study in pediatric patients, the adverse experience profile of TRUSOPT was comparable to that seen in adult patients.
Clinical practice
The following adverse events have occurred either at low incidence (<1%) during clinical trials or have been reported during the use of TRUSOPT in clinical practice where these events were reported voluntarily from a population of unknown size and frequency of occurrence cannot be determined precisely. They have been chosen for inclusion based on factors such as seriousness, frequency of reporting, possible causal connection to TRUSOPT or a combination of these factors: signs and symptoms of systemic allergic reactions including angioedema, bronchospasm, pruritus, and urticaria; Stevens-Johnson syndrome and toxic epidermal necrolysis; dizziness, paresthesia; ocular pain, transient myopia, choroidal detachment following filtration surgery, eyelid crusting; dyspnea; contact dermatitis, epistaxis, dry mouth and throat irritation.

OVERDOSAGE
Electrolyte imbalance, development of an acidotic state, and possible central nervous system effects may occur. Serum electrolyte levels (particularly potassium) and blood pH levels should be monitored.

DOSAGE AND ADMINISTRATION
The dose is one drop of TRUSOPT Ophthalmic Solution in the affected eye(s) three times daily.
TRUSOPT may be used concomitantly with other topical ophthalmic drug products to lower intraocu-

lar pressure. If more than one topical ophthalmic drug is being used, the drugs should be administered at least ten minutes apart.

HOW SUPPLIED

TRUSOPT Ophthalmic Solution is a slightly opalescent, nearly colorless, slightly viscous solution.
No. 3519 — TRUSOPT Ophthalmic Solution 2% is supplied in an OCUMETER®[2] PLUS container, a white, translucent, HDPE plastic ophthalmic dispenser with a controlled drop tip and a white polystyrene cap with orange label as follows:
NDC 0006-3519-36, 10 mL, in an 18 mL capacity bottle.

Storage

Store TRUSOPT Ophthalmic Solution at 15-30°C (59-86°F). Protect from light.

Rx only

[2]Registered trademark of Merck Sharp & Dohme Corp., a subsidiary of **Merck & Co., Inc.**
Manuf. for: Merck Sharp & Dohme Corp., a subsidiary of **MERCK & CO., INC.**, Whitehouse Station, NJ 08889, USA
By: Laboratories Merck Sharp & Dohme-Chibret 63963 Clermont-Ferrand Cedex 9, France
Issued December 2009
221A-12/09 514297Z
9368211

INSTRUCTIONS FOR USE
TRUSOPT®

(dorzolamide hydrochloride ophthalmic solution)
Sterile Ophthalmic Solution 2%
Please follow these instructions carefully when using TRUSOPT[3]. Use TRUSOPT as prescribed by your doctor.

1. If you use other topically applied ophthalmic medications, they should be administered at least 10 minutes before or after TRUSOPT.
2. Wash hands before each use.
3. Before using the medication for the first time, be sure the Safety Strip on the front of the bottle is unbroken. A gap between the bottle and the cap is normal for an unopened bottle.

Opening Arrows ▶

Safety Strip ▶

4. Tear off the Safety Strip to break the seal. See figure at top of next column]
5. To open the bottle, unscrew the cap by turning as indicated by the arrows on the top of the

Gap ▶
Finger Push Area ▶

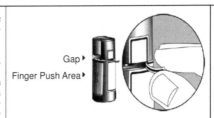

cap. Do not pull the cap directly up and away from the bottle. Pulling the cap directly up will prevent your dispenser from operating properly.

Finger Push Area ▶

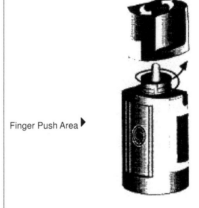

6. Tilt your head back and pull your lower eyelid down slightly to form a pocket between your eyelid and your eye.

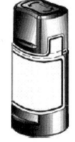

7. Invert the bottle, and press lightly with the thumb or index finger over the "Finger Push Area" (as shown) until a single drop is dispensed into the eye as directed by your doctor. [See figure at top of next column]
DO NOT TOUCH YOUR EYE OR EYELID WITH THE DROPPER TIP.

OPHTHALMIC MEDICATIONS, IF HANDLED IMPROPERLY, CAN BECOME CONTAMINATED BY COMMON BACTERIA KNOWN TO CAUSE EYE INFECTIONS. SERIOUS DAMAGE TO THE EYE AND SUBSEQUENT LOSS OF VISION MAY RESULT FROM USING CONTAMINATED OPHTHALMIC MEDICATIONS. IF YOU THINK YOUR MEDICATION MAY BE CONTAMINATED, OR IF YOU DEVELOP AN EYE INFECTION, CONTACT YOUR DOCTOR IMMEDIATELY CONCERNING CONTINUED USE OF THIS BOTTLE.

8. If drop dispensing is difficult after opening for the first time, replace the cap on the bottle and tighten (DO NOT OVERTIGHTEN) and then remove by turning the cap in the opposite direction as indicated by the arrows on the top of the cap.
9. Repeat steps 6 & 7 with the other eye if instructed to do so by your doctor.
10. Replace the cap by turning until it is firmly touching the bottle. The arrow on the left side of the cap must be aligned with the arrow on the left side of the bottle label for proper closure. Do not overtighten or you may damage the bottle and cap.
11. The dispenser tip is designed to provide a single drop; therefore, do NOT enlarge the hole of the dispenser tip.
12. After you have used all doses, there will be some TRUSOPT left in the bottle. You should not be concerned since an extra amount of TRUSOPT has been added and you will get the full amount of TRUSOPT that your doctor prescribed. Do not attempt to remove excess medicine from the bottle.

WARNING: Keep out of reach of children.
If you have any questions about the use of TRUSOPT, please consult your doctor.

Issued December 2009
Manuf. for: Merck Sharp & Dohme Corp., a subsidiary of **MERCK & CO., Inc.**, Whitehouse Station, NJ 08889, USA
By: Laboratories Merck Sharp & Dohme-Chibret 63963 Clermont-Ferrand Cedex 9, France
9368211

[3]Registered trademark of Merck Sharp & Dohme Corp., a subsidiary of **Merck & Co., Inc.**
Copyright © 2000 Merck Sharp & Dohme Corp., a subsidiary of **Merck & Co., Inc.**
All rights reserved

Shown in Product Identification Guide, page 104

Information on the Merck products listed on these pages is from the prescribing information in use August 1, 2011. For information, please call 1-800-NSC-Merck [1-800-672-6372].

ABBREVIATIONS, ACRONYMS, AND SYMBOLS

ABBREVIATIONS	DESCRIPTIONS
- (eg, 6-8)	to (eg, 6 to 8)
/	per
5-FU	5-fluorouracil
5-HT	5-hydroxytryptamine (serotonin)
ABECB	acute bacterial exacerbation of chronic bronchitis
aa	of each
ac	before meals
ACTH	adrenocorticotrophic hormone
ad	right ear
ADHD	attention-deficit/hyperactivity disorder
A-fib	atrial fibrillation
A-flutter	atrial flutter
AIDS	acquired immunodeficiency syndrome
ALT	alanine transaminase (SGPT)
am	morning
AMI	acute myocardial infarction
ANA	antinuclear antibody
ANC	absolute neutrophil count
APAP	acetaminophen
as	left ear
ASA	aspirin
AST	aspartate transaminase (SGOT)
au	each ear
AUC	area under the curve
AV	atrioventricular
bid	twice daily
BMI	body mass index
BPH	benign prostatic hypertrophy
bpm	beats per minute
BSA	body surface area
BUN	blood urea nitrogen
CABG	coronary arterial bypass graft
CAD(s)	coronary artery disease
Cap	capsule(s) or gelcap(s)
CAP	community-acquired pneumonia
CBC	complete blood count
CF	cystic fibrosis
CHF	congestive heart failure
cm	centimeter

ABBREVIATIONS	DESCRIPTIONS
CMV	cytomegalovirus
C_{max}	peak plasma concentration
CNS	central nervous system
COPD	chronic obstructive pulmonary disease
CrCl	creatinine clearance
Cre	cream
CRF	chronic renal failure
CSF	cerebrospinal fluid
CVA	cerebrovascular accident
CVD	cardiovascular disease
CYP450	cytochrome P450
d(s)	day(s)
d/c or D/C	discontinue
DHEA	dehydroepiandrosterone
DM	diabetes mellitus
DVT	deep vein thrombosis
ECG	electrocardiogram
EEG	electroencephalogram
eg	for example
EPS	extrapyramidal symptom
ESRD	end-stage renal disease
FBS	fasting blood sugar
FPG	fasting plasma glucose
FSH	follicle-stimulating hormone
g	gram
GABA	gamma-aminobutyric acid
GAD	generalized anxiety disorder
GERD	gastroesophageal reflux disease
GFR	glomerular filtration rate
GI	gastrointestinal
GnRH	gonadotropin-releasing hormone
gtt(s)	drop(s)
GVHD	graft versus host disease
hCG	human chorionic gonadotropin
Hct	hematocrit
HCTZ	hydrochlorothiazide
HDL	high-density lipoprotein
Hgb	hemoglobin
HIV	human immunodeficiency virus
HMG-CoA	3-hydroxy-3-methylglutaryl-coenzyme A
HR	heart rate
hr or hrs	hour or hours
hs	at bedtime
HSV	herpes simplex virus
HTN	hypertension
IBD	inflammatory bowel disease

ABBREVIATIONS	DESCRIPTIONS
IBS	irritable bowel syndrome
ICH	intracranial hemorrhage
ICP	intracranial pressure
IM	intramuscular
INH	isoniazid
inj	injection
INR	international normalization ratio
IOP	intraocular pressure
IU	international units
IV	intravenous/intravenously
K^+	potassium
kg	kilogram
kiu	kallikrein inhibitor unit
L	liter
lbs	pounds
LD	loading dose
LDL	low-density lipoprotein
LFT	liver function test
LH	luteinizing hormone
LHRH	luteinizing hormone-releasing hormone
Liq	liquid
Lot	lotion
Loz	lozenge
LVH	left ventricular hypertrophy
M	molar
MAC	mycobacterium avium complex
Maint	maintenance
MAOI	monoamine oxidase inhibitor
Max	maximum
mcg	microgram
mEq	milliequivalent
mg	milligram
MI	myocardial infarction
min(s)	minute(s) (usually as mL/min)
mL	milliliter
mm	millimeter
mM	millimolar
MRI	magnetic resonance imaging
MS	multiple sclerosis
msec	millisecond
MTX	methotrexate
Na	sodium
NaCl	sodium chloride
Ng	nasogastric
NKA	no known allergies
NMS	neuroleptic malignant syndrome

ABBREVIATIONS	DESCRIPTIONS
NPO	nothing by mouth
NSAID	nonsteroidal anti-inflammatory drug
NTE	not to exceed
NV or N/V	nausea and vomiting
OA	osteoarthritis
OCD	obsessive-compulsive disorder
od	right eye
Oint	ointment
OS	left eye
ou	each eye
PAT	paroxysmal atrial tachycardia
pc	after meals
PCN	penicillin
PCP	*Pneumocystis carinii* pneumonia
PD	Parkinson's disease
PID	pelvic inflammatory disease
pkt, pkts	packet, packets
pm	evening
po or PO	orally
PONV	postoperative nausea and vomiting
pr	rectally
prn	as needed
PSA	prostate-specific antigen
PSVT	paroxysmal supraventricular tachycardia
PT	prothrombin time
pt	patient
PTSD	post-traumatic stress disorder
PTT	partial thromboplastin time
PTU	propylthiouracil
PUD	peptic ulcer disease
PVD	peripheral vascular disease
q	every
q4h, q6h, q8h, etc.	every four hours, every six hours, every eight hours, etc.
qd	once daily
qh	every hour
qid	four times daily
qod	every other day
qs	a sufficient quantity
qs ad	a sufficient quantity up to
RA	rheumatoid arthritis
RBC	red blood cells
RDS	respiratory distress syndrome
REM	rapid eye movement
SAH	subarachnoid hemorrhage
SBP	systolic blood pressure

ABBREVIATIONS	DESCRIPTIONS
sec	second(s)
SGOT	serum glutamic oxaloacetic transaminase (AST)
SGPT	serum glutamate-pyruvate transaminase (ALT)
SIADH	syndrome of inappropriate antidiuretic hormone secretion
SLE	systemic lupus erythematosus
SOB	shortness of breath
Sol	solution
SQ, SC	subcutaneous
SrCr	serum creatinine
SSRI	selective serotonin reuptake inhibitor
SSSI	skin and skin structure infection
STD	sexually transmitted disease
Sup	suppository
Sus	suspension
SVT	supraventricular tachycardia
$t_{1/2}$	half-life
Tab	tablet or caplet
Tab, SL	sublingual tablet
TB	tuberculosis
TBG	thyroxine binding globulin
tbsp	tablespoon
TCA	tricyclic antidepressant
TD	tardive dyskinesia
TFT	thyroid function test
TG	triglyceride
tid	three times daily
T_{max}	time to maximum concentration
TNF	tumor necrosis factor
TPN	total parenteral nutrition
TSH	thyroid stimulating hormone (thyrotropin)
tsp	teaspoonful
TTP	thrombotic thrombocytopenic purpura
U	unit(s)
ud	as directed
ULN	upper limit of normal
URTI/URI	upper respiratory tract infection
UTI	urinary tract infection
UV	ultraviolet
WBC	white blood cell count
WNL	within normal limits
Vd	volume of distribution
VTE	venous thromboembolism
X	times (eg, >2X ULN)
yr or yrs	year or years

THE PRESCRIBER'S #1 SOURCE FOR DRUG INFORMATION FOR OVER 66 YEARS

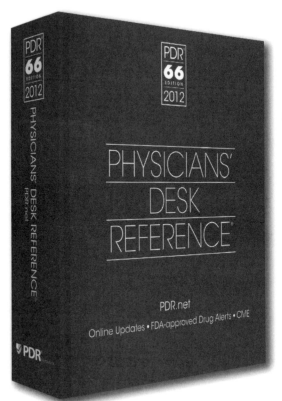

2012 *Physicians' Desk Reference*®

Found in virtually every physician's office, pharmacy, clinic, and library, no medical reference is more current, more user-friendly, or more recognized and respected.

This indispensible reference is even better; with FREE PDR eDrug Updates!

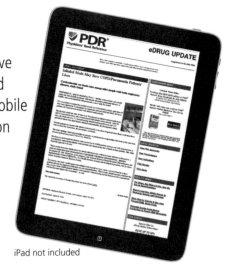

Stay up-to-date with the FREE PDR® eDrug Update ($29.95 value if purchased separately). These time-sensitive email reports deliver news of important label changes and new FDA product approvals directly to your desktop or mobile device, allowing you to have absolutely current information throughout the year without spending valuable time on research every time you write a prescription.

Go to www.PDRbooks.com to order

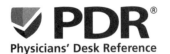

iPad not included

Could your patients use support to start and sustain your therapeutic recommendations?

- **DRUG EDUCATION?**

- **FINANCIAL ASSISTANCE?**

- **MEDICATION SUPPORT?**

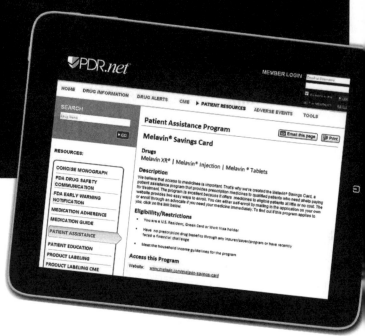

Now the PDR® makes it simple and easy to find and use available programs

Introducing the **PDR® Patient Resource Guide for Physicians**, a comprehensive electronic directory that aggregates information on patient resource programs all in one place for easy access, updates the content continuously, making it easy to compare the current available patient resources so you can provide recommendations accordingly.

PDR® Patient Resource Guide for Physicians supports your efforts to:

- help patients with prescription compliance, medication utilization, regimen adherence and monitoring
- reduce prescribing risks for patients and professionals
- enhance patient satisfaction

These patient programs are compiled by *PDR®*, your most trusted source for drug information, and conveniently delivered into your workflow. Don't spend any more time flipping through the cardboard displays or searching through Pharma company's websites to find the appropriate programs.

Available January 2012 on *PDR.net®*

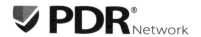